Pharmacogenetics to Avoid Adverse Drug Reactions

Pharmacogenetics to Avoid Adverse Drug Reactions

Editor

Luis A. López-Fernández

MDPI • Basel • Beijing • Wuhan • Barcelona • Belgrade • Manchester • Tokyo • Cluj • Tianjin

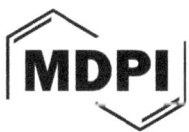

Editor
Luis A. López-Fernández
Servicio de Farmacia
Hospital General Universitario
Gregorio Marañón, Instituto de
Investigación Sanitaria Gregorio
Marañón
Madrid
Spain

Editorial Office
MDPI
St. Alban-Anlage 66
4052 Basel, Switzerland

This is a reprint of articles from the Special Issue published online in the open access journal *Journal of Personalized Medicine* (ISSN 2075-4426) (available at: www.mdpi.com/journal/jpm/special_issues/Pharmacogenetics_Adverse_Drug_Reactions).

For citation purposes, cite each article independently as indicated on the article page online and as indicated below:

LastName, A.A.; LastName, B.B.; LastName, C.C. Article Title. *Journal Name* **Year**, *Volume Number*, Page Range.

ISBN 978-3-0365-3344-5 (Hbk)
ISBN 978-3-0365-3343-8 (PDF)

© 2022 by the authors. Articles in this book are Open Access and distributed under the Creative Commons Attribution (CC BY) license, which allows users to download, copy and build upon published articles, as long as the author and publisher are properly credited, which ensures maximum dissemination and a wider impact of our publications.
The book as a whole is distributed by MDPI under the terms and conditions of the Creative Commons license CC BY-NC-ND.

Contents

About the Editor vii

Preface to "Pharmacogenetics to Avoid Adverse Drug Reactions" ix

Luis A. López-Fernández
Pharmacogenetics to Avoid Adverse Drug Reactions
Reprinted from: *J. Pers. Med.* **2022**, *12*, 159, doi:10.3390/jpm12020159 1

Mariana Angulo-Aguado, Karen Panche, Caroll Andrea Tamayo-Agudelo, Daniel-Armando Ruiz-Torres, Santiago Sambracos-Parrado and Maria Jose Niño-Orrego et al.
A Pharmacogenetic Study of *CYP2C19* in Acute Coronary Syndrome Patients of Colombian Origin Reveals New Polymorphisms Potentially Related to Clopidogrel Therapy
Reprinted from: *J. Pers. Med.* **2021**, *11*, 400, doi:10.3390/jpm11050400 5

Pablo Zubiaur, Maria Dolores Benedicto, Gonzalo Villapalos-García, Marcos Navares-Gómez, Gina Mejía-Abril and Manuel Román et al.
SLCO1B1 Phenotype and CYP3A5 Polymorphism Significantly Affect Atorvastatin Bioavailability
Reprinted from: *J. Pers. Med.* **2021**, *11*, 204, doi:10.3390/jpm11030204 21

Solomon M. Adams, Habiba Feroze, Tara Nguyen, Seenae Eum, Cyrille Cornelio and Arthur F. Harralson
Genome Wide Epistasis Study of On-Statin Cardiovascular Events with Iterative Feature Reduction and Selection
Reprinted from: *J. Pers. Med.* **2020**, *10*, 212, doi:10.3390/jpm10040212 37

Xandra García-González and Sara Salvador-Martín
Pharmacogenetics to Avoid Adverse Reactions in Cardiology: Ready for Implementation?
Reprinted from: *J. Pers. Med.* **2021**, *11*, 1180, doi:10.3390/jpm11111180 51

Johanna Raymond, Laurent Imbert, Thibault Cousin, Thomas Duflot, Rémi Varin and Julien Wils et al.
Pharmacogenetics of Direct Oral Anticoagulants: A Systematic Review
Reprinted from: *J. Pers. Med.* **2021**, *11*, 37, doi:10.3390/jpm11010037 71

Dominic Schaerer, Tanja K. Froehlich, Seid Hamzic, Steven M. Offer, Robert B. Diasio and Markus Joerger et al.
A Novel Nomenclature for Repeat Motifs in the Thymidylate Synthase Enhancer Region and Its Relevance for Pharmacogenetic Studies
Reprinted from: *J. Pers. Med.* **2020**, *10*, 181, doi:10.3390/jpm10040181 83

Ana Rita Simões, Ceres Fernández-Rozadilla, Olalla Maroñas and Ángel Carracedo
The Road so Far in Colorectal Cancer Pharmacogenomics: Are We Closer to Individualised Treatment?
Reprinted from: *J. Pers. Med.* **2020**, *10*, 237, doi:10.3390/jpm10040237 97

Ali Fadhel Ahmed, Chonlaphat Sukasem, Majeed Arsheed Sabbah, Nur Fadhlina Musa, Dzul Azri Mohamed Noor and Nur Aizati Athirah Daud
Genetic Determinants in *HLA* and Cytochrome P450 Genes in the Risk of Aromatic Antiepileptic-Induced Severe Cutaneous Adverse Reactions
Reprinted from: *J. Pers. Med.* **2021**, *11*, 383, doi:10.3390/jpm11050383 137

Shobana John, Karuppiah Balakrishnan, Chonlaphat Sukasem, Tharmarajan Chinnathambi Vijay Anand, Bhutorn Canyuk and Sutthiporn Pattharachayakul
Association of *HLA-B*51:01, HLA-B*55:01, CYP2C9*3*, and Phenytoin-Induced Cutaneous Adverse Drug Reactions in the South Indian Tamil Population
Reprinted from: *J. Pers. Med.* **2021**, *11*, 737, doi:10.3390/jpm11080737 157

Lorena Carrascal-Laso, Manuel Ángel Franco-Martín, María Belén García-Berrocal, Elena Marcos-Vadillo, Santiago Sánchez-Iglesias and Carolina Lorenzo et al.
Application of a Pharmacogenetics-Based Precision Medicine Model (5SPM) to Psychotic Patients That Presented Poor Response to Neuroleptic Therapy
Reprinted from: *J. Pers. Med.* **2020**, *10*, 289, doi:10.3390/jpm10040289 173

Muh. Akbar Bahar, Pauline Lanting, Jens H. J. Bos, Rolf H. Sijmons, Eelko Hak and Bob Wilffert
Impact of Drug-Gene-Interaction, Drug-Drug-Interaction, and Drug-Drug-Gene-Interaction on (es)Citalopram Therapy: The PharmLines Initiative
Reprinted from: *J. Pers. Med.* **2020**, *10*, 256, doi:10.3390/jpm10040256 189

About the Editor

Luis A. López-Fernández

Luis Andrés López Fernández, Senior Researcher, Head of the Pharmacogenetics Laboratory, Instituto de Investigación Sanitaria Gregorio Marañón (IiSGM), Hospital General Universitario Gregorio Marañón. His current lines of research are related to the study of drug response and toxicity in multiple pathologies (cancer, neurology, immunology, psychiatry). He is the author of more than 90 peer-reviewed articles included in the journal citation report. Currently, Dr. López-Fernández is leading studies whose objectives are to identify genetic variants associated with responses to biologic therapy in children with inflammatory bowel disease, to develop a simple and inexpensive pharmacogenetic test to be implemented in countries with limited resources, and to identify genomic biomarkers associated with opioid abuse and dual pathology.

Preface to "Pharmacogenetics to Avoid Adverse Drug Reactions"

Although a cure is the main goal of a treatment, serious adverse reactions associated with treatments are a major problem in clinical practice and cost healthcare systems a lot of money. These adverse reactions limit the success of drugs and can even lead to the death of patients. Identifying the DNA variants associated with adverse drug reactions can help to personalize medicine and sustain healthcare systems. This book focuses on the following topics: the identification of DNA variants associated with adverse drug reactions and their clinical application. It contains seven original papers and four reviews that will spread the knowledge on these critical matters. The pharmacogenetic works presented in this Special Issue can be classified into three major areas: cardiovascular, cancer, and the nervous system.

This book is aimed at cardiologists, oncologists, neurologists, psychiatrists, geneticists, molecular biologists, and hospital pharmacists and other healthcare personnel.

I would like to thank the staff at the Laboratory of Pharmacogenetics of the Hospital Gregorio Marañón for their support, and the patients who have participated in all the research studies shown here.

Luis A. López-Fernández
Editor

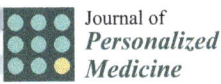

Editorial

Pharmacogenetics to Avoid Adverse Drug Reactions

Luis A. López-Fernández

Servicio de Farmacia, Instituto de Investigación Sanitaria Gregorio Marañón, Hospital General Universitario Gregorio Marañón, 28007 Madrid, Spain; llfernandez@salud.madrid.org

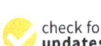

Citation: López-Fernández, L.A. Pharmacogenetics to Avoid Adverse Drug Reactions. *J. Pers. Med.* **2022**, *12*, 159. https://doi.org/10.3390/jpm12020159

Received: 4 January 2022
Accepted: 11 January 2022
Published: 26 January 2022

Publisher's Note: MDPI stays neutral with regard to jurisdictional claims in published maps and institutional affiliations.

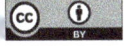

Copyright: © 2022 by the author. Licensee MDPI, Basel, Switzerland. This article is an open access article distributed under the terms and conditions of the Creative Commons Attribution (CC BY) license (https://creativecommons.org/licenses/by/4.0/).

Although a cure is the main goal of a treatment, serious adverse reactions associated with these treatments are a major problem in clinical practice and cost a lot of money for health systems. These adverse reactions limit the success of medicines and can even lead to the death of patients. Identifying the DNA variants associated with adverse drug reactions can help to personalize medicine and sustain health systems. In this way, there are multiple and successful examples of pharmacogenetics to avoid severe adverse drug reactions. Simultaneously, cost-effective studies have confirmed the usefulness of the implementation of pharmacogenetics. This Special Issue focuses on these topics.

In this number, seven original papers and four reviews have spread the knowledge on this critical issue. The pharmacogenetic works presented in this Issue can be classified in three major areas: cardiovascular, cancer, and the nervous system.

Concerning the cardiovascular area, three original research papers and a review are presented. Angulo-Aguado et al., carried out a pharmacogenetic study of *CYP2C19* in acute coronary syndrome patients of Colombian origin that reveals new polymorphisms potentially related to clopidogrel therapy [1]. They established a pharmacogenetic profile of *CYP2C19* in the Colombian population, and identified a new potentially pathogenic mutation (p.L15H) and several intronic variants. Functional and larger studies are necessary to apply these findings.

Zubiaur et al. studied 60 variants in 15 genes in 156 healthy volunteers enrolled in atorvastatin bioequivalence clinical trials [2]. Genetic analyses showed that variants in *SLCO1B1*, *CYP3A5*, *SLC22A1*, and *UGT2B7* are associated with pharmacokinetic variability. This fact suggests that these changes can also affect adverse reactions to this drug.

Statins are used to reduce the risk of adverse cardiovascular events. Solomon et al. analyzed the high-level epistatic risk for on-statin adverse cardiovascular events using genome wide association studies and including up to 5890 individuals [3]. This large study is essential for the progress of this research line. Although the replication of these findings in other populations is desirable, this study opens new ways and will be essential in the future of statins.

In recent years, the biomarkers to avoid adverse reactions in cardiology have been identified and clinical guidelines with recommendations published. In this Issue, a deep and complete review on this subject is presented. The comparison of mainly the Clinical Pharmacogenetics Implementation Consortium and Dutch Pharmacogenetics Working group recommendations is presented and commented on, trying to answer the question: are we ready for implementation? [4]. Thus, drugs, such as acenocoumarol, atorvastatin, clopidogrel, flecainide, metoprolol, phenprocoumon, propafenone, simvastatin, and warfarin, are included in those with recommendations by any of these consortia.

Finally, in the field of cardiovascular diseases, Raymond et al. presented a systematic review about the pharmacogenetics of direct oral anticoagulants [5]. In this work, direct oral anticoagulants, such as dabigatran, rivaroxaban, apixaban, edoxaban, and betrixaban, are reviewed, and the association between polymorphism and the exposure variation to them is presented. Thus, the DNA variants in *CES1*, *ABCB1*, *CYP3A4*, and *CYP3A5* are identified as relevant in the pharmacogenetics of direct anticoagulants.

Another field that is well represented in this Issue is cancer pharmacogenetics. Fluoropyrimidines are the base of the treatment in many solid tumors. However, a high proportion of patients receiving these drugs experience a severe adverse reaction that can even be fatal. Fluoropyrimidines exert their anti-oncogenic activity by inhibiting the thymidylate synthase gene (*TYMS*). A polymorphism in the enhancer region of *TYMS* has been associated with its transcription rate and subsequently with the efficacy and toxicity of these drugs. However, the results are inconclusive. Schaerer et al., after the sequencing of this region in more than 600 patients, suggested a new nomenclature and demonstrated its usefulness, associating the number of upstream stimulatory factor (USF1)-binding sites with 5-fluorouracil-induced gastrointestinal toxicity [6].

In line with this, Simoes et al. suggested that chemotherapy-induced toxicity in colorectal cancer is likely complex and multigenic [7]. For this reason, they summarized the pharmacogenomic data on colorectal cancer, including candidate gene approaches, genome wide association studies, and next-generation sequencing studies. They also reviewed functional studies, mainly for *DPYD* variants and fluoropyrimidine-induced toxicity, and cost-effectiveness analysis for the clinical implementation of pharmacogenetic tests in colorectal cancer pharmacogenetics.

Drugs used in the nervous system can potentially induce adverse reactions. Since the use of these types of drugs is increasing, the identification of the pharmacogenetic biomarkers to prevent adverse reactions is necessary.

Phenytoin is an anti-epileptic drug that causes cutaneous adverse reactions. Two works are presented in this Issue on antiepileptic drugs. Ahmed et al., reviewed the role of DNA variants in HLA and cytochrome P450 genes in the risk of aromatic antiepileptic-induced severe cutaneous adverse reactions [8]. They summarized the knowledge on HLA, *CYP2C9*, and *CYP2C19*, and its role in severe cutaneous adverse reactions, as well as drugs inducing this adverse reaction, such as carbamazepine, phenytoin, lamotrigine, or phenobarbital.

Furthermore, Shobana et al. found an association between *HLA-B*57:01*, *HLA-B*55:01*, *CYP2C9*3*, and phenytoin-induced cutaneous adverse drug reactions in the South Indian Tamil population [9] (Shobana John et al.). The identification of these pharmacogenetic biomarkers in this specific population is highly relevant because it contributes to expand the knowledge and application of pharmacogenetics in poorly studied populations, and it can contribute to the worldwide expansion of pharmacogenetic implementation.

Antipsychotics are extended drugs used for mental disorders. Many of these drugs are metabolized by the genes of cytochrome P450, which are highly polymorphic and well known. Carrascal-Laso et al. developed a pharmacogenetic model to personalize antipsychotic treatments [10]. As a result, the mean daily doses of these drugs and polytherapy is reduced in these patients. It leads to less risk of drug-related adverse events and the reduction of treatment costs.

Polymedication is one of the greatest challenges in pharmacogenetics. To know how drugs interact between them and what the role is of our genes in these interactions is crucial, especially in aged populations in which polytherapy is very common. The PharmLines is an initiative to study drug–gene, drug–drug, and drug–drug–gene interactions in (es)citalopram therapy [11]. *CYP2C19* intermediate metabolizers were associated with an increased need of drug switching and dose reduction, and being an intermediate metabolizer for *CYP3A4* increases these effects.

Funding: This research received no external funding.

Institutional Review Board Statement: Not applicable.

Informed Consent Statement: Not applicable.

Data Availability Statement: Not applicable.

Acknowledgments: I wish to thank all the authors who contributed their work, and in so doing made the Special Issue a success. I wish also to thank Alicia López Salvador for the English editing of this editorial and Sera Li for her support throughout the editorial process.

Conflicts of Interest: The author declares no conflict of interest.

References

1. Angulo-Aguado, M.; Panche, K.; Tamayo-Agudelo, C.A.; Ruiz-Torres, D.-A.; Sambracos-Parrado, S.; Niño-Orrego, M.J.; Páez, N.; Piñeros-Hernandez, L.B.; Castillo-León, L.-F.; Pardo-Oviedo, J.M.; et al. A Pharmacogenetic Study of CYP2C19 in Acute Coronary Syndrome Patients of Colombian Origin Reveals New Polymorphisms Potentially Related to Clopidogrel Therapy. *J. Pers. Med.* **2021**, *11*, 400. [CrossRef] [PubMed]
2. Zubiaur, P.; Benedicto, M.D.; Villapalos-García, G.; Navares-Gómez, M.; Mejía-Abril, G.; Román, M.; Martín-Vílchez, S.; Ochoa, D.; Abad-Santos, F. SLCO1B1 Phenotype and CYP3A5 Polymorphism Significantly Affect Atorvastatin Bioavailability. *J. Pers. Med.* **2021**, *11*, 204. [CrossRef] [PubMed]
3. Adams, S.M.; Feroze, H.; Nguyen, T.; Eum, S.; Cornelio, C.; Harralson, A.F. Genome Wide Epistasis Study of On-Statin Cardiovascular Events with Iterative Feature Reduction and Selection. *J. Pers. Med.* **2020**, *10*, 212. [CrossRef] [PubMed]
4. García-González, X.; Salvador-Martín, S. Pharmacogenetics to Avoid Adverse Reactions in Cardiology: Ready for Implementation? *J. Pers. Med.* **2021**, *11*, 1180. [CrossRef] [PubMed]
5. Raymond, J.; Imbert, L.; Cousin, T.; Duflot, T.; Varin, R.; Wils, J.; Lamoureux, F. Pharmacogenetics of Direct Oral Anticoagulants: A Systematic Review. *J. Pers. Med.* **2021**, *11*, 37. [CrossRef] [PubMed]
6. Schaerer, D.; Froehlich, T.K.; Hamzic, S.; Offer, S.M.; Diasio, R.B.; Joerger, M.; Amstutz, U.; Largiadèr, C.R. A Novel Nomenclature for Repeat Motifs in the Thymidylate Synthase Enhancer Region and Its Relevance for Pharmacogenetic Studies. *J. Pers. Med.* **2020**, *10*, 181. [CrossRef] [PubMed]
7. Simões, A.R.; Fernández-Rozadilla, C.; Maroñas, O.; Carracedo, Á. The Road so Far in Colorectal Cancer Pharmacogenomics: Are We Closer to Individualised Treatment? *J. Pers. Med.* **2020**, *10*, 237. [CrossRef] [PubMed]
8. Ahmed, A.F.; Sukasem, C.; Sabbah, M.A.; Musa, N.F.; Mohamed Noor, D.A.; Daud, N.A.A. Genetic Determinants in HLA and Cytochrome P450 Genes in the Risk of Aromatic Antiepileptic-Induced Severe Cutaneous Adverse Reactions. *J. Pers. Med.* **2021**, *11*, 383. [CrossRef] [PubMed]
9. John, S.; Balakrishnan, K.; Sukasem, C.; Anand, T.C.V.; Canyuk, B.; Pattharachayakul, S. Association of HLA-B*51:01, HLA-B*55:01, CYP2C9*3, and Phenytoin-Induced Cutaneous Adverse Drug Reactions in the South Indian Tamil Population. *J. Pers. Med.* **2021**, *11*, 737. [CrossRef] [PubMed]
10. Carrascal-Laso, L.; Franco-Martín, M.Á.; García-Berrocal, M.B.; Marcos-Vadillo, E.; Sánchez-Iglesias, S.; Lorenzo, C.; Sánchez-Martín, A.; Ramos-Gallego, I.; García-Salgado, M.J.; Isidoro-García, M. Application of a Pharmacogenetics-Based Precision Medicine Model (5SPM) to Psychotic Patients That Presented Poor Response to Neuroleptic Therapy. *J. Pers. Med.* **2020**, *10*, 289. [CrossRef] [PubMed]
11. Bahar, M.A.; Lanting, P.; Bos, J.H.J.; Sijmons, R.H.; Hak, E.; Wilffert, B. Impact of Drug-Gene-Interaction, Drug-Drug-Interaction, and Drug-Drug-Gene-Interaction on (es)Citalopram Therapy: The PharmLines Initiative. *J. Pers. Med.* **2020**, *10*, 256. [CrossRef] [PubMed]

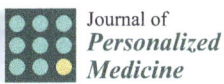
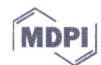

Article

A Pharmacogenetic Study of *CYP2C19* in Acute Coronary Syndrome Patients of Colombian Origin Reveals New Polymorphisms Potentially Related to Clopidogrel Therapy

Mariana Angulo-Aguado [1], Karen Panche [2], Caroll Andrea Tamayo-Agudelo [1], Daniel-Armando Ruiz-Torres [1], Santiago Sambracos-Parrado [1], Maria Jose Niño-Orrego [1], Nathaly Páez [1], Laura B Piñeros-Hernandez [1], Luisa-Fernanda Castillo-León [1], Juan Mauricio Pardo-Oviedo [2], Katherine Parra Abaunza [2], Paul Laissue [1,3], Nora Contreras [1], Carlos Alberto Calderón-Ospina [1] and Dora Janeth Fonseca-Mendoza [1,*]

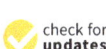

Citation: Angulo-Aguado, M.; Panche, K.; Tamayo-Agudelo, C.A.; Ruiz-Torres, D.-A.; Sambracos-Parrado, S.; Niño-Orrego, M.J.; Páez, N.; Piñeros-Hernandez, L.B.; Castillo-León, L.-F.; Pardo-Oviedo, J.M.; et al. A Pharmacogenetic Study of *CYP2C19* in Acute Coronary Syndrome Patients of Colombian Origin Reveals New Polymorphisms Potentially Related to Clopidogrel Therapy. *J. Pers. Med.* **2021**, *11*, 400. https://doi.org/10.3390/jpm11050400

Academic Editor: Luis A. López-Fernández

Received: 14 March 2021
Accepted: 22 April 2021
Published: 12 May 2021

Publisher's Note: MDPI stays neutral with regard to jurisdictional claims in published maps and institutional affiliations.

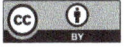

Copyright: © 2021 by the authors. Licensee MDPI, Basel, Switzerland. This article is an open access article distributed under the terms and conditions of the Creative Commons Attribution (CC BY) license (https://creativecommons.org/licenses/by/4.0/).

[1] Center for Research in Genetics and Genomics—CIGGUR, GENIUROS Research Group, School of Medicine and Health Sciences, Universidad Del Rosario, Carrera 24 N° 63C-69, 112111 Bogotá, Colombia; mariana.anguloa@urosario.edu.co (M.A.-A.); caroll.tamayo@urosario.edu.co (C.A.T.-A.); danielar.ruiz@urosario.edu.co (D.-A.R.-T.); santiago.sambracosp@urosario.edu.co (S.S.-P.); mariaj.nino@urosario.edu.co (M.J.N.-O.); Nathalya.paez@urosario.edu.co (N.P.); laurab.pineros@urosario.edu.co (L.B.P.-H.); lu-casti@hotmail.com (L.-F.C.-L.); paullaissue@yahoo.com (P.L.); nora.contreras@urosario.edu.co (N.C.); carlos.calderon@urosario.edu.co (C.A.C.-O.)

[2] Internal Medicine Department, School of Medicine and Health Sciences, Hospital Universitario Mayor-Méderi, Universidad del Rosario, Carrera 24 N° 63C-69, 112111 Bogotá, Colombia; karen.panche@urosario.edu.co (K.P.); juan.pardo@urosario.edu.co (J.M.P.-O.); katherinea.parra@urosario.edu.co (K.P.A.)

[3] Biopas Laboratoires, Orphan Diseases Unit, BIOPAS GROUP, 111111 Bogotá, Colombia

* Correspondence: dora.fonseca@urosario.edu.co; Tel./Fax: +57-12970200

Abstract: Clopidogrel, an oral platelet $P2Y_{12}$ receptor blocker, is used in the treatment of acute coronary syndrome. Interindividual variability in treatment response and the occurrence of adverse effects has been attributed to genetic variants in *CYP2C19*. The analysis of relevant pharmacogenes in ethnically heterogeneous and poorly studied populations contributes to the implementation of personalized medicine. We analyzed the coding and regulatory regions of *CYP2C19* in 166 patients with acute coronary syndrome (ACS) treated with clopidogrel. The allele frequencies of *CYP2C19* alleles *1, *2, *4, *17, *27 and *33 alleles were 86.1%, 7.2%, 0.3%, 10.2%, 0.3% and 0.3%, respectively. A new potentially pathogenic mutation (p.L15H) and five intronic variants with potential splicing effects were detected. In 14.4% of the patients, a new haplotype in strong linkage disequilibrium was identified. The clinical outcome indicated that 13.5% of the patients presented adverse drugs reactions with a predominance of bleeding while 25% of these patients were carriers of at least one polymorphic allele. We propose that new regulatory single-nucleotide variants (SNVs) might potentially influence the response to clopidogrel in Colombian individuals.

Keywords: platelet reactivity; single-nucleotide variants; pharmacogenetics; acute coronary syndrome; clopidogrel; genotype; allele; polymorphism

1. Introduction

Dual antiplatelet therapy with clopidogrel and aspirin has been routinely recommended in the American College of Cardiology/American Heart Association guidelines for patients with acute coronary syndrome to prevent atherothrombotic events [1,2]. Clopidogrel is an inactive prodrug that is converted into an active metabolite by two-step biotransformation. This metabolite binds irreversibly to the purinergic adenosine diphosphate (ADP) platelet receptor $P2Y_{12}$ and inhibits ADP-stimulated platelet aggregation [3,4]. Clopidogrel is one of the most widely used platelet antiaggregant with over 40,000,000 patients prescribed worldwide [5,6]. Although clopidogrel has high clinical efficacy, over 30%

patients exhibit significant interindividual variability in platelet inhibition, which reduces the antithrombotic effect of the medication [7]. Inadequate response to clopidogrel is associated with a higher risk of cardiac events and bleeding in patients that show high platelet reactivity (HPR) or low platelet reactivity (LPR), respectively [4,8]. Interindividual variability in the response to clopidogrel is influenced by clinical and environmental factors such as age, diabetes, body mass index, triglycerides and drug–drug interactions [9,10]. In addition to these clinical factors, genetic polymorphisms implicated in the pharmacokinetics and pharmacodynamics of clopidogrel are considered determinants in the response to anti-aggregation therapy, and heritability appears to be responsible for over 70% of interindividual variability [6,7,11]. To date, association studies between genetic variants, cardiovascular events, HPR and LPR have focused on polymorphisms on *PON1* (p.Q192R), *ABCB1* (C.3435C>T) polymorphisms, and particularly the *CYP2C19* gene [12–15]. CYP2C19, an enzyme of the cytochrome P450 (CYP450) superfamily, is considered the key enzyme related to the bioactivation of clopidogrel through the two-step oxidative process that leads to the formation of 2-oxo-clopidogrel and the active metabolite clopi-H4 [16,17]. Only some genetic variants of *CYP2C19* have been widely explored and their relation to the therapeutic response to clopidogrel has been established. The *CYP2C19*2* (c.681 G>A, rs4244285) and *3 (c.636 G>A, rs4986893) alleles are considered loss-of-function (LOF) alleles and have been associated with higher platelet aggregation induced by ADP and a higher risk of atherothrombotic events [18,19]. The *CYP2C19*17* (c.−806C>T, rs 12248560), a gain-of-function allele has been associated with ultrarapid metabolism that leads to the increase of platelet inhibition and a higher risk of bleeding. Response to clopidogrel can be assessed by determining the platelet function through the quantification of platelet reactivity. Diverse methods such as ADP-induced light transmittance aggregometry (LTA), the Verify Now $P2Y_{12}$ assay and the INNOVANCE PFA-200 system, determine the potential anti-aggregation effectiveness of the drug. Few reports correlating molecular genotype and platelet reactivity, a potential positive association between these two factors has been determined [20]. Variations in gene allele frequencies are common across populations and can contribute to differences in the treatment effectiveness, which impacts the prevalence of HPR due to LOF *CYP2C19* alleles [17,21].

There have been many studies about *CYP2C19* on individuals with predominantly European ancestry, which limits the clinical implementation of pharmacogenetics in understudied populations, such as Latin Americans.

Due to the key role of loss and gain-of-function *CYP2C19* alleles in therapeutic response to clopidogrel, new studies for Latin American subgroups are necessary to identify susceptibility polymorphisms and their association to the response to clopidogrel.

In the present study, in order to assess the potential association of *CYP2C19* polymorphic alleles with platelet reactivity in acute coronary syndrome (ACS) patients, we studied the promoter, coding regions and intron-exon boundaries of the gene. Our results indicated that 33.7% of ACS patients were carriers of at least 1 polymorphic allele in *CYP2C19*, 7.8% of which were loss-of-function variants and 10.2% gain-of-function alleles. Our study identified intronic variants with potential splicing alterations leading to the generation of new predicted cryptic splicing sites or branch point modifications.

To our knowledge, this study is the first analysis of the *CYP2C19* gene and platelet reactivity assessment using the INNOVANCE PFA-200 system in a Latin American Population. These results reveal new polymorphisms worth considering in the implication of pharmacogenetics-based clopidogrel therapy in the Colombian population.

2. Patients and Methods

2.1. Sampling and Data Collection

This study included 166 patients who received care in the Hospital Universitario Mayor-Méderi, located in Bogota (Colombia). Eligible patients were invited to participate in the study. Those who accepted signed informed consent. The study included patients 18 years or older admitted to the hospital due to acute coronary syndrome who received a dose of clopidogrel of 300 mg and then 75 mg dose for at least seven consecutive days. The clinical management of clopidogrel therapy and the dose indicated for the patients were performed according to the guidelines specified in the national clinical practice guide for acute coronary syndrome (http://gpc.minsalud.gov.co/ (accessed on 14 March 2021)). All patients included in the study received treatment with clopidogrel for at least 7 days. However, according to medical criteria, 13 of them subsequently changed their antiplatelet therapy (12 to ticagrelor and 1 to prasugrel).

The study excluded individuals who were using oral anticoagulants and glycoprotein IIb/IIa receptor inhibitors, with hematocrit values <25% or >52%, platelet count <100 × 10^9/L, creatinine >15 mg/dL, clinical evidence of liver damage or profound alteration of platelet function.

Variables in patients were compiled; these variables included information such as demographics characteristics, gender, type of acute coronary syndrome (unstable angina, acute infarction with or without ST elevation) and comorbidities (e.g., diabetes, hypertension and obesity).

All experimental procedures were approved by the Ethics Committee of Universidad del Rosario. The study followed the guidelines of the Declaration of Helsinki. (Approved DVO005 990-CV1018, institutional review board reference IV-FPC015 and ABN062).

2.2. Genotyping of the Promoter and Coding Regions of CYP2C19

Genomic DNA was obtained from blood samples of 166 patients using the Quick-DNA™ Miniprep Plus Kit (Zymo research). Using PCR, the coding region of *CYP2C19* (9 exons), the intron-exon boundaries, and the promoter (−1 to −1500 base pairs relative to transcriptional start site) were amplified. PCR products were purified and sequenced directly using Sanger sequencing. Primers were designed using Primer3 (Supplementary Table S1). The reference sequence was obtained from the Ensembl database (ENST00000371321.9).

To define the *CYP2C19* alleles, we used the information described in The Human CYP allele nomenclature database (http://www.cypalleles.ki.se/ (accessed on 14 March 2021)). Variants were considered novel when they were not previously reported in public databases or literature. We used the PolyPhen2, SIFT, and MutPred software to predict the effect of the amino acid substitution on protein function. Sequences of proteins with modified residues were compared with orthologous proteins of mammalian species using available public database sequences (https://www.uniprot.org/uniprot/ (accessed on 14 March 2021)), to assess evolutionary conservation. For the splice variants, we realized an in silico prediction using Human Splicing Finder v3.1 (http://www.umd.be/HSF/ (accessed on 14 March 2021)) and Alamut software (v2.15) (http://downloads.interactive-biosoftware.com (accessed on 14 March 2021)). Linkage disequilibrium was assessed for variants c.681G>A (rs 4244285), c.819 + 228 A>G (rs12571421) and c. 332-23A>G (rs12769205) using Haploview 4.2 (https://www.broadinstitute.org/ (accessed on 14 March 2021)).

Promoter variants were identified using Ensembl database ENST00000371321.9 (https//www.ensembl.org/ondex.html (accessed on 14 March 2021)). In the cases where the promoter region or intronic variant defined a specific allele, it was assigned according to the information in The Human CYP Allele Nomenclature database (http://www.cypalleles.ki.se/ (accessed on 14 March 2021))

2.3. Platelet Function Test

The platelet function was assessed using the INNOVANCE PFA-200 P2Y system (Siemens Healthcare). Blood samples were obtained at least 4 h after the administration of the loading dose of clopidogrel. The samples were obtained in tubes containing 3.2% sodium citrate. The PFA-200 P2Y is a system used for the assessment of platelet function by simulating the process of primary hemostasis in vitro. The assay simulates in vitro the process of platelet adhesion and aggregation. The PFA-200 P2Y$_{12}$ allows detecting platelet ADP receptor blockades using a membrane covered with 20 ug of ADP, 5 ng PGE1, and

125 ug of calcium. As recommended by the manufacturer we defined HPR as closure time (CT) <106 s (Siemens Healthcare. 2010. Guide insert. Innovance PFA P2Y.)

2.4. Adverse Reactions and Causality Analysis

Patients were prospectively evaluated to establish the phenotypic response to treatment (bleeding or thrombosis). This evaluation was carried out through of periodic phone calls for six months and the completion of a monitoring form for each patient included in the study. At follow-up, the 13 patients who switched their antiplatelet therapy to ticagrelor or prasugrel were excluded.

Each time that an adverse event was aimed to obtain additional information from the patient's medical records and data provided by the treating physician.

Each adverse event consisting of hemorrhage was subsequently evaluated in terms of its causality using the Naranjo algorithm [22]. The Naranjo algorithm was not used to evaluate therapeutic failures since this tool is not designed for this purpose. The Naranjo algorithm is a questionnaire proposed by Naranjo et al. for establishing the probability of whether an adverse drug reaction (ADR) was caused by the suspect drug (clopidogrel in our study) rather than concurrent factors (e.g., comorbidities). Probability was assigned using the following scores: definite, probable, possible, or doubtful. Every time the answer to any of the Naranjo algorithm questions was unknown, a score of "0" was allocated to the corresponding question, as it is established in the algorithm [22].

We defined the occurrence of major bleedings according to the criteria of Schulman et al. [23], these include: (1) fatal bleeding, and/or, (2) symptomatic bleeding in a critical area or organ, such as intracranial, intraspinal, intraocular, retroperitoneal, intra-articular or pericardial, or intramuscular with compartment syndrome, and/or, (3) bleeding causing a fall in hemoglobin level of 20 g L^{-1} (1.24 mmol L^{-1}) or more, or leading to transfusion of two or more units of whole blood or red blood cells [23].

Two independent researchers evaluated the cases separately, and any disagreements were solved by consensus with a third author (pharmacologist).

2.5. Statistical Analysis

Allele and genotype frequencies and Hardy–Weinberg equilibrium were determined using the SNP-Stats software (https://www.snpstats.net/start.htm (accessed on 14 March 2021)). Deviation from HWE was estimated using a χ^2 goodness-of-fit test with 1° of freedom. The χ^2 test was used to compare allele frequencies between the Colombian population and others (a p-value of <0.05 was considered statistically significant). Linkage disequilibrium (LD) between intronic SNVs was determined by applying the LOD and D' value on Haploview v4.2 (https://www.broadinstitute.org/ (accessed on 14 March 2021)). The groups were defined as Non-HPR or HPR based on the CT value obtained using the INNOVANCE PFA-200 P2Y system (Siemens Healthcare). The χ^2 test was used to compare genotype and Non-HPR or HPR condition. Genotypes were categorized into two subgroups: extensive metabolizers (EM, including the diplotypes wild type and diplotypes with at least one allele*17) and intermediate metabolizers (IM, including diplotypes with at least one LOF allele). To compare CT value with EM or IM status, data distribution was evaluated using the Shapiro–Wilk test. Non-normally distributed data was found ($p < 0.05$) and nonparametric Mann–Whitney U test was used to compare groups.

3. Results

3.1. Clinical and Demographic Characteristics

The patients' characteristics are summarized in Table 1. The majority were males (63.8%). Most cases were over 50 years old, and the predominant type of coronary syndrome was acute myocardial infarction with ST elevation (63.2%). 32.5% of patients previously presented one or more ACS when recruited into the study and nearly 30% presented a comorbidity (e.g., diabetes, obesity, or dyslipidemia) (Table 1).

Table 1. Patients' characteristics.

Characteristics	(n)	%
Sex	166	100
Female	60	36.1
Male	106	63.8
Age (years)		
30–50	11	6.6
50–70	88	53
>70	67	40.3
Type of ACS		
UA	25	15
STEMI	105	63.2
NSTEMI	36	21.6
Previous ACS medical history *	54	32.5
Type of intervention current event		
Medical †	44	26.5
PCI	86	51.8
CABG	36	21.6
Stent placement current event	73	43.9
Type 2 Diabetes Mellitus		
Body Mass Index	46	27.7
Underweight	2	1.2
Normal	58	34.9
Overweight	64	38.5
Obese	42	25.3

ACS, acute coronary syndrome; UA, unstable angina; STEMI, ST elevation myocardial infarction; NSTEMI, non-ST myocardial infarction; PCI, percutaneous coronary intervention; CABG, coronary artery bypass grafting. * Patients who had previously presented one or more ACS when recruited into the study. † Medical Management, supportive and pharmacologic care.

3.2. Analysis of Genetic Variants in CYP2C19

CYP2C19 was sequenced in the 166 ACS patients, and we identified a total of 41 single nucleotide variations (SNVs). For the analyzed population, the following allelic frequencies were established: 81.6% CYP2C19*1, 10.2% CYP2C19*17, 7.2% CYP2C19*2, and 0.3% for the *27, *4, and *33 CYP2C19 alleles. (Figure 1A). 18.3% of the population were carriers of alleles that have been related to interindividual variability in response to clopidogrel. Furthermore, 66.3% of the identified genotypes were wild type, CYP2C19*1/*1 and 33.7% had a genotype with at least one polymorphic allele. From the last, 18.1% were ultrarapid metabolizers (*1/*17, *17/*17), 14.4% intermediate metabolizers (*1/*2, *4/*17, *2/*17) and 0.6% to slow metabolizers (*2/*27). There were no patients identified as homozygous for allele*2. One patient was identified as heterozygous for allele*33 (0.6%), whose metabolizer phenotype has not been established. (Figure 1B)

Two novel non-synonymous CYP2C19 variants were identified, both with an allele frequency of 0.3%. These variants correspond to c.44T>A p.L15H and c.1215G>C p.E405D. In silico analysis (SIFT, MutPred, PolyPhen-2) predicted the pathogenic effect of p.L15H, while p.E405D was predicted as benign. Alignment with different species showed evolutionary conservation for these two variants (Supplementary Figure S1).

Twelve intronic variants were identified, in silico analysis predicted a potential splicing alteration for five of them. For c.332-23A>G, c.1292-17A>G and c.634-4 T>A, a branch point modification was identified. The software predicted activation of a cryptic acceptor and donor site for the variants c.643-81 A>T and c.819 + 228 A>G, respectively (Figure 2). Nine variants were identified in the promoter region; these correspond to −1418C>T, −1333C>A, −1163G>A, −1041G>A (*27), −889T>G, −806C>T (*17), −782G>A, −741C>T and −70T>C. From these variants, seven have been reported previously in the literature, while two are novel (−1333C>A, −1163G>A). Only two polymorphisms identified (−1041C>A and −806C>T) have been related to modifications in the CYP2C19 enzyme activity (Figure 2).

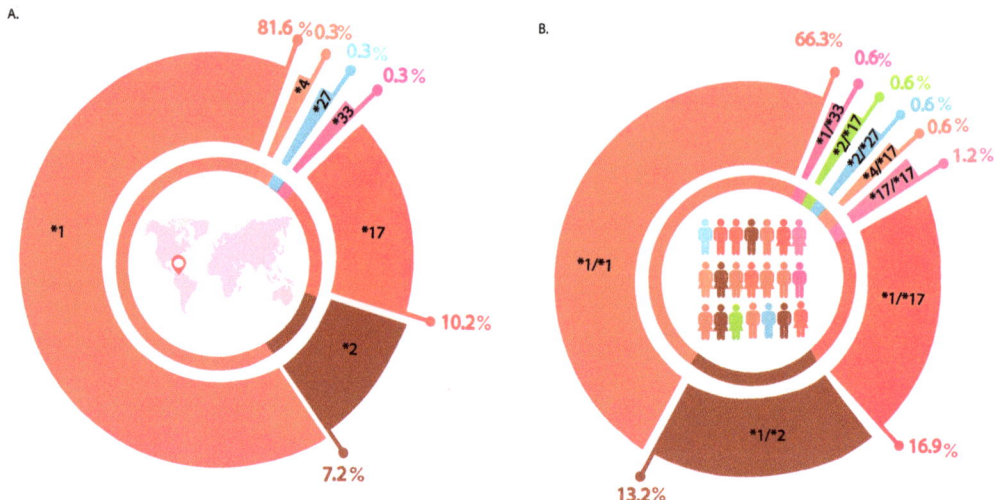

Figure 1. Allele and genotype frequencies. Data for allele and genotype frequencies of *CYP2C19* are illustrated. (**A**) Allele frequency and (**B**) genotype frequency.

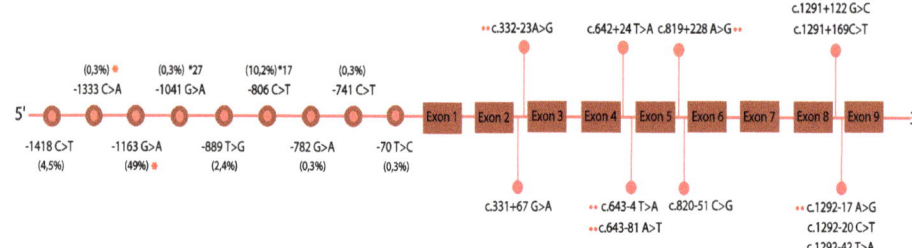

Figure 2. Promoter and intronic variants. *CYP2C19* genetic variants in promoter and intronic regions are described. Numbers in parentheses represent allele frequencies; * indicates novel variants and ¨ illustrates a predicted potential splicing alteration.

LD analysis indicates that rs12769205, rs424428 and rs12571421 exhibit extremely significant linkage disequilibrium (LOD > 2, D'1, R2 ≥ 0.6). The three SNVs were all located in one LD block of 6kb. Haplotype analysis identified two haplotypes: AGA (92.8%) and GAG (6.3%) (Figure 3).

The comparison of allelic frequencies between the Colombian population and other populations showed statistically significant differences between the wild-type and polymorphic alleles (Supplementary Table S2). The Asian, Caucasian, African and Latin America (e.g., Argentina, Brazil) populations have a lower frequency for *CYP2C19*1 compared to our study ($p < 0.00001$). Conversely, Ecuador México and Peru had *CYP2C19*1 frequencies like that described by us ($p = 0.91$). Regarding LOF alleles for *CYP2C19*, our findings demonstrated that allele frequency for *CYP2C19*2 in Colombian patients was significantly lower than that reported for other populations. Strikingly, allele frequency for Asian populations is 0.28 whereas for our population is just 0.7 (p-value < 0.00001). No significant differences were detected with other Latin American populations (Argentina, Brazil, Ecuador, Mexico). *CYP2C19*4 allelic frequency was low in our study (0.3%), consistently with studies in other populations. Other LOF alleles identified in our study (*27) have not been extensively evaluated in other reports. Regarding *CYP2C19*17 allelic frequencies, our data showed differences with most Latin American, Asian, and African populations, where *CYP2C19*17* is more frequent (Supplementary Table S2).

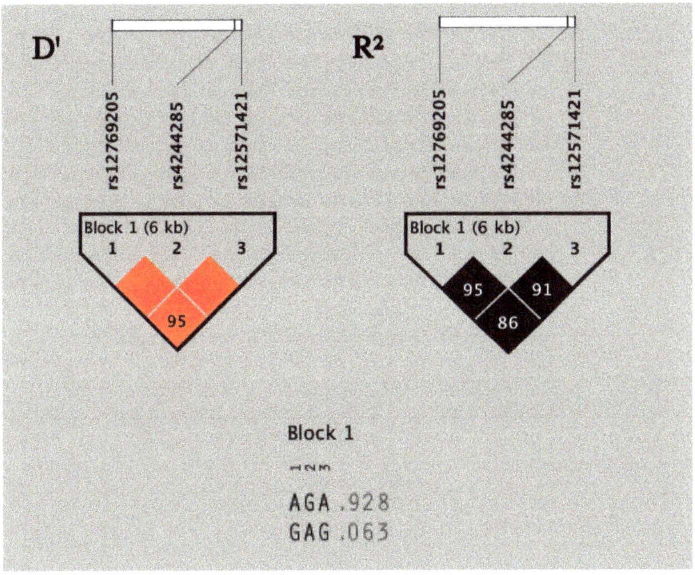

[Figure 3: Linkage disequilibrium plot showing D' and R² values for rs12769205, rs4244285, and rs12571421 in Block 1 (6 kb). R² values: 95, 91, 86. Haplotype frequencies: AGA .928, GAG .063]

Figure 3. Linkage disequilibrium analysis. Linkage disequilibrium among the intronic single nucleotide variations (SNVs) and haplotype block analyzed by Haploview 4.2 software. The D' value is shown within the square (D' = 1, not shown). The three SNVs constitute one haplotype block spanning 6 kb of the *CYP2C19* gene. R^2 value indicates the high correlation coefficients between SNVs.

3.3. Reactivity Platelet Function and Genotype

The mean closure time (CT) values assessed using the INNOVANCE PFA-200 P2Y system (Siemens Healthcare) were 210 +/−110 s (range 37–300). 34% patients showed a CT value suggestive of HPR. Due to the low frequency of polymorphic *CYP2C19* alleles, carriers of at least one LOF variant (*2, *4, *27) and UR variant (*17) were compared with wild-type individuals. The non-HPR and HPR group had not a statistically significant difference between genotype frequencies (Table 2). Corresponding p-values after comparison were $p = 0.21$ for loss-of-function and $p = 0.83$ for gain-of-function.

Table 2. Non-high platelet reactivity (HPR) and HPR statistical comparison.

Genetic Variants Genotypes	All n (%)	HPR n (%)	Non-HPR n (%)	*p*-Value
CYP2C19 Loss function alleles				
Wild type	143 (86)	46 (27.7)	97 (58.4)	0.21
Carrier	23 (14)	11 (6.6)	12 (7.2)	
CYP2C19 Gain function alleles				
Wild type	134 (80.7)	45 (27.1)	89 (53.6)	0.83
Carrier	32 (19.2)	12 (7.2)	20 (12)	

CYP2C19 loss-function-alleles includes *2, *4, *27, *33. *CYP2C19* gain-function-alleles correspond to *17. Values are represented in n (%). Abbreviations: HPR, high platelet reactivity.

Although we did not find a statistically significant difference in ranges between CT vs. EM or IM ($p = 0.315$), the range in EM subgroups was higher than those of IM patients (84.82 and 74.86, respectively).

3.4. Clinical Adverse Reactions and Causality Analysis

We identified 23 patients with adverse events. Considering that some patients had more than one adverse event the total number was 28.

Seven of these events were fatal, but only one of them was related to bleeding/thrombosis. Three therapeutic failures occurred (one case of ischemic stroke and death and two of acute myocardial infarction). Both patients with acute myocardial infarction had stent thrombosis. One of them had a stent in the right coronary artery and in the second case the clinical history indicates the use of a stent in the anterior and posterior descending coronary artery. 19 minor bleedings were considered adverse reactions to clopidogrel (Table 3). No major bleedings were documented in the study according to pre-established criteria. Regarding causality, without considering therapeutic failures, 44% of the ADRs were classified as possible and 32% were probable.

Table 3. Clinical adverse reactions and causality analysis.

Therapeutic failures	3
Acute myocardial infarction	2
Ischemic stroke and death	1
Bleedings (all minor)	19
Ecchymosis	7
Epistaxis	4
Gingivorrhagia	2
Hematemesis	1
Petechiae	1
Rectorrhagia	1
Spontaneous bruising	2
Uterine hemorrhage	1
Causality (ADR excluding FT cases)	
Probable	8
Possible	11
Unclassifiable	(fatal cases)

Causality was evaluated using the Naranjo algorithm. Abbreviations: ADR: adverse drugs reactions, FT; fatal cases.

4. Discussion

Clopidogrel therapy has shown different clinical outcomes that depend on the efficacy of the drug. HPR has been linked to major adverse cardiovascular events (MACE) and LPR with bleeding, both conditions have a great clinical impact and represent a challenge for the safe and effective use of the drug [16]. Clopidogrel is a second-generation thienopyridine widely used to treat the acute coronary syndrome. It is administered as an inactive prodrug that requires hepatic conversion by cytochrome P450 (CYP) enzymes, mainly 2C19 to produce an active metabolite [6]. CYP2C19 polymorphisms are related to the anti-platelet effects of clopidogrel [4,7,13,24]. To the best of our knowledge, this study is the first to assess the variants of the promoter region, the intronic and coding region of CYP2C19 through sequencing in a group of Colombian patients with ACS and determines the association with platelet reactivity. In this study, we identified 41 genetic variants, including new polymorphisms in the coding and regulatory CY2C19 regions.

Allele frequencies of CYP2C19 *1 were up to 1.4 times higher than those assessed in other populations (Caucasian, Asian, African, and Latin American) ($p < 0.05$). Interestingly, CYP2C19*17 has a lower allele frequency (2.1 times) concerning populations of other ethnic origins, including Latin America [2,25]. The main LOF CYP2C19*2 allele, previously related to interindividual variability of response to clopidogrel behaves similarly between Latin American populations but presents significant differences with Asian and European populations, in which this allele reaches values of 28% [26]. These results suggest that the Colombian population presents a pharmacogenetic profile of less susceptibility to low and high platelet reactivity in patients treated with the antiplatelet clopidogrel compared to other Latin American or world populations. Recently the RIBEF (Consortium of the Ibero-American Network of Pharmacogenetics and Pharmacogenomics) analyzed the frequency of *CYP2C19* variants in several Latin American countries, nevertheless, Colombia was not included [25,27]. The results of this study contribute to fill this knowledge gap in the Latin American populations underlining high degree of genetic admixture. Colombia is the country with the highest inter-population variability, described as nearly 49% being of mixed origin, 37% of European origin, 10% of African origin, and 3.4% of Amerindian origin [23].

Regarding the population impact of pharmacogenetic relevant alleles in response to clopidogrel, 33.7% of patients analyzed were carriers of at least one variant in *CYP2C19* related to gain or loss of function (10.2% and 7.8% respectively). These findings allow us to infer that similar to other Latin American countries, the impact of LOF variants is much lower compared to Asian populations where the frequency of these variants is five times higher [26]. The low frequency of *CYP2C19*17* revealed that our population is potentially less susceptible to developing low platelet reactivity during treatment with clopidogrel in relation to Caucasian or African populations, where the frequency of *CYP2C19*17* is 21% and 17%, respectively. These findings emphasize the importance of using population genetic approaches to determine the real impact of specific populations' drug responses.

Loss-of-function alleles represented 7.8% of the total and from these, *CYP2C19*2* represented 7.2% (Figure 1). This allele is most frequently associated with high residual platelet reactivity (HPR) in clopidogrel therapy. HPR is a relevant marker in adverse cardiovascular outcomes and has been used to individualize antiplatelet therapy [28]. Clinical relevance of *CYP2C19*2* has been described as well as association with risk of cardiovascular events, stroke and major bleeding [29,30]. These findings have justified the implementation of clinical management guidelines based on genotype, which suggest that new $P2Y_{12}$ inhibitors such as prasugrel and ticagrelor are alternatives for patients who are carriers of LOF genetic variants for *CYP2C19*. Screening for the presence of loss-of-function alleles could allow more informed decision-making regarding the choice of the P2Y receptor blocker [15,24,31].

The frequency for the gain-of-function allele *CYP2C19*17* was 10.2%. This allele has been widely characterized and related to ultrarapid metabolism of *CYP2C19*. *CYP2C19*17* has been associated to low risk of cardiovascular events, high risk of major bleeding, and lower PR on-treatment [32]. These outcomes are attributed to the fact that patients with the allele *CYP2C19*17* are proportionally more exposed to the active metabolite of clopidogrel, which results in a higher inhibition of platelet aggregation to wild type individuals [33]. According to the results of our study, we can hypothesize that patients under treatment with clopidogrel from our population will have a lower risk of suffering major adverse cardiovascular events and bleeding have a greater impact in antiplatelet treatment. Genotypes related to ultra-rapid or extensive phenotypes (18.1%) were more prevalent respect to the poor (0.6%) or intermediate metabolism (14.4%). *CYP2C19*17* is defined by an SNV located in the promoter region (c.−806C>T), functional validation using electrophoretic mobility shift assays (EMSA) revealed binding of hepatic nuclear proteins at −806T but not at −806C. Increased transcriptional activity of -806T allele was confirmed in murine models [34].

Interestingly, analysis through reporter genes has revealed a remarkable heterogeneity in the luciferase activity in CYP2C19 *1/*1 individuals, attributed to non-identified SNV in the *CYP2C19* 5′upstream region [34]. Our study led to the identification of 9 SNVs in the −1500 pb promoter region, two of which correspond to novel variants (−1333C>A, −1163 G>A). 0.6% of the patients were carriers of the allele *CYP2C19*27* (c.−1041G>A), for which a significantly reduced luciferase activity in transfected constructs in HepG2 cells has been reported [35]. In silico analyses have suggested that this effect is potentially related to the generation of a new repressor transcription factor binding site with the OCT-1 [35]. Interestingly, the SNV −70T>C, identified in 0.6% of patients, is located in a positive regulatory region of *CYP2C19*. Arefayene et al., conducted a functional study using artificially generated nested deletions in the gene promoter and studied the ability of allele series to activate luciferase expression in the HepG2 cell line. The data indicated that deletions in CYP2C19 c- −17 to −153 pb generate a significantly reduced activity. This finding was according with potential alteration of factor transcription binding. [36].

The diversity of SNVs identified in the promoter region of *CYP2C19* [36–38], permit us to infer that genetic variants in this region might contribute to interindividual variation in enzymatic activity in vivo. Functional validation of these SNVs will light in the understanding of the expression and heterogeneous activity of *CYP2C19*. Additionally, future studies are necessary for improved understanding of CYP2C19 expression, heterogeneous activity and the unexplained interindividual variability response to clopidogrel of *CYP2C19 *1/1* subject. High allele-frequency variants (e.g., −889 T>G) are of particular interest due to the magnitude of their potential effect at population level.

Regarding intronic variants, the SNP c.332-23A>G (*CYP2C19*35*) co-segregated with c.681 G>A (*CYP2C19*2*) was identified in 24 patients. Previous studies have indicated a complete linkage disequilibrium between these two markers (LOD>2, D′ = 1) [39]. Additionally, we show that the polymorphism c.819 + 228 A>G is potentially related with a splicing alteration, activation of a cryptic donor site, and was part of the haplotype block formed by the SNVs c.681 G>A (*CYP2C19*2*) and c. 332-23 A>G (*CYP2C19*35*) which indicates a high LD among the three variants (Figure 2). This finding has not been previously reported and is relevant considering the potential functional impact of this co-segregation due to the generation of multiple aberrant transcripts with drastic effects on the protein. Previous reports have shown that the haplotype involving the*2 and*35 variants generate transcripts with total retention of intron 2 (exon 2B), a 40 bp deletion of exon 5 and a 71 bp deletion of exon 4 that creates a premature stop codon in exon 4 [39]. The presence of a third variant with a potential effect on splicing could lead to the generation of additional aberrant transcripts.

The in silico analysis of the intronic SNVs c.1292-17 A>G, c.634-4 T>A and 332-23 A>G (*35) suggest a potential alteration in the branch point site (BPS). These variants generate or eliminate the adenine that is part of a key conserved sequence, critical for the assembly of the spliceosome and lariat intron formation, changes in BPS can result in aberrant pre-mRNA splicing [40]. As previously mentioned, c.332-23 A>G (*35) generates a functional effect in *CYP2C19*, which allows us to hypothesize that new intronic SNVs can generate alleles that affect the protein [39]. Functional validation (e.g., minigenes) will allow to assess the biological effect of haplotypes and intronic variants, which given their molecular involvement would correspond to possible LOF alleles for *CYP2C19*.

Recently, Morales-Rosado et al. conducted a NGS (next generation sequencing) analysis in *CYP2C19*, and reported potentially disruptive intronic alleles in 16% of patients [41]. Similarly to our study, they were located towards the end of the gene. We show that 41.6% of the polymorphisms were found in intron 8 (Figure 2). Usually, these types of variants are not included in pharmacogenetic analyzes but due to their role in the regulation of alternative splicing and gene regulation, they constitute new potential response factors to the interindividual variability of the response to clopidogrel [41].

This study identified two novel exonic variants, c.44T>A (p.L15H) and c.1215G>C (p.E405D). *CYP2C19*-p.L15H was identified in the patient SCA_136; in silico analysis suggested its pathogenicity due to amino acid conservation during mammalian evolution, which might be related to a role in its biological function. Indeed, *CYP2C19* is inserted cotranslationally in the membrane of the endoplasmic reticulum using signals directed by the N-terminal hydrophobic domain of the protein [42,43]. Functional expression and cellular localization studies of plasmids with mutant proteins for the N-terminal (amino acids 3 to 20) showed that changes in this region modify the degree of integration, potentially affecting subcellular localization and enzyme activity [42]. Variants located in N-terminal end such as p.L16F leads to decreased expression level [44]. *CYP2C19*-p.405E is a residue located in the L Helix, implicated in the binding of the heme group [45]. Functional analysis has shown that genetic variants in *CYP2C19* that modify residues located in or near the binding region of the heme group can alter the stability and/or efficiency of the folding of the holoprotein CYP2C19, which leads to the potential degradation of functional proteins [46]. Despite the conservation of E405 residue and, in silico analysis, CYP2C19-p.E405D could have a functional effect that needs to be validated.

Our study determined platelet function using the INNOVANCE PFA-200 system (Siemens Healthcare, Germany) which assesses P2Y12-receptor blockades in patients undergoing therapy with P2Y12-receptor antagonists [47]. Despite some reports indicating a positive correlation between the CT value, HTPR, and MACE frequency [13,20,48,49], our findings failed to associate the molecular genotype and phenotype of HPR. This result can be attributed to several factors; (a) low frequency of LOF alleles (b) absence of patients with the homozygous genotype for LOF alleles (c) high frequency *CYP2C19**1/*1 with CT suggestive of HPR (d) potential overestimation of patients HPR (technical limitation of PFA-200); (e) involvement of new intronic and/or promoter variants and (f) heterogeneity of response to clopidogrel due to genes not evaluated in this study [5,50].

Similarly, it has been established that the use of platelet function tests such as PFA-200, Verify Now P2Y$_{12}$ assay and others are potentially predictive of the clinical response to clopidogrel [20,49]. Although not significant, intermediate metabolizers (at least one loss function allele) showed a trend towards decreasing CT values and therefore are more susceptible to HPR. Possibly the absence of poor metabolizers and the low proportion of carriers in our population are responsible for the observed non-significance. Studies using the PFA-200 platelet function test in Asian population, where 59% of patients had *CYP2C19*-loss-of-function genotypes, found that CT values were significantly different between EM and IM or PM suggesting a significant association between the efficacy of clopidogrel and *CYP2C19* genotypes [20]

The clinical outcome could be evaluated in 97% of the subjects included in the study (with continuous clopidogrel therapy), 24 patients with adverse reactions were identified, with a predominance of bleeding (Table 3). The occurrence of these events is explained mainly at the pathophysiological level by low or high platelet reactivity, attributed in part to alleles related to UR or slow metabolism for *CYP2C19*. The results of the causality analysis evaluated by the Naranjo algorithm estimated that clopidogrel was the probable or possible cause of 76% of the adverse reactions observed in the patients. Despite not reaching statistical significance between polymorphic alleles and platelet reactivity, we observed that 25% of patients with ADR were carriers of genetic variants of known functional impact (*2, *17). The existence of polymorphisms in regulatory regions (introns and promoter) could explain the heterogeneity in the clinical response to clopidogrel observed by us [41]. In addition, if it is considered that the interindividual variability to antiplatelet treatment attributed to CYP2C19 polymorphisms is 12%, variants in other genes not analyzed could influence the appearance of ADR in people with the CYP2C19*1/*1 genotype [4].

In addition to the potential genetic impact on the generation of adverse drug reactions (ADRs) to clopidogrel, the Colombian clinical practice guidelines for acute coronary syndrome (ACS) recommend a lower loading dose that can impact the presentation of ADRs. In this precise manner, the loading dose of 300 mg recommended at the time of hospital admission is lower as compared to the European society of cardiology guidelines (600 mg) [51].

Given the clinical evidence that has found a higher percentage of bleeding with the 600 mg vs. 300 mg dosage of clopidogrel (1·6% vs. 1·1%, $p = 0·009$) [52], it is plausible to think that our patients can present this adverse reaction lower than expected. Even so, most of our ARDS correspond to bleeding; this evidence supports that other factors (ej. UR metabolism allele carrier *17) can influence the presentation of unwanted effects.

The use of 600 mg loading dose for clopidogrel recommended by the European guidelines was justified through the evidence collected mainly on the CURRENT-OASIS 7 trial, which demonstrated a reduction in major cardiovascular events and stent thrombosis as compared to the lower 300 mg loading dose [53]. Our national guidelines take this evidence into consideration and recommend giving 300 mg to every patient with ACS, and an additional 300 mg (completing 600 mg of loading dose) when the patient can be guaranteed an early percutaneous coronary intervention (PCI). In our study, a therapeutic failure was found in the setting of an Acute myocardial infarct secondary to stent thrombosis, this patient did not receive the 600 mg loading dose of clopidogrel. This case evokes the fact that lower doses can be a potential cause for the MACEs previously reported [53,54]. Taking into account the genetic implication existing in our population with a lesser frequency of alleles related to high platelet reaction that potentially favors the lower presentation of MACEs despite the lower dosages recommended for the country.

Regarding the use of other antiplatelet agents such as ticagrelor and prasugrel, despite the evidence found, in terms of effectiveness and security, they are not first-line medications in our country, and they require additional logistic clearance for their use since they are contemplated outside of the national mandatory plan (https://tablas.sispro.gov.co/TestMiPresNopbs/ModTest/Mipres.aspx (accessed on 14 March 2021)). Furthermore, these agents can generate over costs in countries with budget constraints [53]. These observations can explain the low proportion of patients in whom a change of use of Clopidogrel to ticagrelor or prasugrel was seen.

Taken together, our results allowed us to establish the pharmacogenetic profile of *CYP2C19* in Colombian patients with ACS under clopidogrel treatment. Importantly, differences in allele frequencies responsible for the interindividual variability attributed to the safe and effective antiplatelet response were identified in our population. Additionally, *CYP2C19* sequencing identifies intronic variants potentially related with splicing modification, which are not currently covered by pharmacogenetic analysis of clopidogrel therapy. The association of some of these SNVs and clopidogrel pharmacokinetics needs to be further validated.

Our study has several limitations. The low frequency of alleles related to slow and ultra-rapid metabolism together with the absence of homozygous for LOF alleles of CY2C19 limits the power to detect a significant association between molecular genotype and platelet reactivity. Functional validation is required to determine the biological significance of deep intronic variants and promoter region polymorphisms. However, the identification of polymorphisms that are not usually part of the pharmacogenetic analysis of *CYP2C19* is relevant for the identification of new alleles. Finally, clinical follow-up for a six-months period may be insufficient for the detection of major cardiovascular events.

5. Conclusions

In conclusion, the present study allowed us to identify *CYP2C19* variants in patients affected with ACS and treated with clopidogrel. Allele frequencies for some of the polymorphisms identified in the Colombian population were statistically different to those in other populations and globally, which suggests a specific susceptibility. Given our findings regarding allele frequencies of loss or gain of function, we can infer a greater effect of low platelet reactivity in patients treated with clopidogrel. Furthermore, in silico analysis for new variants in the coding and regulatory regions allowed us to propose new molecular mechanisms potentially related to interindividual variability in response to clopidogrel. Ultimately, our results contribute to the understanding of the population pharmacogenetics in Latin America.

Supplementary Materials: The following are available online at https://www.mdpi.com/article/10.3390/jpm11050400/s1, Figure S1: Comparison between sequences of proteins with modified residues and orthologous proteins of mammalian species. Table S1: Primers sequence. Table S2: The comparison of allelic frequencies between the Colombian population and other populations.

Author Contributions: Conceptualization, K.P.A., C.A.C.-O. and D.J.F.-M.; data curation, D.-A.R.-T., N.P., L.B.P.-H. and C.A.C.-O.; formal analysis, M.A.-A., K.P., C.A.T.-A., D.-A.R.-T., S.S.-P., M.J.N.-O., N.P., L.-F.C.-L., N.C., C.A.C.-O. and D.J.F.-M.; funding acquisition, J.M.P.-O., C.A.C.-O. and D.J.F.-M.; investigation, J.M.P.-O., K.P.A., P.L. and D.J.F.-M.; methodology, K.P., C.A.T.-A., D.-A.R.-T., S.S.-P., M.J.N.-O., L.-F.C.-L., K.P.A., P.L. and N.C.; project administration, D.J.F.-M.; software, M.A.-A. and N.P.; supervision, M.A.-A. and D.J.F.-M.; validation, M.A.-A., K.P. and D.J.F.-M.; writing—original draft, M.A.-A.; writing—review and editing, C.A.T.-A., P.L., C.A.C.-O. and D.J.F.-M. All authors have read and agreed to the published version of the manuscript.

Funding: This project was supported by the Universidad del Rosario (Grants CS/ABN062 and IV-FPC015) and Hospital Universitario Mayor MEDERI.

Institutional Review Board Statement: All this study's experimental steps were approved by the Universidad del Rosario's Ethics Committee (DVO005 990-CV1018); the study was conducted in line with the Declaration of Helsinki (approval date: January 2019).

Informed Consent Statement: All the subjects (n = 166) provided their informed consent for their enrolment in the study.

Data Availability Statement: The data presented in this study are available on request from the corresponding author. The data are not publicly available as they correspond to Sanger sequencing and closure times values.

Conflicts of Interest: The authors declare that they have no competing interests.

References

1. Peng, W.; Shi, X.; Xu, X.; Lin, Y. Both CYP2C19 and PON1 Q192R Genotypes Influence Platelet Response to Clopidogrel by Thrombelastography in Patients with Acute Coronary Syndrome. *Cardiovasc. Ther.* **2019**, *2019*, 3470145. [CrossRef]
2. Pereira, N.L.; Rihal, C.S.; So, D.Y.F.; Rosenberg, Y.; Lennon, R.J.; Mathew, V.; Goodman, S.G.; Weinshilboum, R.M.; Wang, L.; Baudhuin, L.M.; et al. Clopidogrel Pharmacogenetics. *Circ. Cardiovasc. Interv.* **2019**, *12*, 1–21. [CrossRef]
3. Savi, P.; Pereillo, J.M.; Uzabiaga, M.F.; Combalbert, J.; Picard, C.; Maffrand, J.P.; Pascal, M.; Herbert, J.M. Identification and biological activity of the active metabolite of clopidogrel. *Thromb. Haemost.* **2000**, *84*, 891–896. [CrossRef] [PubMed]
4. Brown, S.A.; Pereira, N. Pharmacogenomic Impact of CYP2C19 Variation on Clopidogrel Therapy in Precision Cardiovascular Medicine. *J. Pers. Med.* **2018**, *8*, 8. [CrossRef] [PubMed]
5. Hernandez-Suarez, D.F.; Botton, M.R.; Scott, S.A.; Tomey, M.I.; Garcia, M.J.; Wiley, J.; Villablanca, P.A.; Melin, K.; Lopez-Candales, A.; Renta, J.Y.; et al. Pharmacogenetic association study on clopidogrel response in Puerto Rican Hispanics with cardiovascular disease: A novel characterization of a Caribbean population. *Pharmgenom. Pers. Med.* **2018**, *11*, 95–106. [CrossRef] [PubMed]
6. Patti, G.; Micieli, G.; Cimminiello, C. The Role of Clopidogrel in 2020: A Reappraisal. *Cardiovasc. Ther.* **2020**, *2020*, 8703627. [CrossRef]
7. Yin, T.; Miyata, T. Pharmacogenomics of clopidogrel: Evidence and perspectives. *Thromb. Res.* **2011**, *128*, 307–316. [CrossRef]
8. Amin, A.M.; Sheau Chin, L.; Azri Mohamed Noor, D. The Personalization of Clopidogrel Antiplatelet Therapy: The Role of Integrative Pharmacogenetics and Pharmacometabolomics. *Cardiol. Res. Pract.* **2017**, *2017*, 8062796. [CrossRef]
9. Shuldiner, A.R.; O'Connell, J.R.; Bliden, K.P.; Gandhi, A.; Ryan, K.; Horenstein, R.B.; Damcott, C.M.; Pakyz, R.; Tantry, U.S.; Gibson, Q.; et al. Association of cytochrome P450 2C19 genotype with the antiplatelet effect and clinical efficacy of clopidogrel therapy. *JAMA* **2009**, *302*, 849–857. [CrossRef]
10. Singla, A.; Antonino, M.J.; Bliden, K.P.; Tantry, U.S.; Gurbel, P.A. The relation between platelet reactivity and glycemic control in diabetic patients with cardiovascular disease on maintenance aspirin and clopidogrel therapy. *Am. Heart J.* **2009**, *158*, 784.e1–784.e6. [CrossRef]
11. Lewis, J.P.; Shuldiner, A.R. Clopidogrel pharmacogenetics: Beyond candidate genes and genome-wide association studies. *Clin. Pharmacol. Ther.* **2017**, *101*, 323–325. [CrossRef]
12. Xu, J.; Wang, A.; Wangqin, R.; Mo, J.; Chen, Z.; Dai, L.; Meng, X.; Zhao, X.; Wang, Y.; Li, H.; et al. Efficacy of clopidogrel for stroke depends on CYP2C19 genotype and risk profile. *Randomized Control. Trial* **2019**, *86*, 419–426. [CrossRef]
13. Su, Q.; Li, J.; Tang, Z.; Yang, S.; Xing, G.; Liu, T.; Peng, H. Association of CYP2C19 Polymorphism with Clopidogrel Resistance in Patients with Acute Coronary Syndrome in China. *Med. Sci. Monit.* **2019**, *25*, 7138–7148. [CrossRef]
14. Joob, B.; Wiwanitkit, V. CYP2C19*2 polymorphism and clopidogrel resistance. *Arch. Cardiol. Mex.* **2020**, *90*, 544–548. [PubMed]
15. Scott, S.A.; Sangkuhl, K.; Stein, C.M.; Hulot, J.S.; Mega, J.L.; Roden, D.M.; Klein, T.E.; Sabatine, M.S.; Johnson, J.A.; Shuldiner, A.R. Clinical Pharmacogenetics Implementation Consortium guidelines for CYP2C19 genotype and clopidogrel therapy: 2013 update. *Clin. Pharmacol. Ther.* **2013**, *94*, 317–323. [CrossRef] [PubMed]
16. Wiśniewski, A.; Filipska, K. The Phenomenon of Clopidogrel High On-Treatment Platelet Reactivity in Ischemic Stroke Subjects: A Comprehensive Review. *Int. J. Mol. Sci.* **2020**, *21*, 6408. [CrossRef] [PubMed]

17. Pereira, N.L.; Geske, J.B.; Mayr, M.; Shah, S.H.; Rihal, C.S. Pharmacogenetics of Clopidogrel: An Unresolved Issue. *Circ. Cardiovasc. Genet.* **2016**, *9*, 185–188. [CrossRef] [PubMed]
18. Mărginean, A.; Bănescu, C.; Moldovan, V.; Scridon, A.; Mărginean, M.; Bălaşa, R.; Maier, S.; Țăruși, M.; Dobreanu, M. The Impact of CYP2C19 Loss-of-Function Polymorphisms, Clinical, and Demographic Variables on Platelet Response to Clopidogrel Evaluated Using Impedance Aggregometry. *Clin. Appl. Thromb. Hemost.* **2017**, *23*, 255–265. [CrossRef] [PubMed]
19. Paré, G.; Mehta, S.R.; Yusuf, S.; Anand, S.S.; Connolly, S.J.; Hirsh, J.; Simonsen, K.; Bhatt, D.L.; Fox, K.A.; Eikelboom, J.W. Effects of CYP2C19 genotype on outcomes of clopidogrel treatment. *N. Engl. J. Med.* **2010**, *363*, 1704–1714. [CrossRef]
20. Li, S.; Choi, J.L.; Guo, L.Z.; Goh, R.Y.; Kim, B.R.; Woo, K.S.; Kim, M.H.; Han, J.Y. Correlation between the CYP2C19 phenotype status and the results of three different platelet function tests in cardiovascular disease patients receiving antiplatelet therapy: An emphasis on newly introduced platelet function analyzer-200 P2Y test. *Ann. Lab. Med.* **2016**, *36*, 42–48. [CrossRef]
21. Klein, M.D.; Williams, A.K.; Lee, C.R.; Stouffer, G.A. Clinical Utility of CYP2C19 Genotyping to Guide Antiplatelet Therapy in Patients With an Acute Coronary Syndrome or Undergoing Percutaneous Coronary Intervention. *Arterioscler. Thromb. Vasc. Biol.* **2019**, *39*, 647–652. [CrossRef]
22. Naranjo, C.A.; Busto, U.; Sellers, E.M.; Sandor, P.; Ruiz, I.; Roberts, E.A.; Janecek, E.; Domecq, C.; Greenblatt, D.J. A method for estimating the probability of adverse drug reactions. *Clin. Pharmacol. Ther.* **1981**, *30*, 239–245. [CrossRef]
23. Schulman, S.; Kearon, C. Definition of major bleeding in clinical investigations of antihemostatic medicinal products in non-surgical patients. *J. Thromb. Haemost.* **2005**, *3*, 692–694. [CrossRef]
24. Rath, C.L.; Jørgensen, N.R.; Wienecke, T. Clopidogrel responder status is uninfluenced by CYP2C19*2 in Danish patients with stroke. *PLoS ONE* **2020**, *15*, e0236260. [CrossRef]
25. Rodrigues-Soares, F.; Peñas-Lledó, E.M.; Tarazona-Santos, E.; Sosa-Macías, M.; Terán, E.; López-López, M.; Rodeiro, I.; Moya, G.E.; Calzadilla, L.R.; Ramírez-Roa, R.; et al. Genomic Ancestry, CYP2D6, CYP2C9, and CYP2C19 Among Latin Americans. *Clin. Pharmacol. Ther.* **2020**, *107*, 257–268. [CrossRef]
26. Dorji, P.W.; Tshering, G.; Na-Bangchang, K. CYP2C9, CYP2C19, CYP2D6 and CYP3A5 polymorphisms in South-East and East Asian populations: A systematic review. *J. Clin. Pharm. Ther.* **2019**, *44*, 508–524. [CrossRef]
27. Rodeiro, I.; Remírez-Figueredo, D.; García-Mesa, M.; Dorado, P.; LLerena, A.; CEIBA. Pharmacogenetics in Latin American populations: Regulatory aspects, application to herbal medicine, cardiovascular and psychiatric disorders. *Drug Metabol. Drug Interact.* **2012**, *27*, 57–60. [CrossRef] [PubMed]
28. Gurbel, P.A.; Tantry, U.S. Do platelet function testing and genotyping improve outcome in patients treated with antithrombotic agents? *Circulation* **2012**, *125*, 1276–1287. [CrossRef] [PubMed]
29. Holmes, D.R., Jr.; Dehmer, G.J.; Kaul, S.; Leifer, D.; O'Gara, P.T.; Stein, C.M. ACCF/AHA clopidogrel clinical alert: Approaches to the FDA "boxed warning": A report of the American College of Cardiology Foundation Task Force on clinical expert consensus documents and the American Heart Association endorsed by the Society for Cardiovascular Angiography and Interventions and the Society of Thoracic Surgeons. *J. Am. Coll. Cardiol.* **2010**, *56*, 321–341. [PubMed]
30. Wallentin, L.; James, S.; Storey, R.F.; Armstrong, M.; Barratt, B.J.; Horrow, J.; Husted, S.; Katus, H.; Steg, P.G.; Shah, S.H.; et al. Effect of CYP2C19 and ABCB1 single nucleotide polymorphisms on outcomes of treatment with ticagrelor versus clopidogrel for acute coronary syndromes: A genetic substudy of the PLATO trial. *Lancet* **2010**, *376*, 1320–1328. [CrossRef]
31. Notarangelo, F.M.; Maglietta, G.; Bevilacqua, P.; Cereda, M.; Merlini, P.A.; Villani, G.Q.; Moruzzi, P.; Patrizi, G.; Malagoli Tagliazucchi, G.; Crocamo, A.; et al. Pharmacogenomic Approach to Selecting Antiplatelet Therapy in Patients With Acute Coronary Syndromes: The PHARMCLO Trial. *J. Am. Coll. Cardiol.* **2018**, *71*, 1869–1877. [CrossRef]
32. Li, Y.; Tang, H.L.; Hu, Y.F.; Xie, H.G. The gain-of-function variant allele CYP2C19*17: A double-edged sword between thrombosis and bleeding in clopidogrel-treated patients. *J. Thromb. Haemost.* **2012**, *10*, 199–206. [CrossRef]
33. Mega, J.L.; Close, S.L.; Wiviott, S.D.; Shen, L.; Hockett, R.D.; Brandt, J.T.; Walker, J.R.; Antman, E.M.; Macias, W.; Braunwald, E.; et al. Cytochrome p-450 polymorphisms and response to clopidogrel. *N. Engl. J. Med.* **2009**, *360*, 354–362. [CrossRef]
34. Helsby, N.A.; Burns, K.E. Molecular mechanisms of genetic variation and transcriptional regulation of CYP2C19. *Front. Genet.* **2012**, *3*, 206. [CrossRef]
35. Drögemöller, B.I.; Wright, G.E.; Niehaus, D.J.; Koen, L.; Malan, S.; Da Silva, D.M.; Hillermann-Rebello, R.; La Grange, A.M.; Venter, M.; Warnich, L. Characterization of the genetic profile of CYP2C19 in two South African populations. *Pharmacogenomics* **2010**, *11*, 1095–1103. [CrossRef] [PubMed]
36. Arefayene, M.; Skaar, T.C.; Zhao, X.; Rae, J.M.; Tanus-Santos, J.E.; Brinkmann, U.; Brehm, I.; Salat, U.; Nguyen, A.; Desta, Z.; et al. Sequence diversity and functional characterization of the 5′-regulatory region of human CYP2C19. *Pharmacogenetics* **2003**, *13*, 199–206. [CrossRef] [PubMed]
37. Fukushima-Uesaka, H.; Saito, Y.; Maekawa, K.; Ozawa, S.; Hasegawa, R.; Kajio, H.; Kuzuya, N.; Yasuda, K.; Kawamoto, M.; Kamatani, N.; et al. Genetic variations and haplotypes of CYP2C19 in a Japanese population. *Drug Metab. Pharmacokinet.* **2005**, *20*, 300–307. [CrossRef] [PubMed]
38. Satyanarayana, C.R.; Devendran, A.; Jayaraman, M.; Mannu, J.; Mathur, P.P.; Gopal, S.D.; Rajagopal, K.; Chandrasekaran, A. Influence of the genetic polymorphisms in the 5′ flanking and exonic regions of CYP2C19 on proguanil oxidation. *Drug Metab. Pharmacokinet.* **2009**, *24*, 537–548. [CrossRef] [PubMed]

39. Chaudhry, A.S.; Prasad, B.; Shirasaka, Y.; Fohner, A.; Finkelstein, D.; Fan, Y.; Wang, S.; Wu, G.; Aklillu, E.; Sim, S.C.; et al. The CYP2C19 Intron 2 Branch Point SNP is the Ancestral Polymorphism Contributing to the Poor Metabolizer Phenotype in Livers with CYP2C19*35 and CYP2C19*2 Alleles. *Drug Metab. Dispos.* **2015**, *43*, 1226–1235. [CrossRef]
40. Královicová, J.; Lei, H.; Vorechovský, I. Phenotypic consequences of branch point substitutions. *Hum. Mutat.* **2006**, *27*, 803–813. [CrossRef]
41. Morales-Rosado, J.A.; Goel, K.; Zhang, L.; Åkerblom, A.; Baheti, S.; Black, J.L.; Eriksson, N.; Wallentin, L.; James, S.; Storey, R.F.; et al. Next-Generation Sequencing of CYP2C19 in Stent Thrombosis: Implications for Clopidogrel Pharmacogenomics. *Cardiovasc. Drugs Ther.* **2020**. [CrossRef]
42. Shukla, A.; Huang, W.; Depaz, I.M.; Gillam, E.M. Membrane integration of recombinant human P450 forms. *Xenobiotica* **2009**, *39*, 495–507. [CrossRef] [PubMed]
43. Ahn, K.; Szczesna-Skorupa, E.; Kemper, B. The amino-terminal 29 amino acids of cytochrome P450 2C1 are sufficient for retention in the endoplasmic reticulum. *J. Biol. Chem.* **1993**, *268*, 18726–18733. [CrossRef]
44. Xu, R.A.; Gu, E.M.; Liu, T.H.; Ou-Yang, Q.G.; Hu, G.X.; Cai, J.P. The effects of cytochrome P450 2C19 polymorphism on the metabolism of voriconazole in vitro. *Infect. Drug Resist.* **2018**, *11*, 2129–2135. [CrossRef]
45. Hasemann, C.A.; Kurumbail, R.G.; Boddupalli, S.S.; Peterson, J.A.; Deisenhofer, J. Structure and function of cytochromes P450: A comparative analysis of three crystal structures. *Structure* **1995**, *3*, 41–62. [CrossRef]
46. Wang, H.; An, N.; Wang, H.; Gao, Y.; Liu, D.; Bian, T.; Zhu, J.; Chen, C. Evaluation of the effects of 20 nonsynonymous single nucleotide polymorphisms of CYP2C19 on S-mephenytoin 4′-hydroxylation and omeprazole 5′-hydroxylation. *Drug Metab. Dispos.* **2011**, *39*, 830–837. [CrossRef] [PubMed]
47. Koessler, J.; Kobsar, A.L.; Rajkovic, M.S.; Schafer, A.; Flierl, U.; Pfoertsch, S.; Bauersachs, J.; Steigerwald, U.; Rechner, A.R.; Walter, U. The new INNOVANCE® PFA P2Y cartridge is sensitive to the detection of the $P2Y_{12}$ receptor inhibition. *Platelets* **2011**, *22*, 20–27. [CrossRef] [PubMed]
48. Harmsze, A.; van Werkum, J.W.; Bouman, H.J.; Ruven, H.J.; Breet, N.J.; Ten Berg, J.M.; Hackeng, C.M.; Tjoeng, M.M.; Klungel, O.H.; de Boer, A.; et al. Besides CYP2C19*2, the variant allele CYP2C9*3 is associated with higher on-clopidogrel platelet reactivity in patients on dual antiplatelet therapy undergoing elective coronary stent implantation. *Pharm. Genom.* **2010**, *20*, 18–25. [CrossRef] [PubMed]
49. Lim, H.H.; Li, S.; An, G.D.; Woo, K.S.; Kim, K.H.; Kim, J.M.; Kim, M.H.; Han, J.Y. Platelet Function Analyzer-200 P2Y Results Are Predictive of the Risk of Major Adverse Cardiac Events in Korean Patients Receiving Clopidogrel Therapy Following Acute Coronary Syndrome. *Ann. Lab. Med.* **2018**, *38*, 413–419. [CrossRef]
50. Roule, V.; Ardouin, P.; Repessé, Y.; Le Querrec, A.; Blanchart, K.; Lemaitre, A.; Sabatier, R.; Borel-Derlon, A.; Beygui, F. Point of Care Tests VerifyNow P2Y12 and INNOVANCE PFA P2Y Compared to Light Transmittance Aggregometry After Fibrinolysis. *Clin. Appl. Thromb. Hemost.* **2018**, *24*, 1109–1116. [CrossRef]
51. Ibanez, B.; James, S.; Agewall, S.; Antunes, M.J.; Bucciarelli-Ducci, C.; Bueno, H.; Caforio, A.L.P.; Crea, F.; Goudevenos, J.A.; Halvorsen, S.; et al. 2017 ESC Guidelines for the management of acute myocardial infarction in patients presenting with ST-segment elevation: The Task Force for the management of acute myocardial infarction in patients presenting with ST-segment elevation of the European Society of Cardiology (ESC). *Eur. Heart J.* **2018**, *39*, 119–177. [PubMed]
52. Mehta, S.R.; Tanguay, J.F.; Eikelboom, J.W.; Jolly, S.S.; Joyner, C.D.; Granger, C.B.; Faxon, D.P.; Rupprecht, H.J.; Budaj, A.; Avezum, A.; et al. Double-dose versus standard-dose clopidogrel and high-dose versus low-dose aspirin in individuals undergoing percutaneous coronary intervention for acute coronary syndromes (CURRENT-OASIS 7): A randomised factorial trial. *Lancet* **2010**, *376*, 1233–1243. [CrossRef]
53. Nijjer, S.S.; Davies, J.E.; Francis, D.P. Quantitative comparison of clopidogrel 600 mg, prasugrel and ticagrelor, against clopidogrel 300 mg on major adverse cardiovascular events and bleeding in coronary stenting: Synthesis of CURRENT-OASIS-7, TRITON-TIMI-38 and PLATO. *Int. J. Cardiol.* **2012**, *158*, 181–185. [CrossRef]
54. Mehta, S.R.; Bassand, J.P.; Chrolavicius, S.; Diaz, R.; Eikelboom, J.W.; Fox, K.A.; Granger, C.B.; Jolly, S.; Joyner, C.D.; Rupprecht, H.J.; et al. Dose comparisons of clopidogrel and aspirin in acute coronary syndromes. *N. Engl. J. Med.* **2010**, *363*, 930–942. [PubMed]

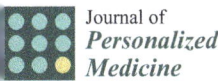 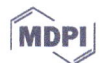

Article

SLCO1B1 Phenotype and CYP3A5 Polymorphism Significantly Affect Atorvastatin Bioavailability

Pablo Zubiaur [1,2,*], Maria Dolores Benedicto [3], Gonzalo Villapalos-García [1], Marcos Navares-Gómez [1], Gina Mejía-Abril [2,4], Manuel Román [5], Samuel Martín-Vílchez [5], Dolores Ochoa [4,5] and Francisco Abad-Santos [1,2,3,4,5,6,*]

1. Pharmacogenetics Unit, Clinical Pharmacology Department, La Princesa University Hospital Research Institute, 28006 Madrid, Spain; g.villapalos@salud.madrid.org (G.V.-G.); marcos.navares@salud.madrid.org (M.N.-G.)
2. Spanish Clinical Research Network (SCReN), La Princesa University Hospital Research Institute, 28006 Madrid, Spain; ginapaola.mejia@scren.es
3. Universidad Autónoma de Madrid (UAM), 28029 Madrid, Spain; lolabenedicto.96@gmail.com
4. Clinical Pharmacology Department, La Princesa University Hospital, 28006 Madrid, Spain; mdolores.ochoa@salud.madrid.org
5. Clinical Trials Unit of La Princesa University Hospital (UECHUP), La Princesa University Hospital Research Institute, 28006 Madrid, Spain; manuel.roman@salud.madrid.org (M.R.); smvilchez@salud.madrid.org (S.M.-V.)
6. Centro de Investigación Biomédica en Red de Enfermedades Hepáticas y Digestivas (CIBERehd), ICIII, 28006 Madrid, Spain
* Correspondence: pablo.zubiaur@salud.madrid.org (P.Z.); francisco.abad@salud.madrid.org (F.A.-S.); Tel.: +34-915202425 (P.Z. & F.A.-S.); Fax: +34-915202540 (P.Z. & F.A.-S.)

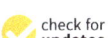

Citation: Zubiaur, P.; Benedicto, M.D.; Villapalos-García, G.; Navares-Gómez, M.; Mejía-Abril, G.; Román, M.; Martín-Vílchez, S.; Ochoa, D.; Abad-Santos, F. SLCO1B1 Phenotype and CYP3A5 Polymorphism Significantly Affect Atorvastatin Bioavailability. *J. Pers. Med.* **2021**, *11*, 204. https://doi.org/10.3390/jpm11030204

Academic Editor: Luis A. López-Fernández

Received: 29 January 2021
Accepted: 9 March 2021
Published: 13 March 2021

Publisher's Note: MDPI stays neutral with regard to jurisdictional claims in published maps and institutional affiliations.

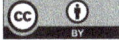

Copyright: © 2021 by the authors. Licensee MDPI, Basel, Switzerland. This article is an open access article distributed under the terms and conditions of the Creative Commons Attribution (CC BY) license (https://creativecommons.org/licenses/by/4.0/).

Abstract: Atorvastatin, prescribed for the treatment of hypercholesterolemia, demonstrated overwhelming benefits in reducing cardiovascular morbidity and mortality. However, many patients discontinue therapy due to adverse reactions, especially myopathy. The Dutch Pharmacogenetics Working Group (DPWG) recommends an alternative agent to atorvastatin and simvastatin or a dose adjustment depending on other risk factors for statin-induced myopathy in SLCO1B1 rs4149056 CC or TC carriers. In contrast, the Clinical Pharmacogenetics Implementation Consortium (CPIC) published their guideline on simvastatin, but not on atorvastatin. In this work, we aimed to demonstrate the effect of SLCO1B1 phenotype and other variants (e.g., in *CYP3A4/5*, *UGT* enzymes or *SLC* transporters) on atorvastatin pharmacokinetics. For this purpose, a candidate-gene pharmacogenetic study was proposed. The study population comprised 156 healthy volunteers enrolled in atorvastatin bioequivalence clinical trials. The genotyping strategy comprised a total of 60 variants in 15 genes. Women showed higher exposure to atorvastatin compared to men ($p = 0.001$), however this difference disappeared after dose/weight (DW) correction. The most relevant pharmacogenetic differences were the following: AUC/DW and C_{max}/DW based on (a) SLCO1B1 phenotype ($p < 0.001$ for both) and (b) *CYP3A5*3* ($p = 0.004$ and 0.018, respectively). As secondary findings: *SLC22A1* *2/*2* genotype was related to higher C_{max}/DW (ANOVA $p = 0.030$) and *SLC22A1* *1/*5* genotype was associated with higher Vd/F (ANOVA $p = 0.032$) compared to *SLC22A1* *1/*1*, respectively. Finally, *UGT2B7* rs7439366 *1/*1* genotype was associated with higher t_{max} as compared with the *1/*3* genotype (ANOVA $p = 0.024$). Based on our results, we suggest that SLCO1B1 is the best predictor for atorvastatin pharmacokinetic variability and that prescription should be adjusted based on it. We suggest that the CPIC should include atorvastatin in their statin-SLCO1B1 guidelines. Interesting and novel results were observed based on *CYP3A5* genotype, which should be confirmed with further studies.

Keywords: atorvastatin; pharmacogenetics; SLCO1B1; precision medicine

1. Introduction

Statins are the most frequently prescribed drugs for the management of hypercholesterolemia, due to their effectiveness and safety profile [1]. They all inhibit the hydroxymethylglutaryl coenzyme A (HMG-CoA) reductase, which reduces cholesterol biosynthesis and modulates lipid metabolism. Statins have an antiatherosclerotic effect correlated with the decrease in LDL cholesterol [2]. Atorvastatin is a member of the statin family with greater effectiveness in cholesterol control compared to other statins, namely lovastatin, pravastatin, simvastatin, and fluvastatin, with a similar tolerability profile [3].

Atorvastatin daily dose ranges between 10 to 80 mg, depending on initial LDL blood levels. After oral administration, atorvastatin is quickly and almost entirely absorbed (95–99%), with maximum concentrations (C_{max}) reached at 1 to 2 h (t_{max}) [4,5]. It suffers pronounced pre-systemic clearance at the gastrointestinal tract and first-pass hepatic clearance, which explains its low systemic bioavailability (around 12%) [5,6]. Atorvastatin binds to plasma proteins (>98%), and its volume of distribution is approximately 38 L. It undergoes cytochrome P450 (CYP) 3A4 (CYP3A4) mediated metabolism to active metabolites [5,7]. Elimination is principally biliary with apparently no significant enterohepatic recirculation. Half-life ($t_{1/2}$) is approximately 14 h for atorvastatin and 20–30 h for its metabolites [5,7]. Atorvastatin is a substrate of the organic anion transporter polypeptides 1B1 (OATP1B1) and 1B3 (OATP1B3), encoded by *SLCO1B1* and *SLCO1B3* genes, respectively [5,8].

Genetic polymorphism is related to variability in atorvastatin pharmacokinetics, pharmacodynamics, drug exposure [9], and effectiveness [10]. However, to date, the only clinical guideline for atorvastatin dose adjustment based on a pharmacogenetic biomarker is the one published by the Dutch Pharmacogenetics Working Group (DPWG) [11]. The use of an alternative statin (e.g., fluvastatin) is recommended for patients with *SLCO1B1* rs4149056 T>C, C/C (*5/*5) or T/C (*1/*5) genotypes and additional significant risk factors for statin-induced myopathy. In other words, therapy must be adjusted in those without the *SLCO1B1* normal function (NF) phenotype (*1/*1), i.e., decreased function (DF) or poor function (PF) phenotypes (*1/*5 and *5/*5 genotypes, respectively). These recommendations are the same for simvastatin (DPWG). In addition, the Clinical Pharmacogenetics Implementation Consortium (CPIC) published their pharmacogenetic guideline for *SLCO1B1* and simvastatin [12], with similar recommendations as those from DPWG.

To confirm the influence of the SLCO1B1 phenotype on atorvastatin exposure, and the need for dose adjustments based on it, we aimed to perform a candidate gene pharmacogenetic study in healthy volunteers enrolled in bioequivalence clinical trials. In addition, we proposed to investigate the influence of single nucleotide polymorphisms (SNPs) in other genes in relation to the disposition of atorvastatin, namely *CYP3A*, other *CYP* enzymes or transporters (e.g., *ABCB1* or *SLC22A1*), as well as on atorvastatin tolerability.

2. Materials and Methods

2.1. Study Population

The study population comprised healthy volunteers enrolled in five different atorvastatin or atorvastatin/ezetimibe bioequivalence clinical trials performed at the Clinical Trial Unit of Hospital Universitario de La Princesa (UECHUP), Madrid, Spain. Study protocols were revised and approved by the Hospital's Research Ethics Committee and by the Spanish Drugs Agency (AEMPS). Complying with Spanish and European legislation on research in humans, all of them were accomplished under the Good Clinical Practice guidelines and endorsing the Declaration of Helsinki. EUDRA-CT numbers were as follows: 2018-000082-37, 2019-002222-67, 2019-000891-41, 2019-001670-29, and 2019-000656-34. All the subjects (n = 178) provided their informed consent for their enrolment in the bioequivalence clinical trial. For the pharmacogenetic study, 156 volunteers signed a specific informed consent.

All the volunteers satisfied the inclusion criteria: being healthy males or females, aged 18 to 55. Exclusion criteria comprised the following: any organic or physical pathology, the use of any pharmacological treatment in the previous 48 h, body mass index (BMI) out of the 18 to 30 range, history of any kind of drug hypersensitivity, positive abuse drug screening, smokers, alcohol addicts or ethylic intoxication in the previous week, having donated blood within the previous month, pregnancy or breastfeeding, having participated in a similar study within the previous 3 months, grapefruit intake in the previous 48 h, swallowing difficulty, and lactose or galactose intolerance.

2.2. Study Design and Procedures

The current observational pharmacogenetic study was based on five independent bioequivalence clinical trials (A, B, C, D, E). In four of them (A, B, C, E), atorvastatin 80 mg film-coated formulations were used. All of them were phase I, single oral dose, open-label, crossover and randomized clinical trials; the reference formulations were Cardyl or Zarator (Pfizer, Spain). Of the latter, three were replicated (B, C, E) (i.e., with four sequences and four periods) and one was not replicated (A) (i.e., with two sequences and two periods). The fifth clinical trial (D) assessed the bioequivalence for atorvastatin/ezetimibe 80/10 mg coated bilayer tablets versus ezetimibe 10 mg tablets (Ezetrol, MSD, Madrid Spain) and atorvastatin 80 mg (Zarator, Pfizer, Spain). It was replicated, with four periods and four sequences.

In all of them, the determination of plasma concentrations was blinded. Volunteers were hospitalized from 10 h before drug intake to 12 or 24 h after dosing. Formulations were administered by oral route under fasting conditions with 240 mL of water. Blood samples were extracted in EDTA K2 tubes (a) at twenty time-points between pre-dose and 48 h after drug intake (A, B, C, E) or (b) at thirty time-points between pre-dose and 72 h after drug intake (D). Plasma was extracted by centrifugation and frozen until its shipment to an external analytical laboratory. The analytical method involved a liquid–liquid extraction procedure with tert-butyl methyl ether after which atorvastatin and an internal standard were determined by reversed phase ultra-high-performance reversed phase liquid chromatography coupled to tandem mass spectrometry (UPLC/MS/MS). Method validation satisfied the European Medicines Agency (EMA) requirements for bioequivalence demonstration.

2.3. Pharmacokinetic Analysis

A non-compartmental approach was used to calculate pharmacokinetic parameters. Following the trapezoidal rule, the area under the curve between pre-dose and the last time-point (t) (AUC_t) was calculated. The terminal rate constant (k_e) was calculated by linear regression of the log-linear part of the concentration–time curve. The AUC between t and infinite was estimated as C_t/k_e ($AUC_{t-\infty}$). The AUC between 0 and ∞ was calculated as $AUC_t + AUC_{t-\infty}$ (AUC_∞). Drug clearance was calculated adjusted for bioavailability (Cl/F) as dose (D) divided by AUC_∞ and weight (W) (i.e., $D/AUC_\infty*W$). Similarly, the volume of distribution was calculated adjusted for bioavailability (Vd/F) as Cl/F divided by k_e. Half-life ($t_{1/2}$) was estimated as $-\ln 2/k_e$. The remaining pharmacokinetic parameters were directly obtained from the concentration–time curves: the maximum concentration (C_{max}) and the time to reach the C_{max} (t_{max}). The CERTARA Phoenix WinNonlin software, version 6.0 (Certara USA, Princeton, NJ, USA) was used.

2.4. Safety

The tolerability assessment consisted of the evaluation of abnormalities in analytical values, blood parameters, physical examination or any other clinically relevant event. Furthermore, to monitor vascular and heart function, a 12-lead electrocardiogram (ECG) was carried out at predose and 1.5 h after drug intake; in all but one study, another ECG was carried out 3–4 h after dosing. Vital signs (VS), i.e., systolic and diastolic blood pressure, heart rate and tympanic temperature, were monitored simultaneously to ECG. For the notation of adverse events (AEs), volunteers were asked for abnormalities in their health status; those reported spontaneously were additionally considered. The Spanish

Pharmacovigilance System algorithm was used for causality determination [13]. Only those AEs with a definite or possible causality were considered adverse drug reactions (ADRs).

2.5. Genotyping, Haplotyping and Phenotyping

DNA was extracted from peripheral blood in a MagNA Pure automatic DNA extractor (Roche Applied Science, Pleasanton, CA, USA). The genotyping strategy comprised the genotyping of 60 variants in 15 genes. However, not all variants could be genotyped for all samples. Firstly, a customized genotyping array was used in an Applied Biosystems QuantStudio 12K flex qPCR instrument with an OpenArray thermal block (ThermoFisher, USA). Table 1 depicts the variants genotyped in four of the five clinical trials (n = 120). The *CYP3A4*20* (rs67666821) polymorphism was genotyped by KASPar SNP Genotyping System (LGC Genomics, Herts, UK) in an ABI PRISM 7900HT Sequence Detection System (Applied Biosystems, Darmstadt, Germany. A *CYP2D6* copy number variation assay (CNV) was performed in a QuantStudio 12k flex thermal cycler with a 96-well thermal block, following the methodology previously reported [14]. The remaining samples (n = 36) could not be genotyped with the OpenArray technology. Their genotyping was outsourced to CEGEN-PRB3-ISCIII (Santiago de Compostela, Galicia, Spain), supported by grant PT17/0019, of the PE I+D+i 2013–2016, funded by ISCIII and ERDF, for the following 24 matching variants: *ABCB1* C1236T (rs1128503), C3435T (rs1045642), G2677TA (rs2032582), *ABCC2* (rs717620), *CYP1A2*1B* (rs2470890), *1F (rs762551), *CYP2A6*9* (rs28399433), *CYP2B6*5* (rs3211371), *CYP2C19*17* (rs12248560) *2 (rs4244285), *3 (rs4986893), *CYP2C8*2* (rs11572103), *3 (rs10509681 and rs11572080), *4 (rs1058930), *CYP2C9*2* (rs1799853), *3 (rs1057910), *CYP3A4*20* (rs67666821), *CYP3A4*22* (rs35599367), *CYP3A5*3* (rs776746), *CYP3A5*6* (rs10264272), *CYP4F2* (rs2108622) and *UGT1A1*28* (rs887829). Another five variants not included in the OpenArray plate were genotyped: *UGT1A1* rs35350960, rs4124874, rs4148323, *UGT2B4* rs4557343 and *UGT2B7* rs7439366.

CYP3A5 (*3, *6), *CYP2D6* (*3, *4, *5, *6, *7, *8, *9, *10, *14, *17, *41 and the gene copy number), *CYP2C19* (*2, *3, *4, *17), *SLCO1B1* (*1B, *5), *CYP2B6* (*5 and *9) and *CYP2C9* (*2, *3) variants were used to infer the enzymatic phenotype according to CPIC guidelines [12,15–19]. Since not all samples were genotyped for the same variants, the absence of genotyping data was assumed to be "not mutated". The same strategy was implemented for genotyping errors (e.g., absence of amplification). *CYP1A2* (*1C, *1F and *1B) variants were used to infer the activity score and phenotype as described in previous publications [20,21]. *SLC22A1* and *ABCB1* variants were merged into haplotypes: the absence of any variant was assigned the wild-type haplotype, the presence of one variant was assigned the heterozygous haplotype and the presence of two or more variants was assigned the mutant haplotype. Another *ABCB1* haplotype was inferred by exclusively considering C3435T, G2677T/A and C1236T variants, as these were elsewhere reported to have a greater impact on the transporter's activity or expression levels [22].

Table 1. Variants/alleles* genotyped with the Open Array/QuantStudio 12k flex platform.

Gene	Allele/SNP	Gene	Allele/SNP
CYP1A2	*1C (rs2069514)	CYP3A4	*22 (rs35599367)
	*1F (rs762551)		rs55785340
	*1B (rs2470890)		rs4646438

Table 1. Cont.

Gene	Allele/SNP	Gene	Allele/SNP
CYP2A6	*9 (rs28399433)	CYP3A5	*3 (rs776746)
	*9 (rs3745274)		*6 (rs10264272)
CYP2B6	*5 (rs3211371)	ABCB1	C3435T (rs1045642)
	*4 (rs2279343)		G2677T/A (rs2032582)
	rs2279345		C1236T (rs1128503)
	rs4803419		1000-44G>T (rs10276036)
CYP2C8	*2 (rs11572103)		2895+3559C>T (rs7787082)
	*3 (rs10509681)		330-3208C>T (rs4728709)
	*4 (rs1058930)		2481+788T>C (rs10248420)
CYP2C9	*2 (rs1799853)		2686-3393T>G (rs10280101)
	*3 (rs1057910)		2320-695G>A (rs12720067)
CYP2C19	*2 (rs4244285)		2482-707A>G (rs11983225)
	*3 (rs4986893)		2212-372A>G (rs4148737)
	*4 (rs28399504)		rs3842
	*17 (rs12248560)	ABCC2	c.1247G>A (rs2273697)
CYP2D6	*3 (rs35742686)		rs717620
	*4 (rs3892097)	SLCO1B1	*1B (rs2306283)
	*6 (rs5030655)		*5 (rs4149056)
	*7 (rs5030867)		c.-910G>A (rs4149015)
	*8 (rs5030865)		rs11045879
	*9 (rs5030656)	SLC22A1	*2 (rs72552763)
	*10 (rs1065852)		*3 (rs12208357)
	*14 (rs5030865)		*5 (rs34059508)
	*17 (rs28371706)	UGT1A1	*28 (rs887829)
	*41 (rs28371725)		

* When the presence of a variant (identified with the RefSeq identifier) unequivocally defines an allele, it is indicated with the *star nomenclature.

2.6. Statistical Analysis

All pharmacokinetic parameters were logarithmically transformed to normalize distributions. Prior to logarithmic transformations, AUC_∞ and C_{max} were divided by the dose/weight ratio (AUC/DW, C_{max}/DW) to correct the differences in weight between sexes or races which can produce pharmacokinetic variability. To avoid random associations, the following statistical analysis strategy was followed: initially, a univariate analysis was performed, where the mean of pharmacokinetic parameters or the incidence of adverse drug reactions (ADRs) were compared according to categorical variables (e.g., sex, race, haplotypes, phenotypes). For the comparison of means, a *t* test (variables with two categories) or an ANOVA test followed by a Bonferroni post-hoc (variables with three or more categories) were used. For the comparison of the incidence of ADRs according to categorical variables, a Chi-squared test was used. Afterwards, each pharmacokinetic parameter or ADR were individually analyzed with a multivariate analysis. Either by linear or logistic regression, pharmacokinetic parameters or ADRs were explored, respectively. As independent variables, only variables with $p < 0.05$ in the univariate analysis were explored; in addition, pharmacokinetic parameters were introduced as independent variables in the logistic regression. A Bonferroni correction for multiple comparisons was carried out; the value of $p < 0.05$ for statistical significance was divided by the number of variables introduced in the multivariate analysis. The Hardy–Weinberg equilibrium (HWE) was calculated for the genotyped variants using the *HardyWeinberg* package [23] and the R-studio v.4.0.3. software. Deviations from the equilibrium were considered Pearson's goodness-of-fit chi-square *p* values below 0.05; other statistics (e.g., Fisher exact test) were calculated with an online software (Institute of Human Genetics, University of Munich, available at https://ihg.gsf.de/cgi-bin/hw/hwa1.pl, accessed on 5 March 2021). The remaining statistical analysis were computed in SPSS v.23.0.

3. Results

3.1. Demographic Characteristics

Study population was composed by 85 women (54%) and 71 men (46%). Men's height, weight and body mass index (BMI) were significantly superior to that of women ($p < 0.0001$, $p < 0.0001$ and $p = 0.005$, respectively) (Table 1). Caucasian was the most prevalent race (52%) compared to Latin-Americans (45%), Black (3%) and Arabic (one male). Demographics also differed significantly according to races (Table 2). The Black or Arabic group was related to higher weight compared to Caucasians and Latin-Americans ($p < 0.0001$ and $p = 0.005$, respectively) and to higher height compared to Latin-Americans ($p = 0.027$). Moreover, Caucasians were younger than Latin-Americans and Black or Arabic volunteers ($p < 0.0001$ and $p = 0.049$, respectively) and showed lower BMI ($p < 0.001$ and $p = 0.001$). Of note, the Black or Arabic group was composed by four men and one woman.

Table 2. Demographic characteristics of the study population.

Sex	n	Weight (kg)	CV%	BMI (kg/m^2)	CV%	Height (m)	CV%	Age (years)	CV%
Women	85	61.5	13.8	23.1	13.4	1.63	3.7	30.1	28.2
Men	71	75.3 *	12.7	24.4 *	10.2	1.75 *	4.0	27.8	27.0
Race									
Caucasian	81	65.5	16.8	22.6 *2	10.6	1.7	5.9	25.5 *2	22.4
Latin-American	70	69.2	15.0	24.8	11.7	1.67	6.0	32.7	26.9
Black or Arabic	5	85.3 *1	15.0	27.0	7.4	1.77 *3	5.6	33.7	18.7
Total	156	67.7	16.8	23.7	12.2	1.69	5.9	29.0	27.9

*: $p < 0.05$ after ANOVA or T-test compared to the other category; *1: $p < 0.05$ after ANOVA and Bonferroni post-hoc (Black or Arabic compared to Caucasians and Latin-Americans); *2: $p < 0.05$ after ANOVA and Bonferroni post-hoc (Caucasians vs. Latin-American and Black or Arabic); *3: $p < 0.05$ after ANOVA and Bonferroni post-hoc (Black or Arabic compared to Latin-Americans).

3.2. Pharmacokinetics

Atorvastatin mean AUC$_\infty$ was 166.6 ± 89.1 ng*h/mL (183.6 ± 90.7 ng*h/mL for females and 146.3 ± 83.4 ng*h/mL for males, $p = 0.001$) and mean C$_{max}$ was 39.0 ± 25.3 ng/mL (44.8 ± 25.5 ng/mL for females and 32.0 ± 23.3 ng/mL for males, $p < 0.001$). After DW correction, the differences disappeared (Table 3).

Eight variables were significantly related to pharmacokinetic variability in the univariate analysis; for multiple-testing correction, the level of significance in the multivariate analysis was set at $p = 0.00625$ ($p < 0.05$ divided by 8, the number of variables introduced in the multivariate analysis). Healthy volunteers enrolled in the "C" clinical trial exhibited lower AUC/DW ($p = 0.010$) and higher Cl/F ($p = 0.007$) than those enrolled in the "B" clinical trial and lower C_{max}/DW ($p = 0.039$) compared to that of volunteers enrolled in the "D" clinical trial. Moreover, Vd/F in "C" was higher than that of "B" and "C" ($p = 0.028$ and $p = 0.037$, respectively), which was confirmed in the multivariate analysis (unstandardized beta coefficient = 0.184, $p = 0.013$, model $R^2 = 0.272$). The use of ezetimibe (i.e., the "D" clinical trial) was associated with higher AUC/DW compared to the other clinical trials, where ezetimibe was not administered (unstandardized beta coefficient = 0.177, $p = 0.048$, model $R^2 = 0.222$), to higher C_{max}/DW (ANOVA $p = 0.029$, unstandardized beta coefficient = 0.288, $p = 0.002$, model $R^2 = 0.225$) and to lower Vd/F (unstandardized beta coefficient = -0.517, $p = 0.001$, model $R^2 = 0.272$). Finally, Caucasians showed higher Vd/F compared to Latin-Americans (ANOVA $p = 0.028$, unstandardized beta coefficient = 0.184, $p = 0.013$, $R^2 = 0.225$) (Table 3).

All variants were in Hardy–Weinberg equilibrium, except for CYP3A4*2 rs55785340, CYP3A4*6 rs4646438, CYP2A6 rs28399433, CYP2C19*3 rs4986893, UGT1A1 rs4124874, UGT1A1 rs4148323, CYP2D6*4 rs3892097, CYP2D6*7 rs5030867, CYP2D6*8 rs5030865, CYP1A2*1F rs762551, CYP2B6*9 rs3745274, and CYP2B6*5 rs2279343. Eight of these SNPs showed no allelic variability (Supplementary Table S1). Genetic polymorphism was associated with atorvastatin pharmacokinetic variability. Carriers of the SLCO1B1 decreased function (DF) and poor function (PF) phenotypes were related to higher AUC/DW, C_{max}/DW and to lower Vd/F and Cl/F compared to carriers of the normal function (NF) phenotype (ANOVA $p < 0.001$, $p < 0.001$, $p = 0.002$, $p < 0.001$, respectively, $p < 0.05$ after Bonferroini post-hoc) which was confirmed by multivariate analysis (unstandardized beta coefficients = 0.365, 0.332, -0.341, -0.357, $p < 0.001$, <0.001, <0.001, <0.001, and $R^2 = 0.222$, 0.225, 0.272 and 0.200, respectively). Moreover, CYP3A5 *1/*3 and *3/*3 genotypes were related to lower AUC/DW, C_{max}/DW and t_{max} and to higher Cl/F compared to the *1/*1 genotype (ANOVA $p = 0.004$, 0.018, <0.001, 0.005, respectively; $p < 0.05$ after Bonferroini post-hoc); the associations for AUC/DW, C_{max}/DW and Cl/F were confirmed by multivariate analysis (unstandardized beta coefficients = -0.208, -0.202, 0.189, $p = 0.007$, 0.009, 0.013 and $R^2 = 0.222$, 0.225 and 0.200, respectively). Moreover, the SLC22A1 *2/*2 genotype was related to higher C_{max}/DW (ANOVA $p = 0.030$, $p > 0.05$ in the multivariate analysis) and SLC22A1 *1/*5 genotype was associated with higher Vd/F (ANOVA $p = 0.032$, unstandardized beta coefficient = 0.535, $p = 0.011$ and $R^2 = 0.272$) compared to SLC22A1 *1/*1, respectively. Finally, UGT2B7 rs7439366 TT genotype was associated with higher t_{max} as compared with the TC genotype (ANOVA $p = 0.024$); this variable could not be analyzed in the multivariate analysis. (Table 4).

3.3. Safety

No serious ADR was reported during any of the five clinical trials. No clinically relevant alteration of VS or ECG was observed. Twenty-one volunteers suffered a total of 27 ADRs. Three types of ADR were reported: first, gastrointestinal symptoms (flatulence, loose stools, or diarrhea) were reported at least once in 13 volunteers; second, headache was reported at least once in 11 volunteers; third, three cases of myalgia or arthralgia were reported at least once in three volunteers. Ten out of 13 cases (76.9%) of gastrointestinal symptoms occurred in the "E" clinical trial compared to two cases in the D clinical trial (15.4%) and one in the B clinical trial (9.8%) ($p < 0.001$). Males were related to a lower risk for developing headache (logOR = -19.054, $p < 0.001$, R^2 (Cox and Snell) = 0.068). Pharmacokinetics or genetic polymorphism were unrelated to occurrence of ADRs.

Table 3. Atorvastatin pharmacokinetic parameters based on sex, study design, use of ezetimibe, and race.

		N	AUC/DW (kg*h*ng/mL*mg)	CV%	C_max/DW (kg*ng/mL*mg)	CV%	t_max (h)	CV%	t_{1/2} (h)	CV%	Vd/F (l/kg)	CV%	Cl/F (L/h*kg)	CV%
Sex	Female	85	142.6	56.7	34.3	61.2	1.4	57.1	9.3	31.2	124.0	66.3	9023.4	49.6
	Male	71	136.6	58.4	29.9	74.9	1.4	57.1	8.7	25.3	117.0	52.3	9248.5	42.7
Clinical trial	A	14	129.2	35.9	22.7	36.1	1.7	88.2	8.1	23.5	103.5	45.1	8745	35.5
	B	30	174.9	63.0	36.1	58.2	1.5	53.3	9.1	23.1	107.3	70.7	7836.7	61.5
	C	39	116.3 *1	59.3	26.6 *2	60.2	1.3	61.5	9.4	28.7	147.1 *1*2	53.0	11,036.7 *1	45.7
	D	37	149.4	46.3	37.4	61.0	1.4	42.9	8.7	33.3	103.9	71.9	8247.0	45.9
	E	36	130.5	57.5	33.7	82.2	1.4	42.9	9.5	30.5	127.7	52.2	9181.5	30.4
Ezetimibe	No	119	136.9	60.9	30.7	69.1	1.4	64.3	9.2	27.2	126.1	57.3	9399.1	46.2
	Yes	37	149.4 !	46.3	37.4 *!	61.0	1.4	42.9	8.7	33.3	103.9	71.9	8247.0	45.9
Race	Caucasian	81	132.5	61.1	33.5	71.6	1.4	50.0	9.5	29.5	138.1 *3!	63.8	9938.9	49.4
	Latin-American	70	147.8	54.2	31.0	62.9	1.5	60.0	8.7	27.6	103.4	45.9	8279.3	38.7
	Black or Arabic	5	148.7	48.4	31.8	34.3	1.6	43.8	7.6	9.2	83.8	33.4	7808.3	36.8

SD: standard deviation; *: $p < 0.05$ after ANOVA or T-test compared to the other category; *1: $p < 0.05$ after ANOVA and Bonferroni post-hoc (C compared to B); *2: $p < 0.05$ after ANOVA and Bonferroni post-hoc (C compared to D); *3: $p < 0.05$ after ANOVA and Bonferroni post-hoc (Caucasians compared to Latin-Americans); Underlined: $p < 0.05$ after multivariate analysis (linear regression, which included the following variables: sex, study design, ezetimibe use, race, SLCO1B1 phenotype, CYP3A5*3, SLC22A1*2, and *5; UGT2B7 rs7439366 was excluded from analysis). ! $p < 0.00625$ after multivariate analysis (Bonferroni correction for multiple testing significance threshold).

Table 4. Atorvastatin pharmacokinetic parameters based on genotypes or phenotypes with significant variability.

		N	AUC/DW (kg*h*ng/mL*mg)	CV%	C_{max} (kg*ng/mL*mg)	CV%	t_{max} (h)	CV%	$t_{1/2}$ (h)	CV%	Vd/F (l/kg)	CV%	Cl/F (L/h*kg)	CV%
SLCO1B1	NF	86	122.6 *1!	44.9	28.5 *1!	59.3	1.4	64.3	9	30.0	127.8 *1!	57.8	9827.4 *1!	43.1
	DF	30	181.5	59.3	37.5	60.0	1.4	57.1	8.7	25.3	99.7	78.0	7680.4	67.0
	PF	4	283.7	41.4	62.4	35.9	1.3	38.5	10.5	9.5	66.4	58.9	4382.7	60.2
CYP3A5*3	*1/*1	5	244.2 *1	21.5	57.1 *1	55.2	1.9 *1	42.1	9.8	26.5	65.2	41.9	4405.1 *1	23.7
	*1/*3	32	153.7	70.3	35.1	75.5	1.4	71.4	8.8	21.6	114.3	60.6	9181.8	55.0
	*3/*3	119	131.8	52.0	30.5	63.0	1.4	50.0	9.1	30.8	124.9	59.9	9309.2	42.7
SLC22A1*2	*1/*1	71	131.8	48.7	28.9	53.6	1.4	57.1	8.9	29.2	121.4	57.5	9393.2	47.7
	*1/*2	41	151.2	66.2	33.5	64.5	1.4	64.3	9	28.9	121.1	72.0	9136.4	54.0
	*2/*2	8	195.7	51.8	49.8 *2	64.7	1.6	68.8	8.9	19.1	83	59.5	6449.1	47.9
SLC22A1*5	*1/*1	114	144.6	57.0	32.3	61.9	1.4	64.3	8.9	28.1	114.8	59.7	8933.1	49.3
	*1/*5	6	105.6	58.4	24.2	34.3	1.6	43.8	10.8	30.6	193.9 *	75.6	12,455.2	56.3
UGT2B7 rs7439366	*1/*1	9	159.6	80.6	44.1	103.9	1.8 *3	44.4	8.2	24.4	106.9	50.4	8821	43.8
	*1/*2	12	108.9	29.5	26.6	35.3	1.1	36.4	9.5	22.1	137.8	35.6	9990.2	22.7
	*2/*2	15	130.4	41.1	33.2	69.3	1.4	28.6	10.1	36.6	132	64.2	8751	28.3
Total		156	139.9	57.3	32.3	67.2	1.4	57.1	9.1	28.6	120.8	60.6	9125.9	46.4

NF: normal function; DF: decreased function; PF: poor function. *$p < 0.05$ after ANOVA or T-test compared to the other category; *1: $p < 0.05$ after ANOVA and Bonferroni post-hoc (NF vs and DF and PF; *1/*1 vs. *1/*3 and *3/*3);*2: $p < 0.05$ after ANOVA and Bonferroni post-hoc (*2/*2 vs. *1/*1);*3: $p < 0.05$ after ANOVA and Bonferroni post-hoc (TT vs. TC). Underlined: $p < 0.05$ after multivariate analysis (linear regression, which included the following variables: sex, study design, ezetimibe use, race, SLCO1B1 phenotype, CYP3A5*3, SLC22A1*2, and *5; UGT2B7 rs7439366 was excluded from analysis). ! $p < 0.00625$ after multivariate analysis (Bonferroni correction for multiple testing significance threshold).

4. Discussion

Statins are widely prescribed for the treatment of hypercholesterolemia, having demonstrated overwhelming benefits in reducing cardiovascular morbidity and mortality. However, a considerable percentage of patients discontinue therapy due to the occurrence of adverse reactions, mainly myopathies [24]. Therefore, the personalized prescription of these drugs is recommended to avoid excessive exposure, which may lead to ADRs. In line with the above, the DPGW published its pharmacogenetic guidelines on atorvastatin and simvastatin, where drug dose adjustment is recommended in relation to the SLCO1B1 phenotype. In contrast, the CPIC published the clinical guideline on SLCO1B1 and simvastatin but not for atorvastatin. Our interest was to demonstrate the effect of SLCO1B1 phenotype on atorvastatin pharmacokinetics, which was certainly observed and reported. Furthermore, we aimed to describe the impact of variants in other genes, demographics and the study design in atorvastatin exposure and safety.

Similar to previous works, men exhibited higher weight, height, and BMI than women [25]. Black (n = 4) and Arabic volunteers (n = 1) had to be merged in a combined group for statistical analysis. The differences related to this group in weight and height may be explained by four of the Black or Arabic volunteers being men and only one being a Black woman.

The observed mean atorvastatin pharmacokinetic parameters, e.g., AUC_∞ = 167 ng*h/mL and C_{max} = 39 ng/mL were consistent with previous works: e.g., after a 40 mg atorvastatin dose, a mean AUC_∞ of 96 ng*h/mL and a C_{max} of 28 ng/mL was previously reported [26]. Because 80 mg fixed-dose formulations were administered in these clinical trials, women received atorvastatin to a higher dose–weight ratio than men, which was evidenced in a significantly higher AUC_∞ (25%) and C_{max} (40%) compared to men. These results contrast with a previous study where an 11% AUC reduction was observed in women compared to men [27]. Nevertheless, after DW correction, these differences disappeared. It could therefore be concluded that dosage strength, and not sex, is related to atorvastatin pharmacokinetic variability. Moreover, the differences observed in Vd/F between Caucasian and Black or Arabic volunteers are likely explained by the different sex distribution in both groups. Hence, again, it would be the dosage strength the responsible for the differences.

The differences observed in drug exposure according to the clinical trial design were expected due to the relatively small sample size of each clinical trial (from n = 14 to n = 39) and the different characteristics (e.g., different number of periods, sequences, reference formulations). The use of ezetimibe was related to an increased atorvastatin exposure. A possible drug–drug interaction between both drugs was interrogated previously [26]. Our results contrast with the previous consensus, in which no such interaction was demonstrated. Of note, the methodology for AUC_∞ extrapolation in the ezetimibe clinical trial was based on $AUC_{0-72\ h}$ compared to the other clinical trials which used $AUC_{0-48\ h}$. Mean atorvastatin $t_{1/2}$ in this study was 9.1 h. Considering five half-lives, the 95% of AUC would be covered 45.5 h after drug intake. Therefore, the sampling time (0 to 48 h vs. 0 to 72 h) will certainly not be a confounding factor. As mentioned before, the relatively small sample size of each clinical trial likely explains the observed differences. Notwithstanding, should ezetimibe increase atorvastatin exposure to the extent observed in this work (i.e., less than 10% of AUC/DW), the effects may not be relevant in the clinical setting.

As expected, SLCO1B1 phenotype was the main pharmacogenetic predictor of atorvastatin pharmacokinetic variability, which justifies a dose reduction or a drug switch in DF and PF phenotype carriers. Consequently, we suggest that the CPIC should extend their pharmacogenetic guideline on simvastatin and SLCO1B1 [12] to atorvastatin, which is congruent with DPWG recommendations [11] and with previous scientific consensus [28–30], and probably to other statins [28] (e.g., fluvastatin, pravastatin).

Moreover, we identified *CYP3A5*3* to be significantly related to atorvastatin pharmacokinetic variability. Our findings are controversial and require an in-depth discussion. As shown in Figure 1, CYP3A4 and CYP3A5 can metabolize atorvastatin in the intestinal and hepatic cells. Based on Ensembl data (available at: https://www.ensembl.org/index.html, accessed on 12 January 2021), the *3 allele (rs776746) has a prevalence of 80–94% in Americans and Europeans, respectively, which is consistent with our findings: approximately 87% of prevalence in a mixed population, with Caucasians, Latin-Americans mainly.

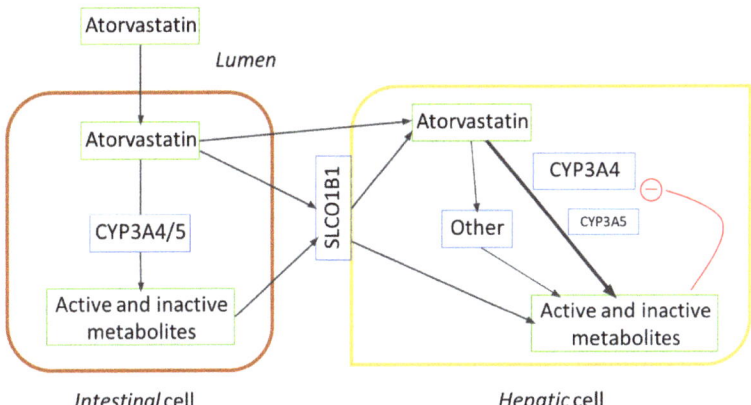

Figure 1. The pharmacokinetic pathway of atorvastatin focused on CYP3A and SLCO1B1.

In theory, the higher metabolic capacity of *CYP3A5* expressers would be expected to result in a lower bioavailability of atorvastatin. Previous works did not observe a clinically relevant interaction [31,32]. However, these were in vitro approaches [31] or clinical observational studies with a low sample size (n = 23) [32]. In contrast, several pharmacodynamic interactions were published. *CYP3A5* *3/*3 subjects were related to higher risk of myalgia and muscle damage compared to *1/*3 subjects [33] and to increased response to atorvastatin compared to *1/*1 + *1/*3 subjects [34]. Moreover, the *3 allele was associated with increased response to statins, including atorvastatin, compared to the *1 allele [35,36]. A higher metabolism of the parent drug, assuming that its metabolites are more active, does not necessarily correlate to a lower risk for toxicity or for drug effectiveness. In contrast, CYP3A4 inhibition relates to toxicity, actually supporting that a higher metabolism indeed relates to lower effectiveness and lower risk for toxicity. Therefore, from these studies, we can conclude that the sum of atorvastatin and atorvastatin active metabolites could be higher in *CYP3A5* non-expressers, and this event relates to a higher risk for toxicity and to a better response to the drug. In our study, *CYP3A5*1 (defined as the absence of *3 and *6 alleles) allele was associated with atorvastatin accumulation (e.g., carriers of *1/*1 exhibited an AUC 1.58 or 1.85 times higher than that of carriers of *1/*3 or *3/*3, respectively, $p = 0.007$). Our study is, to our knowledge, the one with the largest sample size (n = 156) published to date suggesting such an interaction. A possible explanation for this is as follows: atorvastatin, administered in the form of acid, suffers a strong first-pass metabolic effect, involving both intestinal and hepatic CYP3A4 and CYP3A5, with an oral bioavailability of 12–14% [5,6,37]. CYP3A4 is the main enzyme responsible for atorvastatin metabolism, with an intrinsic clearance 2.4 to 5 times higher than that of CYP3A5 [31]. In *CYP3A5* expressers, atorvastatin is metabolized to a wider extent in the gut, leading to active metabolites with CYP3A4 inhibitory effect. These metabolites, together with atorvastatin, reach the liver and inhibit CYP3A4, which is consistent with the previously demonstrated substrate inhibition [31]. Since in our study population a high dose of atorvastatin was administered to healthy subjects without any atorvastatin in the organism, this effect is evident. That is, the inhibitory effect is greater than the enhanced metabolic capacity. Given the high inducibility of CYP3A4, these effects are likely to be normalized over time in patients in steady state. In our study design, however, there was insufficient time for the induction of CYP3A4 expression to compensate for the inhibition associated with the CYP3A5*1 allele. Clearly, considering the controversy with these results, we encourage other researchers to proceed cautiously with them. Further studies are necessary to replicate this effect.

The *SLC22A1* gene encodes for the organic cationic transporter 1 (OCT), a transporter responsible for the hepatic uptake of xenobiotics and for the capture of organic cations from blood to epithelial cells [38]. There is very little information available regarding atorvastatin and *SLC22A1*. Atorvastatin is known to alter the in vitro expression of *SLC22A1* and in rats co-administered with nicotine [39,40]. To date, no study with a robust design or study in humans evaluated if atorvastatin is an OCT1 substrate. This is the first study to date to suggest a similar conclusion. The *SLC22A1**2 allele (rs72552763) or Met420 deletion, was related to a reduced metformin uptake in vitro [41]. Here, *SLC22A1**2 allele was related to a higher C_{max} compared to the *1 allele, which would be consistent with a reduced hepatic uptake and, therefore, to a reduced metabolism; this association disappeared after multivariate analysis. On the other hand, the *SLC22A1**5 allele (rs34059508) was demonstrated to be another reduced-function allele and was related to a reduced metformin uptake in vitro [41]. Here, *1/*5 carriers were related to higher Vd/F. However, this association did not reach the level of significance after Bonferroni correction; these differences were probably explained by the very high standard deviation observed in the *1/*5 group, caused by the presence of outliers.

UGT2B7, among other UDP-glucuroniltransferases, was demonstrated to metabolize statins, including atorvastatin [42]. The *2 allele, defined by the rs7439366 variant, was previously associated with reduced activity in diclofenac and efavirenz acyl glucuronidation [43,44]. However, to the best of our knowledge, this is the first study to report an effect of this variant on atorvastatin pharmacokinetics. Here, the *1/*1 subject exhibited higher t_{max} compared to *1/*2 but not to *2/*2. Unfortunately, the number of samples analyzed for this variant (n = 36) was small and therefore these findings could be spurious.

The scarcity in ADR data is congruent with the study design, i.e., single-dose administrations. Gastrointestinal symptoms, headache and musculoskeletal ADRs are common based on atorvastatin drug label 5 which is consistent with our findings. The lower risk for headache development observed in men compared to women is likely explained by the lower exposure to atorvastatin observed in men, who were dosed to a lower dose–weight ratio.

It would be particularly interesting to validate these results in a cohort of patients chronically treated with atorvastatin for the management of hypercholesterolemia. For instance, it would be of interest to find out whether patients with a poor or reduced-function SLCO1B1 phenotype required lower doses of atorvastatin or had a higher incidence of myalgias.

Limitations

The main limitation of this study is that the administration of a single atorvastatin dose to healthy subjects did not permit drawing any conclusion on long-term effectiveness or safety. Further studies are needed to confirm our hypotheses in a stationary state and in patients treated with atorvastatin. In contrast, bioequivalence clinical trials offer a controlled setting for evaluating pharmacokinetic variability based on genetic polymorphism or demographics as confounding factors are avoided.

5. Conclusions

The best predictor of atorvastatin exposure is SLCO1B1 phenotype. Accordingly, a dose adjustment could be beneficial to avoid toxicities, especially statin-related myalgias, which could lead to interruption of treatment. This conclusion is consistent with DPWG guideline on atorvastatin and SLCO1B1. We suggest that the CPIC should extend their guideline on simvastatin and SLCO1B1 to atorvastatin as the effect of the transporter phenotype on pharmacokinetics is well demonstrated. Moreover, this candidate-gene study is, to the best of our opinion, the most robust one published to date, with the highest sample size (n = 156) and the widest genotyping screening strategy. In this line, a very novel association was observed, between *CYP3A5**1 and a significant increase in atorvastatin exposure. Further studies are warranted to confirm or reject our findings and hypotheses.

Supplementary Materials: The following are available online at https://www.mdpi.com/2075-442 6/11/3/204/s1, Table S1.

Author Contributions: Conceptualization, P.Z. and F.A.-S.; methodology, P.Z.; software, P.Z.; validation, F.A.-S.; formal analysis, P.Z.; investigation, P.Z., M.D.B., G.V.-G., S.M.-V., D.O., F.A.-S.; resources, F.A.-S.; data curation, P.Z.; writing—original draft preparation, P.Z.; writing—review and editing, P.Z., M.D.B., G.V.-G., S.M.-V., D.O., F.A.-S.; visualization, P.Z.; supervision, P.Z., F.A.-S.; project administration, P.Z. and F.A.-S.; funding acquisition, F.A.-S. All authors have read and agreed to the published version of the manuscript.

Funding: G. Villapalos-García is co-financed by Instituto de Salud Carlos III (ISCIII) and the European Social Fund (PFIS predoctoral grant, number FI20/00090). M. Navares-Gómez is financed by the ICI20/00131 grant, Acción Estratégica en Salud 2017-2020, ISCIII.

Institutional Review Board Statement: Study protocols were revised and approved by the Hospital's Research Ethics Committee and by the Spanish Drugs Agency (AEMPS). Complying with Spanish and European legislation on research in humans, all of them were accomplished under the Good Clinical Practice guidelines and endorsing the Declaration of Helsinki. EUDRA-CT numbers were as follows: 2018-000082-37, 2019-002222-67, 2019-000891-41, 2019-001670-29 and 2019-000656-34.

Informed Consent Statement: All the subjects (n = 178) provided their informed consent for their enrolment in the bioequivalence clinical trial. For the pharmacogenetic study, 156 volunteers signed a specific informed consent.

Data Availability Statement: The data presented in this study are available on request from the corresponding author. The data are not publicly available as they belong to the sponsors of the clinical trials.

Conflicts of Interest: F. Abad-Santos and D. Ochoa have been consultants or investigators in clinical trials sponsored by the following pharmaceutical companies: Abbott, Alter, Chemo, Cinfa, FAES, Farmalíder, Ferrer, GlaxoSmithKline, Galenicum, Gilead, Italfarmaco Janssen-Cilag, Kern, Normon, Novartis, Servier, Silverpharma, Teva, and Zambon. The remaining authors declare no conflicts of interest.

References

1. Weng, T.-C.; Yang, Y.-H.K.; Lin, S.-J.; Tai, S.-H. A Systematic Review and Meta-Analysis on the Therapeutic Equivalence of Statins. *J. Clin. Pharm. Ther.* **2010**, *35*, 139–151. [CrossRef]
2. Stancu, C.; Sima, A. Statins: Mechanism of Action and Effects. *J. Cell. Mol. Med.* **2001**, *5*, 378–387. [CrossRef] [PubMed]
3. Malhotra, H.S.; Goa, K.L. Atorvastatin: An Updated Review of Its Pharmacological Properties and Use in Dyslipidaemia. *Drugs* **2001**, *61*, 1835–1881. [CrossRef]
4. Liu, Y.-M.; Pu, H.-H.; Liu, G.-Y.; Jia, J.-Y.; Weng, L.-P.; Xu, R.-J.; Li, G.-X.; Wang, W.; Zhang, M.-Q.; Lu, C.; et al. Pharmacokinetics and Bioequivalence Evaluation of Two Different Atorvastatin Calcium 10-Mg Tablets: A Single-Dose, Randomized-Sequence, Open-Label, Two-Period Crossover Study in Healthy Fasted Chinese Adult Males. *Clin. Ther.* **2010**, *32*, 1396–1407. [CrossRef]
5. Agencia Española del Medicamento y Productos Sanitarios (AEMPS) Cardyl Comprimidos Recubiertos Con Película (Drug Label), Avda. de Europa, 20B, Parque Empresarial La Moraleja, 28108, Alcobendas, Madrid, Spain.
6. García, M.J.; Reinoso, R.F.; Sánchez Navarro, A.; Prous, J.R. Clinical Pharmacokinetics of Statins. *Methods Find. Exp. Clin. Pharmacol.* **2003**, *25*, 457–481. [CrossRef]
7. Schachter, M. Chemical, Pharmacokinetic and Pharmacodynamic Properties of Statins: An Update. *Fundam. Clin. Pharmacol.* **2005**, *19*, 117–125. [CrossRef]
8. Kalliokoski, A.; Niemi, M. Impact of OATP Transporters on Pharmacokinetics: OATP Transporters and Pharmacokinetics. *Br. J. Pharmacol.* **2009**, *158*, 693–705. [CrossRef] [PubMed]
9. DeGorter, M.K.; Tirona, R.G.; Schwarz, U.I.; Choi, Y.-H.; Dresser, G.K.; Suskin, N.; Myers, K.; Zou, G.; Iwuchukwu, O.; Wei, W.-Q.; et al. Clinical and Pharmacogenetic Predictors of Circulating Atorvastatin and Rosuvastatin Concentrations in Routine Clinical Care. *Circ. Cardiovasc. Genet.* **2013**, *6*, 400–408. [CrossRef]
10. Yue, Y.-H.; Bai, X.; Zhang, H.; Li, Y.; Hu, L.; Liu, L.; Mao, J.; Yang, X.; Dila, N. Gene Polymorphisms Affect the Effectiveness of Atorvastatin in Treating Ischemic Stroke Patients. *Cell. Physiol. Biochem.* **2016**, *39*, 630–638. [CrossRef]
11. Dutch Pharmacogenetics Working Group Pharmacogenetic Recommendations. 2005.

12. Ramsey, L.B.; Johnson, S.G.; Caudle, K.E.; Haidar, C.E.; Voora, D.; Wilke, R.A.; Maxwell, W.D.; McLeod, H.L.; Krauss, R.M.; Roden, D.M.; et al. The Clinical Pharmacogenetics Implementation Consortium Guideline for SLCO1B1 and Simvastatin-Induced Myopathy: 2014 Update. *Clin. Pharmacol. Ther.* **2014**, *96*, 423–428. [CrossRef] [PubMed]
13. Aguirre, C.; García, M. Causality assessment in reports on adverse drug reactions. Algorithm of Spanish pharmacovigilance system. *Med. Clin. (Barc)* **2016**, *147*, 461–464. [CrossRef]
14. Belmonte, C.; Ochoa, D.; Román, M.; Saiz-Rodríguez, M.; Wojnicz, A.; Gómez-Sánchez, C.I.; Martín-Vílchez, S.; Abad-Santos, F. Influence of CYP2D6, CYP3A4, CYP3A5 and ABCB1 Polymorphisms on Pharmacokinetics and Safety of Aripiprazole in Healthy Volunteers. *Basic Clin. Pharmacol. Toxicol.* **2018**, *122*, 596–605. [CrossRef]
15. Caudle, K.E.; Sangkuhl, K.; Whirl-Carrillo, M.; Swen, J.J.; Haidar, C.E.; Klein, T.E.; Gammal, R.S.; Relling, M.V.; Scott, S.A.; Hertz, D.L.; et al. Standardizing CYP 2D6 Genotype to Phenotype Translation: Consensus Recommendations from the Clinical Pharmacogenetics Implementation Consortium and Dutch Pharmacogenetics Working Group. *Clin. Transl. Sci.* **2019**. [CrossRef]
16. Scott, S.A.; Sangkuhl, K.; Stein, C.M.; Hulot, J.-S.; Mega, J.L.; Roden, D.M.; Klein, T.E.; Sabatine, M.S.; Johnson, J.A.; Shuldiner, A.R. Clinical Pharmacogenetics Implementation Consortium Guidelines for CYP2C19 Genotype and Clopidogrel Therapy: 2013 Update. *Clin. Pharmacol. Ther.* **2013**, *94*, 317–323. [CrossRef]
17. Caudle, K.E.; Rettie, A.E.; Whirl-Carrillo, M.; Smith, L.H.; Mintzer, S.; Lee, M.T.M.; Klein, T.E.; Callaghan, J.T. Clinical Pharmacogenetics Implementation Consortium Guidelines for CYP2C9 and HLA-B Genotypes and Phenytoin Dosing. *Clin. Pharmacol. Ther.* **2014**, *96*, 542–548. [CrossRef] [PubMed]
18. Desta, Z.; Gammal, R.S.; Gong, L.; Whirl-Carrillo, M.; Gaur, A.H.; Sukasem, C.; Hockings, J.; Myers, A.; Swart, M.; Tyndale, R.F.; et al. Clinical Pharmacogenetics Implementation Consortium (CPIC) Guideline for *CYP2B6* and Efavirenz-Containing Antiretroviral Therapy. *Clin. Pharmacol. Ther.* **2019**, *106*, 726–733. [CrossRef]
19. Birdwell, K.; Decker, B.; Barbarino, J.; Peterson, J.; Stein, C.; Sadee, W.; Wang, D.; Vinks, A.; He, Y.; Swen, J.; et al. Clinical Pharmacogenetics Implementation Consortium (CPIC) Guidelines for *CYP3A5* Genotype and Tacrolimus Dosing. *Clin. Pharmacol. Ther.* **2015**, *98*, 19–24. [CrossRef] [PubMed]
20. Zubiaur, P.; Saiz-Rodríguez, M.; Ochoa, D.; Belmonte, C.; Román, M.; Mejía, G.; Martín-Vilchez, S.; Abad-Santos, F. Influence of CYP2B6 Activity Score on the Pharmacokinetics and Safety of Single Dose Efavirenz in Healthy Volunteers. *Pharmacogenom. J.* **2019**. [CrossRef]
21. Saiz-Rodríguez, M.; Ochoa, D.; Belmonte, C.; Román, M.; Vieira de Lara, D.; Zubiaur, P.; Koller, D.; Mejía, G.; Abad-Santos, F. Polymorphisms in CYP1A2, CYP2C9 and ABCB1 Affect Agomelatine Pharmacokinetics. *J. Psychopharmacol.* **2019**, *33*, 522–531. [CrossRef] [PubMed]
22. Mittal, B.; Tulsyan, S.; Mittal, R. The Effect of ABCB1 Polymorphisms on the Outcome of Breast Cancer Treatment. *Pharmacogenom. Pers. Med.* **2016**, *9*, 47–58. [CrossRef]
23. Graffelman, J.; Weir, B.S. Testing for Hardy–Weinberg Equilibrium at Biallelic Genetic Markers on the X Chromosome. *Heredity* **2016**, *116*, 558–568. [CrossRef]
24. Ward, N.C.; Watts, G.F.; Eckel, R.H. Statin Toxicity: Mechanistic Insights and Clinical Implications. *Circ. Res.* **2019**, *124*, 328–350. [CrossRef]
25. Zubiaur, P.; Soria-Chacartegui, P.; Koller, D.; Navares-Gómez, M.; Ochoa, D.; Almenara, S.; Saiz-Rodriguez, M.; Mejía-Abril, G.; Villapalos-García, G.; Román, M.; et al. Impact of Polymorphisms in Transporter and Metabolizing Enzyme Genes on Olanzapine Pharmacokinetics and Safety in Healthy Volunteer. *Biomed. Pharmacother.* **2021**, *133*, 111087. [CrossRef]
26. Park, J.; Kim, C.O.; Jin, B.H.; Yang, S.; Park, M.S.; Hong, T. Pharmacokinetic Drug Interaction between Atorvastatin and Ezetimibe in Healthy Korean Volunteers. *Transl. Clin. Pharmacol.* **2017**, *25*, 202. [CrossRef]
27. Gibson, D.M.; Bron, N.J.; Richens, M.A.; Hounslow, N.J.; Sedman, A.J.; Whitfield, L.R. Effect of Age and Gender on Pharmacokinetics of Atorvastatin in Humans. *J. Clin. Pharmacol.* **1996**, *36*, 242–246. [CrossRef]
28. Romaine, S.P.R.; Bailey, K.M.; Hall, A.S.; Balmforth, A.J. The Influence of SLCO1B1 (OATP1B1) Gene Polymorphisms on Response to Statin Therapy. *Pharmacogenom. J.* **2010**, *10*, 1–11. [CrossRef] [PubMed]
29. He, Y.-J.; Zhang, W.; Chen, Y.; Guo, D.; Tu, J.-H.; Xu, L.-Y.; Tan, Z.-R.; Chen, B.-L.; Li, Z.; Zhou, G.; et al. Rifampicin Alters Atorvastatin Plasma Concentration on the Basis of SLCO1B1 521T>C Polymorphism. *Clin. Chim. Acta* **2009**, *405*, 49–52. [CrossRef] [PubMed]
30. Rodrigues, A.C.; Perin, P.M.S.; Purim, S.G.; Silbiger, V.N.; Genvigir, F.D.V.; Willrich, M.A.V.; Arazi, S.S.; Luchessi, A.D.; Hirata, M.H.; Bernik, M.M.S.; et al. Pharmacogenetics of OATP Transporters Reveals That SLCO1B1 c.388A>G Variant Is Determinant of Increased Atorvastatin Response. *Int. J. Mol. Sci.* **2011**, *12*, 5815–5827. [CrossRef] [PubMed]
31. Park, J.-E.; Kim, K.-B.; Bae, S.K.; Moon, B.-S.; Liu, K.-H.; Shin, J.-G. Contribution of Cytochrome P450 3A4 and 3A5 to the Metabolism of Atorvastatin. *Xenobiotica* **2008**, *38*, 1240–1251. [CrossRef] [PubMed]
32. Shin, J.; Pauly, D.F.; Pacanowski, M.A.; Langaee, T.; Frye, R.F.; Johnson, J.A. Effect of Cytochrome P450 3A5 Genotype on Atorvastatin Pharmacokinetics and Its Interaction with Clarithromycin. *Pharmacotherapy* **2011**, *31*, 942–950. [CrossRef]
33. Wilke, R.A.; Moore, J.H.; Burmester, J.K. Relative Impact of CYP3A Genotype and Concomitant Medication on the Severity of Atorvastatin-Induced Muscle Damage. *Pharmacogenet. Genom.* **2005**, *15*, 415–421. [CrossRef] [PubMed]
34. Willrich, M.A.V.; Hirata, M.H.; Genvigir, F.D.V.; Arazi, S.S.; Rebecchi, I.M.M.; Rodrigues, A.C.; Bernik, M.M.S.; Dorea, E.L.; Bertolami, M.C.; Faludi, A.A.; et al. CYP3A53A Allele Is Associated with Reduced Lowering-Lipid Response to Atorvastatin in Individuals with Hypercholesterolemia. *Clin. Chim. Acta* **2008**, *398*, 15–20. [CrossRef]

35. Kivistö, K.T.; Niemi, M.; Schaeffeler, E.; Pitkälä, K.; Tilvis, R.; Fromm, M.F.; Schwab, M.; Eichelbaum, M.; Strandberg, T. Lipid-Lowering Response to Statins Is Affected by CYP3A5 Polymorphism. *Pharmacogenetics* **2004**, *14*, 523–525. [CrossRef]
36. Thompson, J.F.; Man, M.; Johnson, K.J.; Wood, L.S.; Lira, M.E.; Lloyd, D.B.; Banerjee, P.; Milos, P.M.; Myrand, S.P.; Paulauskis, J.; et al. An Association Study of 43 SNPs in 16 Candidate Genes with Atorvastatin Response. *Pharmacogenom. J.* **2005**, *5*, 352–358. [CrossRef]
37. Lennernäs, H. Clinical Pharmacokinetics of Atorvastatin. *Clin. Pharmacokinet.* **2003**, *42*, 1141–1160. [CrossRef]
38. Goswami, S.; Gong, L.; Giacomini, K.; Altman, R.B.; Klein, T.E. PharmGKB Summary: Very Important Pharmacogene Information for SLC22A1. *Pharmacogenet. Genom.* **2014**, *24*, 324–328. [CrossRef] [PubMed]
39. Rodrigues, A.C.; Curi, R.; Genvigir, F.D.V.; Hirata, M.H.; Hirata, R.D.C. The Expression of Efflux and Uptake Transporters Are Regulated by Statins in Caco-2 and HepG2 Cells. *Acta Pharmacol. Sin.* **2009**, *30*, 956–964. [CrossRef]
40. Syam Das, S.; Nair, S.S.; Indira, M. Atorvastatin Modulates Drug Transporters and Ameliorates Nicotine-Induced Testicular Toxicity. *Andrologia* **2018**, *50*, e13029. [CrossRef]
41. Shu, Y.; Sheardown, S.A.; Brown, C.; Owen, R.P.; Zhang, S.; Castro, R.A.; Ianculescu, A.G.; Yue, L.; Lo, J.C.; Burchard, E.G.; et al. Effect of Genetic Variation in the Organic Cation Transporter 1 (OCT1) on Metformin Action. *J. Clin. Investig.* **2007**, *117*, 1422–1431. [CrossRef]
42. Sakaeda, T.; Fujino, H.; Komoto, C.; Kakumoto, M.; Jin, J.; Iwaki, K.; Nishiguchi, K.; Nakamura, T.; Okamura, N.; Okumura, K. Effects of Acid and Lactone Forms of Eight HMG-CoA Reductase Inhibitors on CYP-Mediated Metabolism and MDR1-Mediated Transport. *Pharm. Res.* **2006**, *23*, 506–512. [CrossRef]
43. Haas, D.W.; Kwara, A.; Richardson, D.M.; Baker, P.; Papageorgiou, I.; Acosta, E.P.; Morse, G.D.; Court, M.H. Secondary Metabolism Pathway Polymorphisms and Plasma Efavirenz Concentrations in HIV-Infected Adults with CYP2B6 Slow Metabolizer Genotypes. *J. Antimicrob. Chemother.* **2014**, *69*, 2175–2182. [CrossRef] [PubMed]
44. Lazarska, K.E.; Dekker, S.J.; Vermeulen, N.P.E.; Commandeur, J.N.M. Effect of UGT2B7*2 and CYP2C8*4 Polymorphisms on Diclofenac Metabolism. *Toxicol. Lett.* **2018**, *284*, 70–78. [CrossRef] [PubMed]

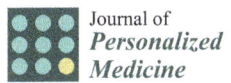

Article

Genome Wide Epistasis Study of On-Statin Cardiovascular Events with Iterative Feature Reduction and Selection

Solomon M. Adams *[ ], Habiba Feroze [†], Tara Nguyen [†], Seenae Eum, Cyrille Cornelio and Arthur F. Harralson [ ]

Department of Pharmacogenomics, Shenandoah University School of Pharmacy, Fairfax, VA 22031, USA; hferoze17@su.edu (H.F.); tnguyen174@su.edu (T.N.); seum@su.edu (S.E.); ccorneli1@su.edu (C.C.); aharrals@su.edu (A.F.H.)
* Correspondence: sadams07@su.edu; Tel.: +1-540-542-6237
† These authors contributed equally to this work.

Received: 10 September 2020; Accepted: 4 November 2020; Published: 7 November 2020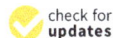

Abstract: Predicting risk for major adverse cardiovascular events (MACE) is an evidence-based practice that incorporates lifestyle, history, and other risk factors. Statins reduce risk for MACE by decreasing lipids, but it is difficult to stratify risk following initiation of a statin. Genetic risk determinants for on-statin MACE are low-effect size and impossible to generalize. Our objective was to determine high-level epistatic risk factors for on-statin MACE with GWAS-scale data. Controlled-access data for 5890 subjects taking a statin collected from Vanderbilt University Medical Center's BioVU were obtained from dbGaP. We used Random Forest Iterative Feature Reduction and Selection (RF-IFRS) to select highly informative genetic and environmental features from a GWAS-scale dataset of patients taking statin medications. Variant-pairs were distilled into overlapping networks and assembled into individual decision trees to provide an interpretable set of variants and associated risk. 1718 cases who suffered MACE and 4172 controls were obtained from dbGaP. Pathway analysis showed that variants in genes related to vasculogenesis (FDR = 0.024), angiogenesis (FDR = 0.019), and carotid artery disease (FDR = 0.034) were related to risk for on-statin MACE. We identified six gene-variant networks that predicted odds of on-statin MACE. The most elevated risk was found in a small subset of patients carrying variants in *COL4A2*, *TMEM178B*, *SZT2*, and *TBXAS1* (OR = 4.53, $p < 0.001$). The RF-IFRS method is a viable method for interpreting complex "black-box" findings from machine-learning. In this study, it identified epistatic networks that could be applied to risk estimation for on-statin MACE. Further study will seek to replicate these findings in other populations.

Keywords: pharmacogenomics; epistasis; random forest; statin; cardiovascular disease

1. Introduction

Predicting risk for Cardiovascular Disease (CVD) is a mainstay of primary care and cardiology. Patients who develop CVD are at risk for major adverse cardiovascular events (MACE), such as myocardial infarction, stroke, or unstable angina. Risk assessments for CVD include clinical biomarkers, family history, lifestyle, co-morbidities and biometrics. Routine risk assessments for CVD risk guide major therapeutic and lifestyle decisions.

Hyperlipidemia is a risk factor for CVD and MACE, and the American College of Cardiology (ACC) guidelines on the management of blood cholesterol recommend statins as the cornerstone pharmacotherapy [1]. CVD risk reduction from statins might be population specific and shows diversity among different patient groups. Ramos and colleagues found that the incidence of MACE was 19.7 (statin-users) and 24.7 (statin non-users) events per 1000 person-years in patients with asymptomatic peripheral artery disease [2]. Another study concluded that statin therapy had no major benefit on stroke in women [3]. Overall, however, statins reduce the risk for MACE proportional to the magnitude of cholesterol lowering in all ages [4].

The clinical pharmacogenetics implementation consortium guidelines support the use of pharmacogenomics (PGx) assessment for prevention of myopathy with simvastatin based on patients' *SLCO1B1* genotype [5]. Additionally, statin biochemical response (e.g., PK, Lipid Lowering Efficacy) is associated with numerous genomic variations. Ruiz-Iruela and colleagues found that decreased lipid lowering of rosuvastatin, atorvastatin, and simvastatin is predicted by *ABCA1* rs2230806 and *CYP2D6*. They also found that *CETP* variants rs708272 and rs5882 were associated with decreased and increased LDL lowering with rosuvastatin, respectively [6]. These variations, however, have not been found to be associated with higher level outcomes like prevention of CVD-related events. Low-effect size risk variants also provide insight into pathogenesis of CVD. Genetic variations in apolipoprotein C-III (*APOC3*) and angiopoietin-like 4 (*ANGPTL4*) have been associated with risk for coronary artery disease (CAD) [7]. Roguin and colleagues found that the Haptoglobin (*HP*) genotype was a significant independent predictor of MACE in patients with diabetes [8]. The PROSPER study found that *SURF6* rs579459 was associated with CAD, stroke and large artery stroke. It also found that *TWIST1* rs2107595 was associated with an increased risk of MACE such as large artery stroke, CAD, and ischemic stroke [9]. Routine genetic testing for hyperlipidemia and CVD risk is limited to patients with history of familial hypercholesterolemia (FH), predicted by variation in *LDLR*, *APOB*, or *PCSK9* [1]. CVD nevertheless shows strong heritability in patients without FH, suggesting an underlying genetic component [7]. Genome-Wide Association Studies (GWAS) have identified over 50 genetic variants that are associated with risk for CVD and MACE. Clinical translation of these genetic risk factors is challenged by individual variants with small effect sizes and poor understanding of the interplay between multiple genetic variants and risk for MACE. These genetic factors might help explain cases in which patients still experience MACE in spite of adequate phamacologic response to statin therapy and other risk reduction strategies.

PGx is exemplified in variations among drug-metabolizing genes, including phase I (oxidation, reduction, hydrolysis), phase II (conjugation), and phase III (transport). In these cases, functional genetic variations can have catastrophic effects on pharmacokinetics [10]. While some evidence supports PGx for pharmacodynamic markers, PGx outside of pharmacokinetics has been limited by relatively low effect-size of individual variants, and the inability to consistently apply multiple gene effects. This is partially addressed by the growing use of polygenic risk scores (PRS) to pool effects from unrelated variants [11]; however, little has been done to incorporate the effects of epistasis (i.e., gene-gene interactions) to create novel predictors of drug response.

The objective of this research was to stratify the risk of on-statin MACE based on polygenic epistatic predictors. We applied a step-wise, interpretable, machine-learning (ML) driven ensemble method for feature reduction and determination of epistasis to a GWAS-scale dataset. We expect that application of this method will drive novel insight into genetic interactions that drive risk for complex cardiovascular phenotypes and statin PGx.

2. Results

2.1. Demographics

Demographic data are summarized in Table 1. Our analysis incorporated genetic variant data and sex, which were available for all subjects. Random forest models do not tolerate missing values and require either imputation or exclusion to include variables with missing data. Given the focus on epistasis in this analysis, non-genetic variables were only included if they were defined in all cases and controls. Weight, and height were frequently missing in controls, and were therefore not used.

Age was only available as "age of first event", which limited its utility in comparing cases and controls. More than 99% of subjects in this population are reported as white. Sex is also a well-established predictor of risk for MACE and was thus included in the model.

Table 1. Population demographics.

Variable	Control	Case	p
Female(%)	38.0%	31.2%	<0.001
White(%)	99.3%	99.4%	0.507
BMI(Mean ± SD)	29.03 ± 7.37	28.57 ± 7.035	0.253
Age First MACE (Median ± IQR)	N/A	65 ± 16	1

2.2. Feature Selection with RF-IFRS

After pruning, there were 637,732 variants and 5890 subjects in the cohort. Of the subjects, there were 1718 cases and 4172 controls. Evaluation of additive statistical association did not identify any variants that met genome-wide significance. The RF with the corrected impurity importance measure identified 6688 variants with a corrected-impurity p value less than 0.01. As with statistical association, no variants met genome-wide significance. The 6688 initially selected variants were extracted from the full dataset and analyzed with r2VIM. This identified 49 genetic variants in addition to sex with a minimum permutation importance value of at least one. Results from these analyses are shown in Figure 1.

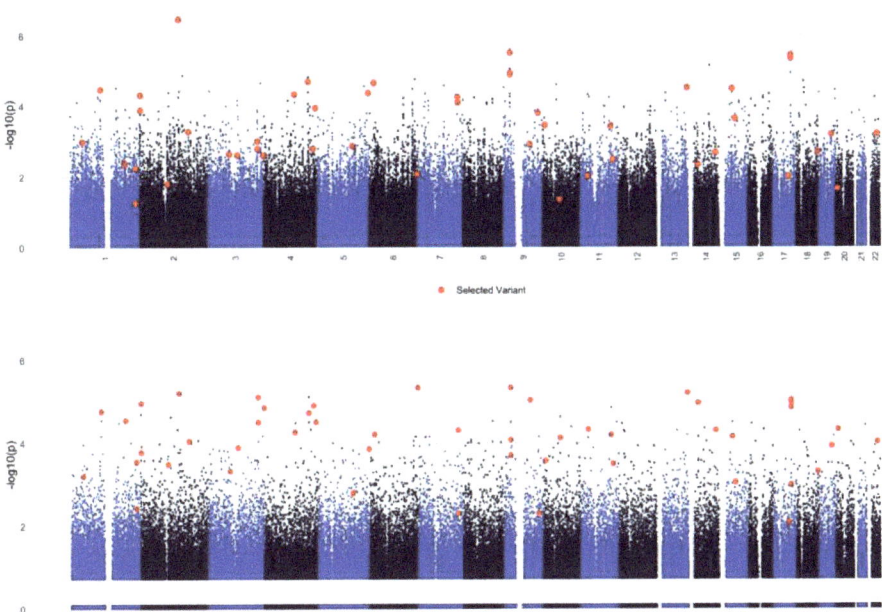

Figure 1. Manhattan plots for statistical GWAS analysis with PLINK (**top**) vs. the initial RF model with ranger (**bottom**). Red dots correspond to variants that were selected with r2VIM, and show that a purely statistical approach fails to identify variants that are likely relevant to the outcome due to interactions.

2.3. Epistasis Screening

Paired selection frequency results identify variant-pairs that co-occur in decision trees more often, as often, or less often than predicted based on individual variant selection. Variants that are selected together more often than expected suggests a greater phenotype prediction from both variants together, and selection less often than expected suggests that co-occurrence comes at a cost to phenotype prediction (i.e., variants are correlated and/or in linkage disequilibrium).

Figure 2 shows the distribution of expected tree co-occurrence for each variant pair. Using an alternative hypothesis of "greater than expected" in a binomial test allows sensitive selection of variant pairs that are chosen more often than predicted (red). We found evidence of epistasis in 16 variant-variant pairs Table 2. Additionally, five variants showed significant interaction with sex.

Condensing variant-pairs based on overlap resulted in six variant networks Figure 3. We found networks that involved intergenic variants, for which the functional consequence is not clear. This is evident in network 1, where sex precedes four intergenic variants, most of which are more than 100 kb away from the nearest gene. Gene-variant networks show diversity in odds for experiencing MACE, with individual node odds ratios reflecting the contribution of multiple variant effects through additive and non-additive relationships.

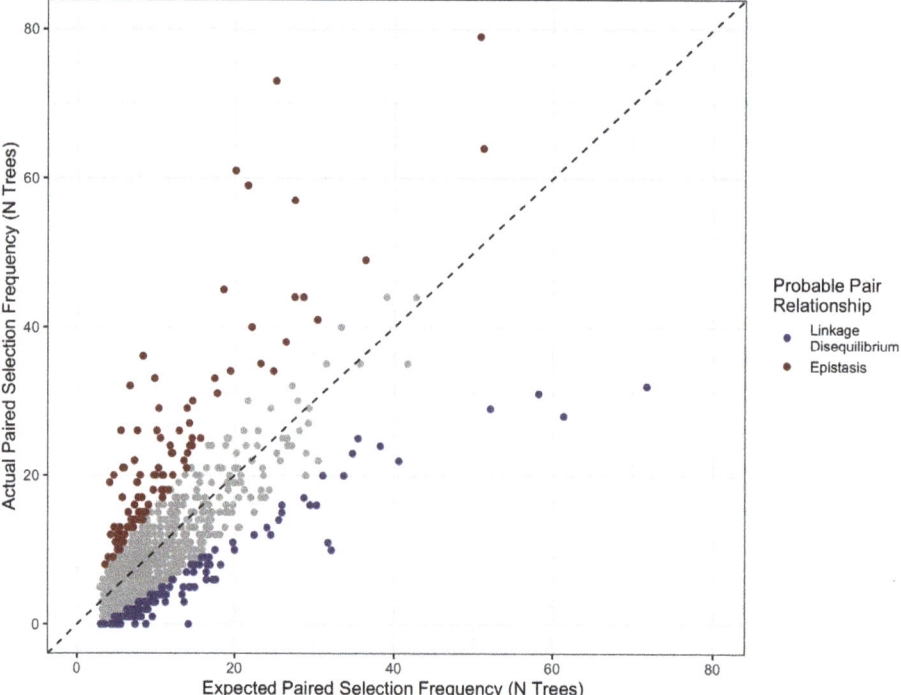

Figure 2. Paired selection frequency based on the combined independent variant probabilities (X axis) vs. the actual frequency of variants being selected together in a decision tree. Variants that are selected together at a lower-than-expected frequency are expected to be correlated with respect to the outcome, suggesting that they are in linkage disequilibrium (blue). Variants selected together more often than expected (red) are predicted to exhibit epistasis with respect to the phenotype.

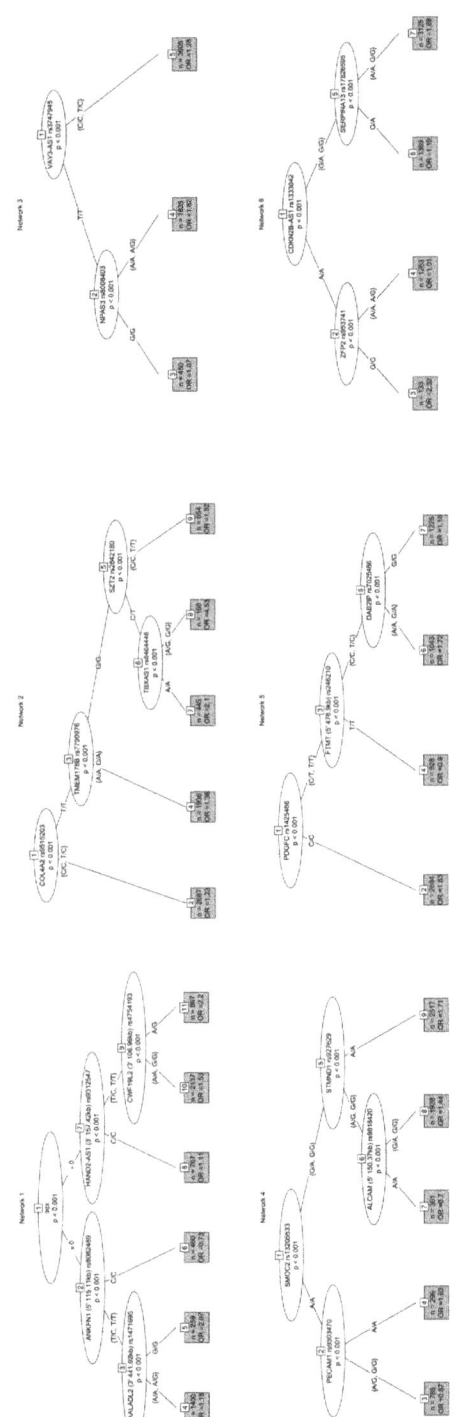

Figure 3. Decision trees incorporating overlapping epistasis-variant-pairs show six unique networks of genes and variants. Odds ratios in terminal nodes represent subject odds of on-statin MACE in someone carrying the collection of alleles shown in the network relative to those who did not carry those variants. This shows a practical interpretation of epistasis findings that might be more practical to incorporate into clinical practice, though validation and replication in independent populations will be necessary to drive clinical translation.

Table 2. Significant Ensemble and Regression Variant Pairs.

Variant 1	Variant 2	$FDR_{ensemble}$	$FDR_{interaction}$
sex	CDCA7 (3′ 242.48 kb) rs6731912	0.001	0.029
sex	NAALADL2 (3′ 441.92 kb) rs1471695	<0.001	0.082
sex	HAND2-AS1 (3′ 157.42 kb) rs9312547	<0.001	0.007
sex	NNMT (5′ 4.01 kb) rs2244175	0.021	0.016
sex	ANKFN1 (5′ 115.11 kb) rs8082489	<0.001	0.007
SZT2 rs2842180	COL4A2 rs9515203	<0.001	0.004
VAV3-AS1 rs3747945	NPAS3 rs8008403	0.001	0.011
KCNT2 (3′ 1239.56 kb) rs6693848	PECAM1 rs2812	<0.001	0.004
KCNT2 (3′ 1239.56 kb) rs6693848	PECAM1 rs9303470	<0.001	0.004
KCNT2 (3′ 1239.56 kb) rs6693848	PECAM1 (5′ 1.22 kb) rs6504218	0.032	0.004
ALCAM (5′ 150.37 kb) rs9818420	STMND1 rs927629	<0.001	0.001
NAALADL2 (3′ 441.92 kb) rs1471695	RFX7 (5′ 10.73 kb) rs2713935	<0.001	0.005
PDGFC rs1425486	FTMT (5′ 478.9 kb) rs246210	<0.001	0.001
FTMT (5′ 478.9 kb) rs246210	DAB2IP rs7025486	<0.001	0.001
ZFP2 rs953741	CDKN2B-AS1 rs1333042	0.011	0.004
STMND1 rs927629	SMOC2 rs13205533	<0.001	0.004
SMOC2 rs13205533	PECAM1 rs2812	0.043	0.016
TBXAS1 rs6464448	COL4A2 rs9515203	0.014	0.009
TMEM178B rs7790976	COL4A2 rs9515203	0.043	0.004
CDKN2B-AS1 rs2383207	SERPINA13 rs17826595	0.001	0.016
SFMBT2 rs10453997	CWF19L2 (3′ 106.96 kb) rs4754193	<0.001	0.001
CWF19L2 (3′ 106.96 kb) rs4754193	NNMT (5′ 4.01 kb) rs2244175	0.006	0.011
GATM (3′ 12.69 kb) rs2461700	ZNF404 rs1978723	<0.001	0.005

We found that a small subset of subjects carrying *COL4A2* rs9515203 (T/T), *TMEM178B* rs7790976 (G/G), *SZT2* rs2842180 (C/T), and *TBXAS1* rs6464448 (G Allele) showed the highest increase in MACE risk (Network 2, OR = 4.53, $p < 0.001$). Variant effects analysis showed evidence of gene networks associated with angiogenesis, endothelial cell development and function, carotid artery disease, and development of vasculature (minimum FDR = 0.019) Table 3.

Table 3. Gene network associated disease processes

Diseases or Functions	Genes	FDR
Angiogenesis	ALCAM CDKN2B COL4A2 DAB2IP PDGFC PECAM1 SMOC2 VAV3	0.0188
Carotid artery disease	NNMT VAV3	0.034
Development of vasculature	ALCAM CDKN2B COL4A2 DAB2IP NPAS3 PDGFC PECAM1 SMOC2 VAV3	0.0188
Endothelial cell development	COL4A2 PDGFC PECAM1 SMOC2	0.0291
Formation of blood vessel	CDKN2B COL4A2 PECAM1	0.0242
Formation of endothelial tube	COL4A2 PECAM1	0.0291
Function of endothelial tissue	PECAM1 VAV3	0.0188
Migration of endothelial cells	ALCAM COL4A2 PECAM1 SMOC2 VAV3	0.0188
Quantity of endothelial cells	ALCAM PDGFC	0.023
Vasculogenesis	ALCAM CDKN2B COL4A2 PDGFC PECAM1 SMOC2	0.0242

3. Discussion

3.1. Risk Variants and Interactions for CVD

This study was a genome-wide study for variant-variant interactions (epistasis) associated with on-statin MACE. We found six variant networks that show a diverse range of genetic interactions that predict increased or decreased risk for on-statin MACE. Our findings show that RF-IFRS produces polygenic predictors of risk for on-statin MACE, suggesting that limitations of low effect-sizes can be overcome by studying variant networks to produce a final odds ratio.

3.2. Novelty and Application to Clinical Practice

Machine learning techniques based on RF have been commonplace in the evaluation of gene-gene interactions in genomic data [12]. The novelty of the RF-IFRS method primarily derives from the direct analysis of forest structure to estimate epistasis, with application to clinical data. This method shows similarity to work by Li and colleagues, who used a permutation-based RF method to find networks of gene-gene interactions in simulated and real data [13]. While our approach is similar, RF-IFRS scales to GWAS-sized data and corrects for case-control imbalance and variable allele frequency, which is a challenge in many other RF implementations [14]. These studies should ultimately seek clinical translation, and is reflected in this study of a highly relevant clinical phenotype (on-statin MACE). Nevertheless, it is critical that readers recognize that this work and gene/variant-interaction networks are preliminary and have not been evaluated *in vitro*.

3.3. Angiogenesis, Endothelial Function, and Vasculogenesis in CVD

Angiogenesis refers to the formation of new capillary beds from existing vasculature, whereas vasculogenesis refers to the formation of *de novo* vascular networks (i.e., during embryonic development) [15]. Among others, *ALCAM*, *CDKN2B*, *COL4A2*, *DAB2IP*, *PECAM1*, *SMOC2*, *VAV3*, and *PDGFC* are related to either angiogenesis and/or vasculogenesis. These genes were included in five out of six networks that we identified, suggesting that these processes are relevant to risk for MACE and on-statin MACE.

3.4. RF-IFRS Replicates Existing Gene Associations with CVD and Incorporates Novel Interactions

Network one incorporated interactions with sex and variants in four intergenic regions. These variants flanked the nearest genes (*NAALADL2*, *HAND2-AS1*, *NNMT*, and *ANKFN1*) by up to 450 kb. Drawing mechanistic insight from these interactions is not practical or necessarily advisable without further mechanistic analysis. However, this finding suggests that the association of male sex with higher risk for on-statin MACE is connected to diverse genetic components that might connect to chromatin structure, un-annotated regulatory RNA genes (e.g., lncRNA, Micro-RNA, etc).

Network two shows a relationship between *COL4A2* rs9515203, *TMEM178B* rs7790976, *SZT2* rs2842184, and *TBXAS1* rs6464448. *COL4A2*. (Collagen Type IV Alpha 2 Chain) codes for the collagen IV peptide α 2 chain, which is a component of the basement membrane surrounding the endothelium of blood vessels [16]. *COL4A2* rs9515203 has previously shown association with sub-clinical atherosclerosis [17], and coronary artery disease [18,19]. Other variants in *COL4A2* and *COL4A1* show associations with risk for MI, atheroslcerotic plaque stability, and vascular stability [16]. The role of *SZT2* (Seizure threshold 2 homolog) rs2842184 in CVD is not clear, and may not indicate a direct mechanism. A recent proteomic study of plasma protein expression in patients with CVD found decreased plasma levels of SZT2 in patients with CVD. The authors suggested that this might be connected to increased mTORC1 signalling in patients with CVD, but this mechanism has not been tested [20]. *TMEM178B* (Transmembrane Protein 178B) codes for a transmembrane protein that is highly expressed in cardiac tissue, among others. The role of the rs7790976 variant is not clear in this network. *TBXAS1* (Thromboxane A synthase 1) codes for Thromboxane A Synthase 1, which is expressed in several tissues including platelets. Thromboxane is a potent vasoconstrictor that causes vasoconstriction and platelet aggregation. The rs6464448 variant has not been previously associated with a phenotype, and the role of genetic variation connecting *TBXAS1* to CVD outcomes is not clear. However, *TBXAS1* has been recently proposed as a potential drug target for CVD [21].

Network three is comprised of an interaction between *VAV3-AS1* rs3747945 and *NPAS3* rs8008403. *VAV3* (Vav Guanine Nucleotide Exchange Factor 3) is important to the migration of smooth muscle cells, which suggests that it has a role in vascular proliferation [22]. *VAV3-AS1* is an RNA gene coding for anti-sense *VAV3*, which might regulate expression of *VAV3* [23]. *VAV3-AS1* rs3747945 has not been previously associated with cardiovascular disease related outcomes, but further supports the role for vasculogenesis in risk for MACE. *NPAS3* (Neuronal PAS Domain Protein 3) rs8008403 has not been previously associated with cardiovascular disease related outcomes, but another variant in *NPAS3* (rs17460823) was associated with C-reactive protein in patients taking fenofibrate [24]. The mechanistic connection of these variants/genes is difficult to determine, but might be linked to development of gross anatomy of the cardiovascular system, or to remodeling associated with CVD.

Network four connects *SMOC2* rs13205533, *PECAM1* rs9303470, *STMND1* rs927629, and a variant (rs9818420) approximately 150 kb upstream from *ALCAM*. This network appears to be related to vascular homeostasis and proliferation. *SMOC2* (SPARC-related modular calcium-binding protein 2) modulates calcium homeostasis, and might be relevant to blood vessel calcification [25]. *SMOC2* rs13205533 has not been previously associated with cardiovascular disease related outcomes. *PECAM1* (Platelet And Endothelial Cell Adhesion Molecule 1) is important for the maintenance of vascular endothelial integrity, and endothelial cells that express PECAM1 are more resilient to the inflammatory response from vascular barrier damage [26,27]. *PECAM1* rs9303470 has not been previously associated with cardiovascular disease related outcomes, but other variants in *PECAM1* have been found to be associated with CAD [26]. *PECAM1* shares similar function with *ALCAM* (Activated leukocyte cell adhesion molecule), and both seem to play roles in CVD [28]. Higher levels of the ALCAM protein have been associated with poor CV outcomes including CV death in patients presenting with ACS [28]. *STMND1* (Stathmin Domain Containing 1) Variants in *STMND1* have been associated with stroke in African Americans, though rs927629 has not been previously reported with CVD [29].

Network five shows interactions between genes relevent to angiogenesis, including *PDGFC* rs1425486 and *DAB2IP* rs7025486. Variants in *PDGFC* (Platelet Derived Growth Factor C) and other *PDGF* genes have been associated with angiogenesis and CVD [30]. PDGFC likely promotes angiogenesis independently of VEGF, which might support a role in CVD development and/or vascular remodeling [31]. *PDGFC* rs1425486 has not been previously associated with cardiovascular disease related outcomes. *DAB2IP* (DAB2-interacting protein) is expressed widely in the cardiovascular system and it is believed to be an inhibitor of VEGF-2 signalling and thus an inhibitor of angiogenesis [32]. Multiple variants in *DAB2IP* have been associated with CAD,[33] and rs7025486 is associated with abdominal aortic aneurysm [34].

Network six includes interactions between *CDKN2B-AS1* rs1333042, *ZFP2* rs953741, and *SERPINA13* rs17826595. *CDKN2B-AS1* (cyclin-dependent kinase inhibitor 2B antisense RNA 1) is an RNA gene that regulates the expression of *CDKN2B*. CDKN2B is an inhibitor of cellular proliferation, though its direct role in CVD is not clear. Numerous variants in *CDKN2B-AS1*, including rs1333042, have been associated with CHD [35]. *ZFP2* (Zinc Finger Protein) is a regulator protein. Variants in *ZFP2* are associated with MI in African Americans[29], though *ZFP2* rs953741 has not been previously associated with cardiovascular disease related outcomes. *SERPINA13* (Serpin Family A Member 13) is a pseudogene, and it is not clear what its role is in CVD. *SERPINA13* rs17826595 has not been previously associated with cardiovascular disease related outcomes. Other members of the *SERPIN* gene superfamily are related to cardiovascular system development and regulation [36].

3.5. Limitations

The RF-IFRS method is a novel approach to genome-wide epistasis that incorporates statistics and interpretable ML methods. The definition of MACE used in this study is less broad than is commonly used in the CVD literature. Notably, ischemic stroke and CV death are not included in the definitions, which is relevant to the generalizability of these findings to other studies that evaluate MACE as an outcome. This study was carried out in a single cohort of patients without replication, however, the RF procedure performs thousands of random samples from the dataset to determing feature importance. While this is not as robust as independent replication, it might help mitigate the bias associated with genetic association studies carried out in a single cohort. We did not split the cohort into training and testing groups or perform hyperparameter tuning, which are often done when developing a predictive

ML model. However, the objective was not to generate a highly predictive ML model, but rather to use the organic structure of the RF approach to identify important variants and interactions. This is also relevant to statistical power, and given that this study found no significant variants with traditional GWAS we opted to keep the entire cohort together to maximize power. Due to the RF inclination to discover LD organically, we did not perform LD pruning. We also did not perform imputation to limit the computational overhead required for the RF model training. This study does not include causal analysis of individual SNPs, thus we do not suggest that the reported variants are necessarily causal. Finally, we did not have access to more extensive clinical data. Further analysis and replication ought to evaluate if findings correspond to degree of lipid control.

4. Materials and Methods

4.1. Clinical Dataset

The data/analyses presented in the current publication are based on the use of controlled-access study data downloaded with permission from the dbGaP web site, under phs000963.v1.p1 (https://www.ncbi.nlm.nih.gov/projects/gap/cgi-bin/study.cgi?study_id=phs000963.v1.p1). This dataset was assembled through Vanderbilt University Medical Center's BioVU repository and clinical data was extracted from the electronic medical record. All subjects gave their informed consent for inclusion before they participated in the study. The study was conducted in accordance with the Declaration of Helsinki, and the protocol was approved by the Vanderbilt Institutional Review Board. These data correspond to 5890 subjects of European descent taking HMG-Coa Reductase Inhibitors (statins) who were genotyped with the Illumina HumanOmniExpressExome 8v1-2_A array by the RIKEN Integrative Medical Sciences Center (IMS) and supported by the Pharmacogenomics Research Network (PGRN)-RIKEN IMS Global Alliance. Inclusion and exclusion criteria for cases and controls is described in Table 4. The primary outcome is on-statin MACE, defined as any revascularization event (e.g., stent placement, bypass) and/or acute myocardial infarction. The case group contains 1718 subjects, and the control group contains 4172 subjects. Case and control status was determined with Vanderbilt's BioVU DNA databank and associated Synthetic Derivative database of clinical information, and software tools developed to identify drugs and clinical events using Electronic Health Record-derived structured and unstructured ("free text") data.

Table 4. Inclusion and Exclusion Criteria.

MACE on statin, defined as either AMI or revascularization on statin
AMI on statins: Case definition (all three conditions required): - At least two ICD9 code for AMI or other acute and subacute forms of ischemic heart disease within a five-day window - Confirmed lab within the same time window - Statin prescribed prior to the AMI event in medical records at least 180 days *Revascularization while on statin: Case definition (both conditions required):* - At least one revascularization CPT code - Statin prescribed prior to the revascularization event in medical records at least 180 days
Case Exclusion: - No diagnosis code for AMI, other acute and subacute forms of ischemic heart disease, or historical AMI assigned previously - No revascularization CPT codes assigned previously - No MACE (Major Adverse Cardiovascular Events) found in previous problem list by NLP
Control definition: - Statin prescribed - No diagnosis code for AMI, other acute and subacute forms of ischemic heart, or historical AMI assigned previously - No revascularization CPT codes assigned previously - No MACE found in previous problem list by NLP - Controls match cases by age, gender, statin type (e.g., simvastatin), and statin exposure

4.2. Data Pre-Processing

Data obtained from dbGaP were in Plink format. The XY pseudo-autosomal region was recoded, and then the resulting file was converted to a multi-sample VCF file. The VCF file chromosome and positions were recoded based on the Illumina variant IDs from the HumanOmniExpressExome manifest file Infinium OmniExpressExome-8 v1.6 for GRCh38. Positions with ambiguous chromosome or positions were filtered from the resulting VCF file. Finally, filters were applied so that variants included in the final analysis were autosomal variants with a minor allele frequency of at least one percent. A PLINK format phenotype file was created from the original phenotype file from dbGaP. This created the necessary ID columns and selects the phenotype column corresponding to MACE. The resulting VCF file was converted to the transposed PLINK (tped) format with PLINK and carried forward for additional analyses.

4.3. Random Forest Iterative Feature Reduction and Selection (RF-IFRS)

Code corresponding to methods is available at https://github.com/sadams-lab/manuscript_onstatin-mace-GWES. PLINK format files were read into an R environment with the GenABEL package [37]. To account for the sensitivity of random forest (RF) models to group imbalance, we weighted cases and controls so that the probability of selecting either from a bootstrapped population was equivalent. To provide a reference comparison, we performed genome-wide association (GWA) analysis on the data with Plink version 1.9 using an additive model with no covariates [38]. We used a two-step process for feature selection that sought to overcome computational limits of analyzing highly dimensional GWAS data. The first stage of feature reduction was performed using the Ranger package for R, in which the forest was grown with a mtry fraction of 1/3, and 1000 trees [39] Considering that this method incorporates the full breadth of data, we used the corrected impurity score implemented by Nembrini and colleagues, which overcomes the sensitivity of GINI importance to allele frequency while allowing a practical computing time compared to the more robust permutation score [14]. This method is computationally fast, but relatively non-specific and produces false-positives similar to that of a traditional GWAS.

Features with p values of < 0.01 were selected for secondary feature selection with r2VIM, which incorporates multiple RF models to build a consensus permutation importance [40]. It was re-implemented by Degenhardt and colleagues to support the ranger package, which allows for parallel tree building and much faster execution in the Pomona package [41]. For our implementation, we cloned the Pomona repository and modified it so that it would accept input from a GenABEL object. The resulting custom r2VIM implementation was run with 11 sequentially grown RF models with 10,000 trees per forest using, an mtry fraction of 1/3, and nodes were limited to a maximum of 10% of the total population to limit tree depth. Features from the first forests with a minimum permutation importance of at least one in each forest were selected for estimation of association and interaction. The final (11th) forest was saved for the ensemble-method for epistasis selection.

4.4. Testing for Epistasis

The ensemble method for epistasis estimation was implemented based on the work by Schmalohr and colleagues [42]. We implemented methods for testing paired selection frequency (i.e., the probability that a variable will be included in the same decision tree) and selection asymmetry (i.e., the probability of a variant favoring a particular node when following another variant) [42]. These methods provides the means to detect AND and XOR epistasis. To create a final estimate for the presence of an interaction, p values from each method were combined using the Fisher method [43].

Variant-pair p values were adjusted with the Benjamini-Hochberg FDR method, and pairs with FDR of less than 0.05 were retained for further analysis [44]. Selected variant pairs were converted to dummy variables, and all pair-wise genotype permutations were compared with logistic regression. The minimum pairwise interaction p value was retained for each variant pair. Interaction p values were adjusted with the Benjamini-Hochberg FDR method.

4.5. Poly-Epistatic Risk and Pathway Analysis

To extend beyond pair-wise interactions, pairwise interacting variants were condensed based on overlap. For example, $A|B$ and $A|C$ -> $A|B|C$. Decision trees were built from the resulting variant interaction networks to visualize relationships and odds ratios based on multiple variants. Decision trees were built with the ctree function in the Party package for R [45] Odds ratios for terminal nodes were normalized to the overall odds of being a case.

To incorporate basic mechanistic insight, data were analyzed through the use of Ingenuity® Variant Analysis™ version 1.18.06(https://www.qiagenbioinformatics.com/products/ingenuity-variant-analysis) from QIAGEN, Inc. (Hilden, Germany). Top diseases and bio-functions relevant to MACE and CVD were reported with correlation to identified decision trees, then filtered for at least two genes involved and a FDR corrected p value of less than 0.05.

5. Conclusions

A RF driven method for feature reduction and selection applied to a GWAS-scale dataset identified six epistasis-networks that may provide insight into the risk for on-statin MACE. This method also provides interpretable results, which may produce a more physiologically relevant assessment of odds and risk for an outcome than PRS. We found that variants related to angiogenesis and vasculogenesis are associated with odds of on-statin MACE. These findings present a unique opportunity for the incorporation of multiple low-effect size variants in the prediction of drug success in preventing CVD events. Future research should seek method-replication in diverse populations to determine the broad reproducibility of these findings and potential clinical application.

Author Contributions: Conceptualization, S.M.A., C.C., S.E., and A.F.H.; methodology, S.M.A., S.E., A.F.H.; software, S.M.A.; resources, S.M.A.; writing–original draft preparation, S.M.A., T.N., H.F.; writing–review and editing, S.M.A., C.C., S.E., A.F.H.; supervision, S.M.A. All authors have read and agreed to the published version of the manuscript.

Funding: Vanderbilt University Medical Center's BioVU is supported by institutional funding and by the Vanderbilt CTSA grant UL1 TR000445 from NCATS/NIH. This study was supported by an NIH Pharmacogenomics Research Network (PGRN)—RIKEN Center for Integrative Medical Sciences (IMS) Global Alliance, and genome-wide genotyping was funded and performed by the IMS. This study was also supported by NHLBI/NIH grants U19 HL065962 and U01 HL069757. The authors of this study are also supported by a grant from the Andrew W. Mellon Foundation (SMA) and U5 4MD010723 (AFH).

Conflicts of Interest: The authors declare no conflict of interest.

References

1. Grundy, S.M.; Stone, N.J.; Bailey, A.L.; Beam, C.; Birtcher, K.K.; Blumenthal, R.S.; Braun, L.T.; de Ferranti, S.; Faiella-Tommasino, J.; Forman, D.E.; et al. 2018 AHA/ACC/AACVPR/AAPA/ABC/ACPM/ADA/AGS/APhA/ASPC/NLA/PCNA Guideline on the Management of Blood Cholesterol: A Report of the American College of Cardiology/American Heart Association Task Force on Clinical Practice Guidelines. *Circulation* **2019**, *139*, e1082–e1143. [CrossRef] [PubMed]
2. Ramos, R.; García-Gil, M.; Comas-Cufí, M.; Quesada, M.; Marrugat, J.; Elosua, R.; Sala, J.; Grau, M.; Martí, R.; Ponjoan, A.; et al. Statins for Prevention of Cardiovascular Events in a Low-Risk Population With Low Ankle Brachial Index. *J. Am. Coll. Cardiol.* **2016**, *67*, 630–640. [CrossRef] [PubMed]
3. Gutierrez, J.; Ramirez, G.; Rundek, T.; Sacco, R.L. Statin therapy in the prevention of recurrent cardiovascular events: A sex-based meta-analysis. *Arch. Intern. Med.* **2012**, *172*, 909–919. [CrossRef] [PubMed]
4. Efficacy and safety of statin therapy in older people: A meta-analysis of individual participant data from 28 randomised controlled trials. *Lancet* **2019**, *393*, 407–415. [CrossRef]

5. Ramsey, L.B.; Johnson, S.G.; Caudle, K.E.; Haidar, C.E.; Voora, D.; Wilke, R.A.; Maxwell, W.D.; McLeod, H.L.; Krauss, R.M.; Roden, D.M.; et al. The clinical pharmacogenetics implementation consortium guideline for SLCO1B1 and simvastatin-induced myopathy: 2014 update. *Clin. Pharmacol. Ther.* **2014**, *96*, 423–428. [CrossRef] [PubMed]
6. Ruiz-Iruela, C.; Candás-Estébanez, B.; Pintó-Sala, X.; Baena-Díez, N.; Caixàs-Pedragós, A.; Güell-Miró, R.; Navarro-Badal, R.; Calmarza, P.; Puzo-Foncilla, J.L.; Alía-Ramos, P.; et al. Genetic contribution to lipid target achievement with statin therapy: A prospective study. *Pharm. J.* **2020**, *20*, 494–504. [CrossRef] [PubMed]
7. Kessler, T.; Vilne, B.; Schunkert, H. The impact of genome-wide association studies on the pathophysiology and therapy of cardiovascular disease. *EMBO Mol. Med.* **2016**, *8*, 688–701. [CrossRef] [PubMed]
8. Roguin, A.; Koch, W.; Kastrati, A.; Aronson, D.; Schomig, A.; Levy, A.P. Haptoglobin genotype is predictive of major adverse cardiac events in the 1-year period after percutaneous transluminal coronary angioplasty in individuals with diabetes. *Diabetes Care* **2003**, *26*, 2628–2631. [CrossRef] [PubMed]
9. Zhao, C.; Zhu, P.; Shen, Q.; Jin, L. Prospective association of a genetic risk score with major adverse cardiovascular events in patients with coronary artery disease. *Medicine* **2017**, *96*, e9473. [CrossRef]
10. Wang, L.; McLeod, H.L.; Weinshilboum, R.M. Genomics and drug response. *N. Engl. J. Med.* **2011**, *364*, 1144–1153. [CrossRef]
11. Gibson, G. On the utilization of polygenic risk scores for therapeutic targeting. *PLoS Genet.* **2019**, *15*, e1008060. [CrossRef] [PubMed]
12. Jiang, R.; Tang, W.; Wu, X.; Fu, W. A random forest approach to the detection of epistatic interactions in case-control studies. *BMC Bioinform.* **2009**, *10* (Suppl. S1), S65. [CrossRef] [PubMed]
13. Li, J.; Malley, J.D.; Andrew, A.S.; Karagas, M.R.; Moore, J.H. Detecting gene-gene interactions using a permutation-based random forest method. *BioData Min* **2016**, *9*, 14. [CrossRef] [PubMed]
14. Nembrini, S.; König, I.R.; Wright, M.N. The revival of the Gini importance? *Bioinformatics* **2018**, *34*, 3711–3718. [CrossRef] [PubMed]
15. Vailhé, B.; Vittet, D.; Feige, J.J. In vitro models of vasculogenesis and angiogenesis. *Lab. Investig.* **2001**, *81*, 439–452. [CrossRef]
16. Yang, W.; Ng, F.L.; Chan, K.; Pu, X.; Poston, R.N.; Ren, M.; An, W.; Zhang, R.; Wu, J.; Yan, S.; et al. Coronary-Heart-Disease-Associated Genetic Variant at the COL4A1/COL4A2 Locus Affects COL4A1/COL4A2 Expression, Vascular Cell Survival, Atherosclerotic Plaque Stability and Risk of Myocardial Infarction. *PLoS Genet.* **2016**, *12*, e1006127. [CrossRef] [PubMed]
17. Vargas, J.D.; Manichaikul, A.; Wang, X.Q.; Rich, S.S.; Rotter, J.I.; Post, W.S.; Polak, J.F.; Budoff, M.J.; Bluemke, D.A. Common genetic variants and subclinical atherosclerosis: The Multi-Ethnic Study of Atherosclerosis (MESA). *Atherosclerosis* **2016**, *245*, 230–236. [CrossRef]
18. Dehghan, A.; Bis, J.C.; White, C.C.; Smith, A.V.; Morrison, A.C.; Cupples, L.A.; Trompet, S.; Chasman, D.I.; Lumley, T.; Völker, U.; et al. Genome-Wide Association Study for Incident Myocardial Infarction and Coronary Heart Disease in Prospective Cohort Studies: The CHARGE Consortium. *PLoS ONE* **2016**, *11*, e0144997. [CrossRef]
19. Vargas, J.D.; Manichaikul, A.; Wang, X.Q.; Rich, S.S.; Rotter, J.I.; Post, W.S.; Polak, J.F.; Budoff, M.J.; Bluemke, D.A. Detailed analysis of association between common single nucleotide polymorphisms and subclinical atherosclerosis: The Multi-ethnic Study of Atherosclerosis. *Data Brief* **2016**, *7*, 229–242. [CrossRef]
20. Lygirou, V.; Latosinska, A.; Makridakis, M.; Mullen, W.; Delles, C.; Schanstra, J.P.; Zoidakis, J.; Pieske, B.; Mischak, H.; Vlahou, A. Plasma proteomic analysis reveals altered protein abundances in cardiovascular disease. *J. Transl. Med.* **2018**, *16*, 104. [CrossRef]
21. Mesitskaya, D.F.; Syrkin, A.L.; Aksenova, M.G.; Zhang, Y.; Zamyatnin, A.A.; Kopylov, P.Y. Thromboxane A Synthase: A New Target for the Treatment of Cardiovascular Diseases. *Cardiovasc. Hematol. Agents Med. Chem.* **2018**, *16*, 81–87. [CrossRef]
22. Toumaniantz, G.; Ferland-McCollough, D.; Cario-Toumaniantz, C.; Pacaud, P.; Loirand, G. The Rho protein exchange factor Vav3 regulates vascular smooth muscle cell proliferation and migration. *Cardiovasc. Res.* **2010**, *86*, 131–140. [CrossRef]
23. Xu, J.Z.; Zhang, J.L.; Zhang, W.G. Antisense RNA: The new favorite in genetic research. *J. Zhejiang Univ. Sci. B* **2018**, *19*, 739–749. [CrossRef] [PubMed]

24. Aslibekyan, S.; Kabagambe, E.K.; Irvin, M.R.; Straka, R.J.; Borecki, I.B.; Tiwari, H.K.; Tsai, M.Y.; Hopkins, P.N.; Shen, J.; Lai, C.Q.; et al. A genome-wide association study of inflammatory biomarker changes in response to fenofibrate treatment in the Genetics of Lipid Lowering Drug and Diet Network. *Pharm. Genom.* **2012**, *22*, 191–197. [CrossRef]
25. Peeters, T.; Monteagudo, S.; Tylzanowski, P.; Luyten, F.P.; Lories, R.; Cailotto, F. SMOC2 inhibits calcification of osteoprogenitor and endothelial cells. *PLoS ONE* **2018**, *13*, e0198104. [CrossRef] [PubMed]
26. Howson, J.M.M.; Zhao, W.; Barnes, D.R.; Ho, W.K.; Young, R.; Paul, D.S.; Waite, L.L.; Freitag, D.F.; Fauman, E.B.; Salfati, E.L.; et al. Fifteen new risk loci for coronary artery disease highlight arterial-wall-specific mechanisms. *Nat. Genet.* **2017**, *49*, 1113–1119. [CrossRef] [PubMed]
27. Privratsky, J.R.; Paddock, C.M.; Florey, O.; Newman, D.K.; Muller, W.A.; Newman, P.J. Relative contribution of PECAM-1 adhesion and signaling to the maintenance of vascular integrity. *J. Cell Sci.* **2011**, *124*, 1477–1485. [CrossRef]
28. Ueland, T.; Åkerblom, A.; Ghukasyan, T.; Michelsen, A.E.; Becker, R.C.; Bertilsson, M.; Budaj, A.; Cornel, J.H.; Himmelmann, A.; James, S.K.; et al. ALCAM predicts future cardiovascular death in acute coronary syndromes: Insights from the PLATO trial. *Atherosclerosis* **2020**, *293*, 35–41. [CrossRef] [PubMed]
29. Shendre, A.; Irvin, M.R.; Wiener, H.; Zhi, D.; Limdi, N.A.; Overton, E.T.; Shrestha, S. Local Ancestry and Clinical Cardiovascular Events Among African Americans From the Atherosclerosis Risk in Communities Study. *J. Am. Heart Assoc.* **2017**, *6*. [CrossRef] [PubMed]
30. Folestad, E.; Kunath, A.; Wågsäter, D. PDGF-C and PDGF-D signaling in vascular diseases and animal models. *Mol. Aspects Med.* **2018**, *62*, 1–11. [CrossRef]
31. Moriya, J.; Wu, X.; Zavala-Solorio, J.; Ross, J.; Liang, X.H.; Ferrara, N. Platelet-derived growth factor C promotes revascularization in ischemic limbs of diabetic mice. *J. Vasc. Surg.* **2014**, *59*, 1402–1409. [CrossRef]
32. Zhang, H.; He, Y.; Dai, S.; Xu, Z.; Luo, Y.; Wan, T.; Luo, D.; Jones, D.; Tang, S.; Chen, H.; et al. AIP1 functions as an endogenous inhibitor of VEGFR2-mediated signaling and inflammatory angiogenesis in mice. *J. Clin. Invest.* **2008**, *118*, 3904–3916. [CrossRef]
33. Harrison, S.C.; Cooper, J.A.; Li, K.; Talmud, P.J.; Sofat, R.; Stephens, J.W.; Hamsten, A.; Sanders, J.; Montgomery, H.; Neil, A.; et al. Association of a sequence variant in DAB2IP with coronary heart disease. *Eur. Heart J.* **2012**, *33*, 881–888. [CrossRef] [PubMed]
34. Gretarsdottir, S.; Baas, A.F.; Thorleifsson, G.; Holm, H.; den Heijer, M.; de Vries, J.P.P.M.; Kranendonk, S.E.; Zeebregts, C.J.A.M.; van Sterkenburg, S.M.; Geelkerken, R.H.; et al. Genome-wide association study identifies a sequence variant within the DAB2IP gene conferring susceptibility to abdominal aortic aneurysm. *Nat. Genet.* **2010**, *42*, 692–697. [CrossRef]
35. Xu, J.J.; Jiang, L.; Xu, L.J.; Gao, Z.; Zhao, X.Y.; Zhang, Y.; Song, Y.; Liu, R.; Sun, K.; Gao, R.L.; et al. Association of CDKN2B-AS1 Polymorphisms with Premature Triple-vessel Coronary Disease and Their Sex Specificity in the Chinese Population. *Biomed. Environ. Sci.* **2018**, *31*, 787–796. [CrossRef]
36. Heit, C.; Jackson, B.C.; McAndrews, M.; Wright, M.W.; Thompson, D.C.; Silverman, G.A.; Nebert, D.W.; Vasiliou, V. Update of the human and mouse SERPIN gene superfamily. *Hum. Genomics* **2013**, *7*, 22. [CrossRef] [PubMed]
37. Aulchenko, Y.S.; Ripke, S.; Isaacs, A.; van Duijn, C.M. GenABEL: An R library for genome-wide association analysis. *Bioinformatics* **2007**, *23*, 1294–1296. [CrossRef]
38. Chang, C.C.; Chow, C.C.; Tellier, L.C.; Vattikuti, S.; Purcell, S.M.; Lee, J.J. Second-generation PLINK: Rising to the challenge of larger and richer datasets. *Gigascience* **2015**, *4*, 7. [CrossRef] [PubMed]
39. Wright, M.; Ziegler, A. ranger: A Fast Implementation of Random Forests for High Dimensional Data in C++ and R. *J. Stat. Softw. Artic.* **2017**, *77*, 1–17. [CrossRef]
40. Szymczak, S.; Holzinger, E.; Dasgupta, A.; Malley, J.D.; Molloy, A.M.; Mills, J.L.; Brody, L.C.; Stambolian, D.; Bailey-Wilson, J.E. r2VIM: A new variable selection method for random forests in genome-wide association studies. *BioData Min.* **2016**, *9*, 7. [CrossRef]
41. Degenhardt, F.; Seifert, S.; Szymczak, S. Evaluation of variable selection methods for random forests and omics data sets. *Brief. Bioinform.* **2019**, *20*, 492–503. [CrossRef]
42. Lewis Schmalohr, C.; Grossbach, J.; Clément-Ziza, M.; Beyer, A. Detection of epistatic interactions with Random Forest. *bioRxiv* **2018**. [CrossRef]
43. Berger, A. FUNDAMENTALS OF BIOSTATISTICS. *Am. J. Public Health Nat. Health* **1969**, *59*, 1266–1266. [CrossRef]

44. Benjamini, Y.; Hochberg, Y. Controlling the False Discovery Rate: A Practical and Powerful Approach to Multiple Testing. *J. Royal Stat. Soc. Ser. B (Methodological)* **1995**, *57*, 289–300. [CrossRef]
45. Hothorn, T.; Hornik, K.; Zeileis, A. Unbiased Recursive Partitioning: A Conditional Inference Framework. *J. Comput. Graph. Stat.* **2006**, *15*, 651–674. [CrossRef]

Publisher's Note: MDPI stays neutral with regard to jurisdictional claims in published maps and institutional affiliations.

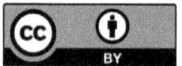

© 2020 by the authors. Licensee MDPI, Basel, Switzerland. This article is an open access article distributed under the terms and conditions of the Creative Commons Attribution (CC BY) license (http://creativecommons.org/licenses/by/4.0/).

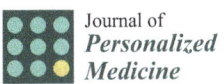

Journal of Personalized Medicine

Review

Pharmacogenetics to Avoid Adverse Reactions in Cardiology: Ready for Implementation?

Xandra García-González *,† and Sara Salvador-Martín †

Instituto de Investigación Sanitaria Gregorio Marañón (IiSGM), Hospital General Universitario Gregorio Marañón, 28007 Madrid, Spain; sara.salvador@iisgm.com
* Correspondence: xandra.garcia@salud.madrid.org
† Both authors contributed equally to this manuscript.

Abstract: Cardiovascular Diseases (CVs) are one of the main causes of mortality and disability around the world. Advances in drug treatment have greatly improved survival and quality of life in the past decades, but associated adverse events remain a relevant problem. Pharmacogenetics can help individualize cardiovascular treatment, reducing associated toxicities and improving outcomes. Several scientific societies and working groups periodically review available studies and provide consensus recommendations for those gene-drug pairs with a sufficient level of evidence. However, these recommendations are rarely mandatory, and the indications on how to adjust treatment can vary between different guidelines, which limits their clinical applicability. The aim of this review is to compile, compare and discuss available guidelines and recommendations by the main Pharmacogenetics Consortiums (Clinical Pharmacogenetics Implementation Consortium (CPIC); Dutch Pharmacogenetics Working Group (DPWG); the French Network of Pharmacogenetics (Réseau national de pharmacogénétique (RNPGx) and The Canadian Pharmacogenomics Network for Drug Safety (CPNDS) regarding how to apply pharmacogenetic results to optimize pharmacotherapy in cardiology. Pharmacogenetic recommendations included in European or American drug labels, as well as those included in the European Society of Cardiology (ESC) and the American College of Cardiology (ACC) and the American Heart Association (AHA) treatment guidelines are also discussed.

Keywords: pharmacogenetics; cardiology; adverse events; guidelines

1. Introduction

Cardiovascular Diseases (CVDs) are one of the main public health challenges of our time. They are currently the leading cause of death in the world and a major contributor to disability [1]. They include numerous entities among which Ischemic Heart Disease (IHD) and stroke are the most common.

CVDs were responsible for 18.6 million deaths in 2019 and prevalent cases reached 523 million. The global trends for Disability-Adjusted Life Years (DALYs) and years of life lost also increased significantly, and years lived with disability have almost doubled in the last three decades [2].

Thankfully, patient life expectancy and quality of care has significantly improved over the years thanks to prevention strategies, advances in surgery and other intervention techniques and of course, drug treatment. Anticoagulant and antiplatelet agents, beta-blockers, antihypertensive drugs, and lipid-lowering therapies are commonly used for the treatment and prevention of CVDs, accompanied by the modification of behavioral risk factors, such as tobacco and alcohol use, diet, and physical activity.

Despite their proven effectiveness and safety, drugs used in cardiology, as any drug, can also cause significant adverse reactions. Different factors influence interindividual variability in drug response and tolerance, but one of the most relevant is undoubtedly genetic variability [3].

The association between genetic variations and drug effectiveness and safety have been studied, although only a few are now being translated to clinical practice [4]. Several Scientific Societies and working groups periodically review available studies and provide consensus recommendations for those drug-gene pairs with a sufficient level of evidence to consider therapy modifications according to patient genotype. The Clinical Pharmacogenetics Implementation Consortium (CPIC) is probably the most influential one, but national guidance is also provided by the Dutch Pharmacogenetics Working Group (DPWG), the French Network of Pharmacogenetics (RNPGx) within the French Society of Pharmacology and Therapeutics (SFPT) and the Canadian Pharmacogenomics Network for Drug Safety (CPNDS) amongst others [5–8]. The Spanish Society of Pharmacogenetics and Pharmacogenomics has also included in its strategic plan the publication of practice guidelines for relevant drug-gene pairs [9]. Recently, the European Society of Cardiology issued a position statement on the role of Pharmacogenomics in contemporary cardiovascular therapy [10]. However, in most cases there are no official recommendations provided by the drug agencies. This together with the fact that recommendations from different Societies often differ from one another, makes the implementation into clinical practice challenging.

The aim of this review is to compile, compare and discuss available guidelines and recommendations regarding how to apply pharmacogenetic results to optimize pharmacotherapy in cardiology.

Reviewing the evidence supporting pharmacogenetic testing in cardiovascular medicine including available clinical trials that constitute the basis for the recommendations included in these guidelines falls beyond the scope of this article. An excellent review on this issue has been recently published by Duarte et al. [11].

2. Cardiovascular Drugs in Pharmacogenetics Guidelines

The most recent guidelines and publications by the Clinical Pharmacogenetics Implementation Consortium (CPIC); Dutch Pharmacogenetics Working Group (DPWG); the French Network of Pharmacogenetics (Réseau national de pharmacogénétique (RNPGx) and The Canadian Pharmacogenomics Network for Drug Safety (CPNDS) were reviewed and compared for drugs pertaining to therapeutic groups B01 ANTITHROMBOTIC AGENTS and C CARDIOVASCULAR SYSTEM of the Anatomical Therapeutic Chemical Classification System (ATC) of the World Health Organization (WHO) [12]. Table 1 includes all drug-gene pairs in these categories mentioned in the guidelines until 30 September 2021. The left row includes those drug-gene pairs for which a therapeutic recommendation (action recommended based on patient genotype such us dose adjustment or use of alternative treatment) has been issued by at least one of these organizations. Currently, it includes those drug-gene pairs that are reviewed but considered not to be a relevant drug-gene interaction at this time based on available evidence.

Table 1. Cardiovascular drug-gene pairs reviewed in main pharmacogenetic guidelines.

Reviewed with Recommendation	Reviewed with No Recommendation
Acenocoumarol-*VKORC1* (DPWG [13], RNPGx [14]) Atorvastatin-*SLCOB1* (DPWG [15]) Clopidogrel-*CYP2C19* (CPIC [16], DPWG [17], RNPGx [14]) Flecainide-*CYP2D6* (DPWG [18]) Metoprolol-*CYP2D6* (DPWG [19]) Phenprocoumon-*VKORC1* (DPWG [20]) Propafenone-*CYP2D6* (DPWG [21]) Simvastatin-*SLCOB1* (CPIC [22], DPWG [23], RNPGx [14]) Warfarin-*CYP2C9* (CPIC [24], DPWG [25], CPNDS [26], RNPGx [14]) Warfarin-*VKORC1* (CPIC [24], DPWG [27], RNPGx [14]) Warfarin-*CYP4F2* (CPIC [24])	Acenocoumarol-*CYP2C9* (DPWG [28]) Amiodarone-*CYP2D6* (DPWG [29]) Aspirin-*CYP2C9* (CPIC [30]) Atenolol-*CYP2D6* (DPWG [31]) Bisoprolol-*CYP2D6* (DPWG [32]) Carvedilol-*CYP2D6* (DPWG [33]) Clonidine-*CYP2D6* (DPWG [34]) Disopyramide-*CYP2D6* (DPWG [35]) Fluvastatin-*SLCOB1* (DPWG [36]) Phenprocoumon-*CYP2C9* (DPWG [37]) Prasugrel-*CYP2C19* (DPWG [38]) Quinidine-*CYP2D6* (DPWG [39]) Sotalol-*CYP2D6* (DPWG [40]) Ticagrelor-*CYP2C19* (DPWG [41])

CPIC, Clinical Pharmacogenetics Implementation Consortium; DPWG, Dutch Pharmacogenetics Working Group; RNPGx, French Network of Pharmacogenetics (Réseau national de pharmacogénétique); CPNDS, Canadian Pharmacogenomics Network for Drug Safety.

Additionally, the European Medicines Agency (EMA) and FDA drug labels were reviewed in search of any recommendations based on patient genotype. Any pharmacogenetic recommendations included in relevant treatment guidelines, such as those published by the European Society of Cardiology (ESC), the American College of Cardiology (ACC) and the American Heart Association (AHA) are also discussed below.

By 30 September 2021, 25 cardiovascular drug-gene pairs had been reviewed by at least one of the main groups issuing Pharmacogenetics guidelines (CPIC, DPWG, RNPGx and CPNDS). Eleven drug-gene pairs had therapeutic recommendations published by at least one of these groups. In more than half of the cases (6/11), therapeutic recommendations were made by just one of these groups, in one case (Acenocoumarol-VKORC1) recommendations were made by two groups and in two cases (Clopidogrel-CYP2C19, Simvastatin-SLCOB1 and Warfarin-VKORC1) by three of the four groups. Warfarin-CYP2C9 was the only drug-gene pair for which all four groups have issued therapeutic recommendations.

DPWG is by far the group that reviewed more cardiovascular drug-gene pairs [23] and also the one that has issued more therapeutic recommendations [10].

Published recommendations on how to avoid adverse reactions and increase treatment effectiveness based on patient genotype for drugs in the following therapeutic groups: anticoagulants, antiplatelet, statins, beta-blockers and antiarrhythmic, are reviewed below.

2.1. Anticoagulants

Three drugs in the ATC group B01AA Vitamin K antagonists are reviewed in the guidelines: warfarin, acenocoumarol and phenprocoumon. Different drug-gene pairs are reviewed and published recommendations vary between groups (Table 2): Warfarin-CYP2C9 is the drug-gene pair considered essential by the four groups; the CPIC, DPWG, RNPGx and CPNDS recommend therapeutic adjustment. Warfarin-VKORC1 has additional recommendations (always combined with CYP2C9 genotype) by CPIC, DPW and RNPGx. The CPIC is the only group that considers CYP4F2 genotype to further adjust warfarin dosage. Specific recommendations for other coumarin derivatives (acenocoumarol and phenprocoumon) and VKORC1 are only available by the DPWG, although these drugs are also mentioned in the RNPGx guidelines.

Coumarin derivatives, warfarin, acenocoumarol and phenprocoumon are Vitamin K antagonists (VKAs) used to prevent or treat thromboembolism. The dose of coumarin required to maintain an International Normalized Ratio (INR) between 2.0 and 3.0 is highly variable between individuals due to the narrow therapeutic window and significant inter- and intra-individual variability in a response that may be associated with over-anticoagulation (and thus risk of bleeding) or resistance to treatment.

Table 2. Drug-gene pairs and dose recommendations by different clinical guidelines. Anticoagulants.

Drug	Gene	Guideline	Genotype/Phenotype	Therapeutic Recommendation	Level of Evidence
Warfarin	CYP2C9 Combined with VKORC1 and CYP4F2	CPIC 2017	*1/*2 *1/*3 *2/*2 *2/*3 *3/*3	Use validated pharmacogenetics algorithms to calculate initial dose	Strong (Non-African) Moderate (African)
Warfarin	CYP2C9	DPWG 2018	*1/*2 (IM)	Use initial standard dose	4A
			*1/*3 (IM)	Use 65% of the standard initial dose. Specific dose can be calculated using an algorithm	4D
			*2/*2 (PM)	Use 65% of the standard initial dose. Specific dose can be calculated using an algorithm	4A
			*2/*3 (PM)	Use 45% of the standard initial dose. Specific dose can be calculated using an algorithm	4A
			*3/*3 (PM)	Use 20% of the standard initial dose. Specific dose can be calculated using an algorithm	4C

Table 2. Cont.

Drug	Gene	Guideline	Genotype/Phenotype	Therapeutic Recommendation	Level of Evidence
Warfarin	CYP2C9 Combined with VKORC1	RNPGx 2017	*1/*1	Suggested initial dose between 5 and 7 mg or 3 and 4 mg depending on VKORC1 genotype	A priori genotyping: advisable A posteriori: advisable
			*1/*2 (IM)	Suggested initial dose between 5 and 7 mg or 3 and 4 mg depending on VKORC1 genotype	
			*1/*3 (IM)	Suggested initial dose between 3 and 4 mg or 0.5 and 2 mg depending on VKORC1 genotype	
			*2/*2 (PM)	Suggested initial dose between 3 and 4 mg or 0.5 and 2 mg depending on VKORC1 genotype	
			*2/*3 (PM)	Suggested initial dose between 3 and 4 mg or 0.5 and 2 mg depending on VKORC1 genotype	
			*3/*3 (PM)	Suggested initial dose between 0.5 and 2 mg	
Warfarin	CYP2C9 Combined with VKORC1	CPNDS 2015	*2 *3	Use pharmacogenetic dosing algorithm to estimate the required dose	Strong A
Warfarin	VKORC1 Combined with CYP2C9 and CYP4F2	CPIC 2017	−1639 AG −1639 GG	Use validated pharmacogenetics algorithms to calculate initial dose	Strong (Non-African) Moderate (African)
Warfarin	VKORC1	DPWG 2018	−1639 AG	Use initial standard dose	4A
			−1639 GG	Use 60% of the standard initial dose. Specific dose can be calculated using an algorithm	4A
Warfarin	VKORC1 Combined with CYP2C9	RNPGx 2017	−1639 GG	Suggested initial dose between 5 and 7, 3 and 4 or 0.5 and 2 mg depending on VKORC1 genotype	1A
			−1639 AG	Suggested initial dose between 5 and 7, 3 and 4 or 0.5 and 2 mg depending on VKORC1 genotype	
			−1639 AA	Suggested initial dose between 5–7, 3–4 or 0.5–2 mg depending on VKORC1 genotype	
Warfarin	VKORC1 Combined with CYP2C9	CPNDS 2015	−1639 AG −1639 GG	Use pharmacogenetic dosing algorithm to estimate the required dose	Strong A
Warfarin	CYP4F2 Combined with CYP2C9 and VKORC1	CPIC 2017	rs2108622 T	Increase initial dose calculated with algorithm by 5–10%	Optional
Acenocoumarol	VKORC1	DPWG 2018	−1639 AG	Use initial standard dose	4C
			−1639 AA	Use 50% of the standard initial dose. Recommend more frequent INR monitoring	4F
Phenprocoumon	VKORC1	DPWG 2018	−1639 AG	Use initial standard dose	4D
			−1639 AA	Use 50% of the standard initial dose. Recommend more frequent INR monitoring	4D

CPIC, Clinical Pharmacogenetics Implementation Consortium; DPWG, Dutch Pharmacogenetics Working Group; RNPGx, French Network of Pharmacogenetics (Réseau national de pharmacogénétique); CPNDS, Canadian Pharmacogenomics Network for Drug Safety; IM, Intermediate metabolizer; PM, Poor metabolizer; INR, international normalized ratio.

Warfarin

Common genetic variants in CYP2C9, VKORC1, CYP4F2, in addition to known non-genetic factors, account for 50–60% of the variability in warfarin dosage [10].

- Warfarin and CYP2C9

CYP2C9 is the enzyme primarily responsible for the metabolic clearance of the S-warfarin [42].

In the Caucasian population, there are two main genetic variants associated with deficient CYP2C9 activity: polymorphism rs1799853 (CYP2C9*2 or c.430C>T) and rs1057910 (CYP2C9*3 or c.1075A>C) [43]. CYP2C9 allele frequencies differ between racial/ethnic groups; in fact, these alleles are significantly less prevalent in African-American and Asian populations [44].

The polymorphisms CYP2C9*2 and *3 compromise S-warfarin metabolism by 30–40% and 80–90%, respectively [44]. Compared to patients homozygous for CYP2C9*1, individuals with one or two copies of CYP2C9*2 or *3 may have an increased risk of bleeding when treated with warfarin as compared to patients with two normally- functioning alleles [45]. They require lower doses to achieve similar levels of anticoagulation and need more time to achieve a stable INR [44].

Other CYP2C9 alleles (CYP2C9*5, *6, *8 and *11), especially in the African population, are also associated with decreased CYP2C9 enzyme function and contribute to the variability of warfarin doses, requiring lower doses [46].

- Warfarin and VKORC1

VKORC1 encodes a key enzyme of the vitamin K cycle and is the pharmacological target of coumarinic anticoagulants, whose inhibitory action blocks vitamin K-dependent coagulation factors (factors II, VI, IX and X).

The c.−1639G>A variant (rs9923231) results in altered warfarin sensitivity, lower VKORC1 expression, and lower warfarin dose requirement during long-term treatment [47,48].

The −1639 AA genotype results in an increased sensitivity to warfarin. This results in an increased risk of an excessively severe inhibition of blood coagulation (INR > 4) during the first month of treatment, while the −1639 AG genotype results in a reduction in the required dose and an increase in the risk of an excessively severe inhibition of blood clotting during the first month of treatment. However, the effect is small and GA is the most common genotype, meaning that the standard treatment will primarily be based on patients with this genotype. As with the CYP2C9 variants, the frequency of the −1639G>A variant differs among ethnic groups, occurring most frequently in Asians.

- Warfarin and CYP4F2

CYP4F2 is an enzyme involved in vitamin K metabolism. It acts as an important counterpart of VKORC1 to limit excessive vitamin K accumulation [49]. CYP4F2 activity is decreased in the presence of the *3 allele (c.1297G>A; p.Val433Met; rs2108622). This *3 allele is associated with a higher bleeding risk and therefore, with lower warfarin dose requirements than the *1 allele to obtain the same anticoagulant response in European and Asian populations [50,51]. Moreover, inclusion of this CYP4F2 variant in warfarin dosing algorithms that included CYP2C9, VKORC1, and clinical factors improved the accuracy of dose prediction [50].

Both the DPWG and CPIC provide recommendations for CYP2C9 and VKORC1 gene pairs and warfarin. The CPIC calculates the recommended daily dosage for warfarin in mg/day based on specific algorithms including genotype (VKORC1−1639G>A, CYP2C9*2 and CYP2C9*3 alleles) and clinical variables that influence the response to warfarin [52,53]. Importantly, neither published algorithm includes the CYP2C9*5, *6, *8, *11, rs12777823 variant or the CYP4F2*3 allele, although, the CPIC provides separate guidance for patients of African and non-African descent. For populations of non-African ancestry, it recommends estimating the dose based on CYP2C9*2 and *3 and VKORC1 variants with the use of one of the available dosing algorithms. CYP4F2*3 genotyping is considered optional, but if detected, a dose increase of 5–10% is recommended. However, for persons of African descent, genotype-guided dosing is recommended only if information on CYP2C9*5, *6, *8 and *11 genotyping is available, and in this case, genotyping of rs12777823 is considered optional. If this additional genotype information is available, the warfarin dose should first be estimated with the use of a warfarin dosing algorithm and then reduced by 15–30% for each CYP2C9*5, *6, *8 or *11 allele, with an additional 15–30% reduction if the rs12777823 variant is detected.

On the other hand, the DPWG guidelines limit recommendations to VKORC1 −1639G>A and CYP2C9*2 and *3 alleles and only provide a decrease in the loading dose. The use of a different starting dose of warfarin is somewhat controversial and plays different roles in different regions of the world, depending on local experience and standards.

The RNPGx group have recommendations for CYP2C9 and VKORC1 gene pairs and warfarin [14]. Their recommendations correspond to international guidelines issued by the CPIC. Thus, they recommend genotyping the variants: VKORC1 −1639G>A, CYP2C9*2 and CYP2C9*3 alleles, on the one hand, before initiating VKA treatment to determine the optimal dose or to guide the prescription of an alternative therapeutic option; and on the other hand, after initiating treatment to explain a bleeding event or resistance to VKAs.

The Canadian Pharmacogenomics Network for Drug Safety (CPNDS) also recommends that VKORC1 (21639G.A), CYP2C9*2, and CYP2C9*3 testing be considered for all patients, including paediatric patients, within the first 2 weeks of therapy or after a bleeding event. Genotyping results should be interpreted using a pharmacogenetic dosing algorithm to estimate the dose needed [26]. The CPNDS clinical recommendation group, in the order of the RNPGx, recommend testing before initiating therapy. If this is not feasible, they recommend that testing be considered if results can be obtained in the first 2 weeks of therapy, as genetic information may still be useful in estimating the maintenance dose. After 2 weeks, the benefits derived from genetic testing diminish.

The recently published ESC position paper states that prospective genotyping prior to warfarin initiation is advisable. Their recommendation is to genotype for all the relevant CYP2C9, VKORC1 and CYP4F2 alleles irrespective of patient's ethnicity and adjust the initial dosage with a universal algorithm, that still needs to be developed and properly validated [10].

- Acenocoumarol/phenprocoumon and VKORC1

Same as warfarin, other coumadin derivatives, such as acenocoumarol, phenprocoumon or fluindione, exert their anticoagulant action by inhibiting VKORC1. Therefore, mutations in the VKORC1 gene that lead to reduced production of the VKORC1 protein would also require lower VKA doses needed to achieve the desired INR. However, available pharmacogenetic studies are limited compared to warfarin, due to the fact that the use of these derivatives is highly variable across different countries. In Europe for instance, warfarin has been reported to be used predominantly in the UK and Italy, phenprocoumon in Germany, acenocoumarol in Spain, and fluindione in France [54]. Contrarily, in the US, warfarin is the only VKA commercialized.

For this reason, recommendations on other VKAs are only provided by the European consortia. The DPWG provides therapeutic recommendations for acenocoumarol and fenprocoumon [13]. For both drugs, patients with VKORC1 −1639 AA genotype should receive 50% of the standard initial dose and undergo more frequent INR monitoring. RNPGx extends the recommendation to consider genetic factors to establish warfarin dosage to other VKAs but makes no specific statement regarding treatment adjustment.

Spain's summary of product characteristics for acenocoumarol (in Spain acenocoumarol is the most commonly used VKA) does advise that patients with CYP2C9 variants *2 and *3 have diminished clearance and can consequently need lower acenocoumarol doses, but again no specific dose adjustments are recommended [55].

2.2. Antiplatelets

Four antiplatelet agents in the ATC group B01AC (platelet aggregation inhibitors excluding heparin) are reviewed in the guidelines: acetylsalicylic acid, clopidogrel, prasugrel and ticagrelor. Based on available evidence, therapeutic recommendations are only made for clopidogrel and the CYP2C19 gene by three groups: the CPIC [16], DPWG [17] and RNPGx [14] (Table 3).

Table 3. Drug-gene pairs and dose recommendations by different clinical guidelines. Antiplatelets.

Drug	Gene	Guideline	Genotype/Phenotype	Therapeutic Recommendation	Level of Evidence
Clopidogrel	CYP2C19	CPIC 2013	UM (*1/*17 or *17/*17)	Label recommended dosage and administration	Strong
			EM (*1/*1)	Label recommended dosage and administration	Strong
			IM (*1/*2; *1/*3 or *2/*17)	Alternative antiplatelet therapy (if no contraindication)	Moderate
			PM (*2/*2; *2/*3 or *3/*3)	Alternative antiplatelet therapy (if no contraindication)	Strong
Clopidogrel	CYP2C19	DPWG 2018	UM (*17/*17)	Label recommended dosage and administration	4A
			IM (*1/*2; *1/*3; *2/*17 or *3/*17)	Percutaneous coronary intervention, stroke or TIA: choose an alternative or double the dose to 150 mg/day (600 mg loading dose). Other indications: no action required	4F
			PM (*2/*2; *2/*3 or *3/*3)	Percutaneous coronary intervention, stroke or TIA: choose an alternative or double the dose to 150 mg/day (600 mg loading dose). Other indications: determine the level of inhibition of platelet aggregation by clopidogrel. Consider an alternative in poor responders	4F
Clopidogrel	CYP2C19	RNPGx 2017	UM (*1/17 or *17/*17)	Label recommended dosage and administration	A priori genotyping: Coronary angioplasty: *essential* Other: *potentially useful* A posteriori: *advisable*
			EM (*1/*1)	Label recommended dosage and administration	
			IM (*1/*2 or *1/*3)	Alternative antiplatelet therapy	
			PM (*2/*2; *3/*3)	Alternative antiplatelet therapy	

CPIC, Clinical Pharmacogenetics Implementation Consortium; DPWG, Dutch Pharmacogenetics Working Group; RNPGx, French Network of Pharmacogenetics (Réseau national de pharmacogénétique); UM, Ultrarapid metabolizer; EM, Extensive metabolizer; IM, Intermediate metabolizer; PM, Poor metabolizer; TIA, Transient ischaemic attack.

- Clopidogrel and CYP2C19

CYP2C19 is the main enzyme involved in the conversion of clopidogrel into its active form that acts irreversibly inhibiting the P2Y12 receptor, thus preventing platelet activation and aggregation [56]. CYP2C19 presents significant genetic variation, with approximately 30% of individuals presenting reduced or absent enzyme activity due to genetic polymorphisms. The most frequent no-function alleles are *2 (~15% in Caucasians and Africans, and 29–35% in Asians) and *3 (2–9% in Asians) (others include *4, *5, *6, *7 and *8 but are very rare). There are also alleles associated with increased enzyme function, among which the most common is *17 (3–21% in different ethnicities) [16]. Alleles *2, *3 and *17 are those backed up by a bigger body of scientific evidence, which is why they are the ones considered essential for testing by the US Association for Molecular Pathology [57]. Both the DPWG and RNPgx base their recommendations on the metabolic status inferred by the determination of these three alleles. CPIC considers other possible no-function alleles in case they are present, but recognizes they are rarely determined and even more rarely found.

The Dutch Pharmacogenetics Working Group considers genotyping before starting clopidogrel to guide drug and dose selection in percutaneous coronary intervention or stroke patients to be essential for drug efficacy. The RNPGx considers that a priori genotyping is essential for coronary angioplasty with stenting and potentially useful in other indications.

All three groups agree to recommend the switch to an alternative platelet inhibitor not metabolized by CYP2C19 (e.g., prasugrel, ticagrelor) for both the intermediate (IM) and poor metabolizer (PM) status, due to the risk of treatment ineffectiveness and consequent thrombotic events.

Prasugrel and ticagrelor also act by inhibiting the P2Y12 receptor but have significantly different pharmacokinetic and pharmacodynamic characteristics, with a quicker and more potent antiplatelet effect and less variability in response. However, they are also associated with a higher risk of bleeding when compared with clopidogrel [58]. An important limitation to the clopidogrel switching recommendation is that all three P2Y12 inhibitors are not interchangeable in all clinical situations. For example, the more potent alternatives (prasugrel, ticagrelor) are usually preferred in high-risk patients undergoing Percutaneous Coronary Intervention (PCI), whereas clopidogrel is the only P2Y12 antagonist indicated for established peripheral artery disease and long-term secondary prevention of stroke, and also the only one that can be used in combination with anticoagulant therapy [59–61]. For this reason, the CPIC guidelines focus their recommendations on patients with acute coronary syndrome undergoing PCI, for whom more evidence is available. The DPWG considers that alternative agents should be used in CYP2C19 IM and PM for stroke and transient ischemic attack as well as PCI. It should be noted that prasugrel and ticagrelor cannot be used in these circumstances and alternatives to clopidogrel are limited (e.g., dipyridamole). For other indications, measuring the level of platelet inhibition may be considered in PM to warrant minimal drug effectiveness. In the case of intermediate metabolizers, doubling the dose to 150 mg/day and a 600 mg loading dose can also be considered. The 2010 FDA Drug Safety Communication on the use of clopidogrel in PM warns that although the use of a higher dose regimen increases antiplatelet response, the appropriateness of this regimen has not been established in a clinical outcome trial [62]. The RNPgx recommends testing for the main CYP2C19 deficiency alleles before instituting clopidogrel treatment (a test is essential for coronary angioplasty with stenting and based on the current state of knowledge this test is potentially useful in the other indications). For patients carrying at least one deficiency allele, the recommendation is to use an alternative treatment that is not a CYP2C19 substrate [14].

Clopidogrel's European and American SPCs state that alternative treatments may be considered in patients who are CYP2C19 PM due to the risk of treatment failure [59,63]. However, this is not listed as a specific contraindication and no recommendations are made on how to best determine the patient's metabolic status.

The latest position statement from the ESC on the role of pharmacogenomics in contemporary cardiovascular therapy insists that CYP2C19 genotyping is only recommended in high-risk cardiovascular situations (e.g., ACS undergoing percutaneous intervention, patients at a high risk of thrombosis or bleeding or patients with recurrent adverse events) and not to systematically tailor the selection of antiaggregation therapy [10]. However, it does recognize that clopidogrel should be avoided in those patients that are known to be intermediate or poor metabolizers due to the risk of ineffectiveness. The 2020 ESC Guidelines for the management of acute coronary syndrome in patients presenting without persistent ST-segment elevation also recognize that CYP2C19 genotyping may be useful to de-escalate P2Y12 receptor inhibitor treatment (e.g., in patients deemed unsuitable for potent platelet inhibition) with a Class IIB, level A evidence [64].

2016. ACC/AHA Guideline focused update on duration of dual antiplatelet therapy in patients with coronary artery disease recommends against routine pharmacogenetic testing for clopidogrel on the base no randomized controlled trials have demonstrated that testing improves patients' outcomes [65]. However, it must be noted that this guideline was published before relevant evidence from randomized control trials was available and is probably due for actualization soon [66–68].

2.3. Statins

Three drugs pertaining to the ATC group C10AA HMG CoA reductase inhibitors are reviewed in the guidelines: atorvastatin, simvastatin and fluvastatin. Based on available evidence, therapeutic recommendations are made for simvastatin and the SLCO1B1 gene by three groups: the CPIC [22], DPWG [23] and RNPGx [14]. The DPWG group also has recommendations for Atorvastatin and SLCO1B1 [15] (Table 4).

Table 4. Drug-gene pairs and dose recommendations by different clinical guidelines. Statins.

Drug	Gene	Guideline	Genotype/Phenotype	Therapeutic Recommendation	Level of Evidence
Simvastatin	SLCO1B1	CPIC 2014	IM (CT)	Lower dose or consider an alternative statin (consider routine CK surveillance)	Strong
			PM (CC)	Lower dose or consider an alternative statin (consider routine CK surveillance)	Strong
Simvastatin	SLCO1B1	DPWG 2020	521 CT	1. Choose an alternative 2. If not possible: (a) Avoid simvastatin doses exceeding 40mg/day. (b) Advise the patient to contact their doctor in the event of muscle symptoms.	4D
			521 CC	Choose an alternative drug	4D
Simvastatin	SLCO1B1	RNPGx 2017	521 TT	Avoid maximum dose (80 mg) during the first year of treatment	A priori genotyping: *no indication* A posteriori: *potentially useful*
			521 CT	Reduce the dose to max. 20 mg per day. Close CPK monitoring and avoid OATP1B1 inhibitors	
			521 CC	Reduce the dose to max. 20 mg per day. Close CPK monitoring and avoid OATP1B1 inhibitors	
Atorvastatin	SLCO1B1	DPWG 2020	521 CT	Additional risk factors for myopathy: 1. Choose an alternative 2. If not possible: Advise the patient to contact their doctor in the event of muscle symptoms. No additional risk factors for myopathy: Advise the patient to contact their doctor in the event of muscle symptoms.	4C
			521 CC	Additional risk factors for myopathy: 1. Choose an alternative 2. If not possible: Advise the patient to contact their doctor in the event of muscle symptoms. No additional risk factors for myopathy: Advise the patient to contact their doctor in the event of muscle symptoms.	4C

CPIC, Clinical Pharmacogenetics Implementation Consortium; DPWG, Dutch Pharmacogenetics Working Group; RNPGx, French Network of Pharmacogenetics (Réseau national de pharmacogénétique); IM, Intermediate metabolizer; PM, Poor metabolizer; CPK, Creatine Phosphokinase.

- Simvastatin and SLCO1B1

Statins are the most widely prescribed cholesterol-lowering drugs for the treatment and prevention of cardiovascular disease. These drugs decrease endogenous cholesterol synthesis by inhibiting the enzyme HMG-CoA reductase and the systemic concentration of low-density lipoprotein cholesterol (LDL-C) [69].

The most commonly prescribed is simvastatin. Despite the success of this drug, the use of simvastatin has been associated with an increased risk of myopathy, which is estimated to occur in 1–5% of patients treated with this drug [70].

The risk of myopathy may be partly explained by a genetic variation in the SLCO1B1 gene. This gene encodes organic anion transporter polypeptide 1B1 (OATP1B1), a transporter that is essential for hepatic uptake and subsequent elimination of statins [71]). A genetic polymorphism in SLCO1B1, c.521T>C (rs4149056), is associated with a significant reduction in transporter activity [72], with significantly lower LDL-C reductions and a higher risk of myopathy, especially in homozygous patients [73]. The minor C allele at rs4149056 is contained within SLCO1B1*5, as well as the *15 and *17 haplotypes and is associated with lower plasma clearance of simvastatin [74].

All groups recommend reducing the dose of simvastatin to no more than 20 mg per day or prescribing another statin for patients carrying at least one C allele of the reduced-function rs4149056. If the homozygous variant (CC) is present, the DPWG directly recommends prescribing an alternative drug [23].

The RNPGx considers rs4149056 genotyping potentially useful before starting statin treatment, especially in patients at high risk of myopathy and also when muscle toxicity appears. However, the ESC considers that routine pharmacogenetic testing before statin initiation is not necessary. Only if patients are known homozygous carriers of allele SLCO1B1*5, the maximum simvastatin dosage (80 mg) must be avoided and an alternative statin used whenever possible.

The simvastatin European summary of product characteristics advises that carriers of the SLC01B1 gene c.521T>C allele have lower OATP1B1 activity. The mean exposure (AUC) of the main active metabolite, simvastatin acid, is 120% in heterozygote carriers (CT) of the C allele and 221% in homozygote (CC) carriers relative to that of patients who have the most common genotype (TT). The C allele has a frequency of 18% in the European population. In patients with SLC01B1 polymorphism there is a risk of increased exposure of simvastatin which may lead to an increased risk of rhabdomyolysis. The FDA drug label only states that simvastatin is a substrate of the transport protein OATP1B1.

- Atorvastatin and SLCO1B1

Regarding atorvastatin, evidence has shown associations between the C allele variant and higher rates of intolerance and muscle-associated adverse effects [75]. Therefore, the DPWG guidelines extend their simvastatin recommendation and advise that atorvastatin should also be avoided in C allele carriers with substantial additional risk factors for myopathy.

2.4. Beta-Blockers

Five drugs pertaining to the ATC group C07A BETA BLOCKING AGENTS are reviewed in the DPWG guidelines: atenolol, bisoprolol, carvedilol, metoprolol and sotalol. Among them, recommendations are only published for metoprolol and CYP2D6 (2018) (Table 5).

Table 5. Drug-gene pairs and dose recommendations by different clinical guidelines. Beta-blockers.

Drug	Gene	Guideline	Genotype/Phenotype	Therapeutic Recommendation	Level of Evidence
Metoprolol	CYP2D6	DPWG 2018	UM	1. Use the maximum dose for the relevant indication as a target dose. 2. If effectiveness is still insufficient: increase the dose based on effectiveness and side effects to 2.5 times the standard dose or select an alternative.	4D
			IM	Gradual reduction of heart rate or in the event of symptomatic bradycardia: 1. increase the dose in smaller steps and/or prescribe no more than 50% of the standard dose. Other cases: no action required.	4A
			PM	Gradual reduction of heart rate or in the event of symptomatic bradycardia: 1. increase the dose in smaller steps and/or prescribe no more than 25% of the standard dose. Other cases: no action required.	4C

DPWG, Dutch Pharmacogenetics Working Group; UM, Ultrarapid metabolizer; IM, Intermediate metabolizer; PM, Poor metabolizer.

- Metoprolol and CYP2D6

CYP2D6 is the main enzyme involved in the catabolism of most beta-blockers including carvedilol, metoprolol, nevibolol, propranolol and timolol, and has a relevant role in the metabolism of 20–25% of prescribed drugs [76].

The CYP2D6 gene is highly polymorphic and there is wide interindividual variability in the associated enzyme activity. Specifically, several alleles (*3, *4, *5, etc.) condition null enzyme activity. In contrast, patients with more than two copies of functional alleles (*1/*2) have increased CYP2D6 activity.

The percentage of ultra-rapid metabolizers is variable and depends on ethnic origin.

In addition, CYP2D6 is a gene susceptible to metabolic induction and inhibition by other drugs and compounds which makes phenotype determination even more difficult.

It has been reported that due to increased metoprolol concentrations, CYP2D6 IM and especially PM experience lower heart rates and an increased incidence of bradycardia [77–79]. However, this does not seem to relevantly impact drug safety and tolerability in most cases.

The DPWG recommends that when a gradual reduction in heart rate is desired in IM and PM, dose titration should be carried out slowly. If symptomatic bradycardia occurs, it is recommended to use not more than 25–50% of the standard dose.

In the case of UM, targeting the maximum standard dosage is recommended. When the desired effect is not achieved, increasing the dose up to 2.5× the standard dose can be considered with careful motorization of possible adverse events. Use of other beta-blockers not metabolized by CYP2D6 (e.g., atenolol, bisoprolol) or metabolized to a lesser extent (carvedilol) can be considered in these cases depending on indication and other clinical considerations.

At this time, the CPIC considers that evidence supporting the use of genetic evidence to make treatment recommendations for beta-blockers and CYP2D6 is weak (B/C) and has not yet published any guidelines on this issue. No recommendations by the RNPGx are available either.

The ESC working group on cardiovascular pharmacotherapy states that for patients known to be CYP2D6 PM or UM, avoiding metoprolol when starting beta-blocker treatment seems prudent since there are multiple alternatives to choose from. However, no clear statement on when and which patients to genotype is made besides for those patients that suffer metoprolol-related adverse events. They also advise prescribers to be cautious when concomitant treatment with CYP2D6 inhibitors (e.g., bupropion, fluoxetine, paroxetine, and quinidine) is used due to the risk of phenoconversion from the baseline genotype-inferred metabolic status.

European and US metoprolol drug labels acknowledge that CYP2D6 PM show plasmatic metoprolol concentrations significantly higher than normal metabolizers but state that this shows little to no effect in the drug´s safety and tolerability [80].

2.5. Antiarrithmics

Four drugs in the ATC group C01B ANTIARRHYTHMICS, CLASS I AND III (disopyramide, flecainide, propafenone and quinidine) are reviewed in the guidelines. Treatment recommendations are available for flecainide and propafenone by the DPWG (2018) (Table 6).

Table 6. Drug-gene pairs and dose recommendations by different clinical guidelines. Antiarrythmics.

Drug	Gene	Guideline	Genotype/Phenotype	Therapeutic Recommendation	Level of Evidence
Flecainide	CYP2D6	DPWG 2018	UM	Monitor the plasma concentration as a precaution and record an ECG or select an alternative	NA
			IM	Indications other than diagnosis of Brugada syndrome: reduce the dose to 75% of the standard dose and record an ECG and monitor the plasma concentration. Provocation test for diagnosis of Brugada syndrome: No action required.	3A
			PM	Reduce the dose to 50% of the standard dose and record an ECG and monitor the plasma concentration.	4F
Propafenone	CYP2D6	DPWG 2018	UM	Monitor the plasma concentration as a precaution and record an ECG or select an alternative (possible reduced efficacy)	3D
			IM	Monitor the plasma concentration as a precaution and record an ECG or select an alternative (be alert to side effects)	3A
			PM	Reduce the dose to 30% of the standard dose, perform an ECG and monitor plasma concentrations.	4C

DPWG, Dutch Pharmacogenetics Working Group; UM, Ultrarapid metabolizer; IM, Intermediate metabolizer; PM, Poor metabolizer; ECG, electrocardiogram; NA, not applicable.

- Flecainide and CYP2D6

Flecainide is indicated for the treatment and prevention of several types of arrhythmias including supraventricular tachicardias and ventricular arrhythmias. It is also used for pharmacological cardioversion and as a provocation test to diagnose Brugada syndrome. It belongs to class IC antiarrhythmic agents, and works by blocking the cardiac fast inward sodium (Na+) current resulting, thus slowing cardiac conduction. Andrikopoulos 25717355.

Flecainide is mainly metabolized via CYP2D6 which is why IM and PM are at risk of drug accumulation and adverse events, due to the drug´s relatively narrow therapeutic range (plasma concentration 200–1000 ng/mL) [18].

Due to this increased risk of adverse events, the DPWG recommends reducing the flecainide dose by half in PM, and by 25% in IM, and monitoring the effect via ECG and plasma levels if possible. The indication for the diagnosis of Brugada syndrome is excluded from this recommendation. In UM caution is advised although data is lacking, and ECG monitoring, plasma levels or the use of alternatives that are not CYP2D6 substrates (e.g., sotalol, disopyramide, quinidine) is recommended.

CPIC has not yet issued a guideline, but the clinical annotation on CYP2D6*1, CYP2D6*4, CYP2D6*5, CYP2D6*10, CYP2D6*21, CYP2D6*36 and flecainide is assigned to level 1A of evidence. It recognizes that patients carrying one or more no function or decreased function alleles may have lower clearance of flecainide but advises that other genetic and clinical factors may also influence flecainide metabolism. The annotation only covers the pharmacokinetic relationship, and due to conflicting evidence on clinical outcomes, no treatment recommendations are made. https://www.pharmgkb.org/clinicalAnnotation/1183621726 (accessed on 6 October 2021).

No relevant pharmacogenetic information is included in flecainide drug labels besides that its metabolism appears to involve the cytochrome P450 isoenzyme CYP2D6, which shows genetic variation.

- Propafenone and CYP2D6

Same as flecainide, the propafenone antiarrhythmic effect is mediated by blockage of the fast sodium current. It is also a weak potassium channel blocker and can exert beta-blocking effects. It works by slowing conduction and prolonging refractoriness of cardiac conduction tissue. Propafenone is indicated for life-threatening ventricular arrhythmias, various supraventricular arrhythmias, and atrial fibrillation and has a therapeutic range between 0.2 and 1.5 µg/mL. (Kaplan's Essentials of Cardiac Anesthesia).

Propafenone is metabolized by CYP2D6, CYP3A4, and CYP1A2 enzymes. Standard doses of propafenone will lead to higher plasma drug concentrations in poor metabolizers, compared to normal metabolizers. In addition, drugs that inhibit CYP2D6, CYP3A4, and CYP1A2 may also increase propafenone levels, which may lead to cardiac arrhythmia episodes [81].

The DPWG recommends a 70% reduction of the standard dose in PM. For IM and UM, data is lacking in order to recommend specific dose adjustments but the use of an antiarrhythmic drug that is not a CYP2D6 substrate is recommended if possible. The use of ECG and measurement of plasma drug concentrations is recommended in all three cases to monitor adverse events or possible inefficacy [21].

The FDA-approved drug label for propafenone states that administration of the drug to CYP2D6's slow and extensive metabolizers resulted in significant differences in plasma concentrations, but that no dose adjustments are needed.

ESC guidelines for the diagnosis and management of atrial fibrillation only mention that CYP2D6 inhibitors increase flecainide concentrations but do not mention any effect of genetic variations on treatment effectiveness and safety. No specific mention of propafenone and CYP2D6 is included [82].

Drug labels acknowledge that in CYP2D6 PM propafenone clearance is impaired and plasma half-life is significantly longer. However, no dosing adjustments are recommended in PM patients [83].

2.6. Other Drugs Used in Cardiology

One antihypertensive agent in the group C02 ANTIHYPERTENSIVES (clonidine) is reviewed in the guidelines in regard to CYP2D6, but no recommendations are made based on available evidence.

Research for new biomarkers to decrease adverse events of other drugs frequently used in cardiology is ongoing. Many studies have found significant associations between genetic variants and drug toxicity and effectiveness, but in most cases available evidence does not reach the established threshold to warrant publication of specific therapeutic recommendations and pharmacogenetic guidelines.

For instance, CES1 rs2244613 has been associated to higher dabigatran plasma levels and an increased risk of bleeding [84]. Dabigatran is a direct oral anticoagulant widely used for atrial fibrillation instead of vitamin k antagonists. Polymorphisms in CYP2C9 and ABCB1 have been associated to response to angiotensin receptor blocker losartan, since these proteins participate in the drug's metabolism and transport [85,86]. Also, variant rs1799752 in the gene coding for the Angiotensin Converting Enzyme (ACE) has been linked to the effectiveness of some ACE inhibitors, such as captopril [87] and enalapril, [88] and to spironolactone; patients with del/del genotype and chronic heart failure may have less improvement in left ventricular ejection fraction, end-systolic and end-diastolic volume [89]. Variants in the ACE gene have also been proposed as potential predictors of susceptibility to COVID-19 [90]. A significant association between alpha-adducin gene1 (ADD1) Gly460Trp polymorphism and blood pressure change with hydrochlorothiazide has also been reported [91]. In regard to antiarrhythmics, a polygenic risk score has been proposed to predict the risk of QT prolongation or torsade the pointe induced by quinidine or dofetilide [92].

All these drug-gene pairs are currently assigned a level of evidence that ranges between 2A and 3 according to the PharmGKB scoring system.

3. Differences in Therapeutic Recommendations

Genetic information on drug labels is often unspecific or vague and does not usually include recommendations on how to adjust treatment accordingly. Different national and international groups provide evidence-based guidelines to help drug selection and dosage adjustment according to pharmacogenetic results in order to avoid unnecessary adverse events and optimize response.

The US Clinical Pharmacogenetics Implementation Consortium (CPIC), the Dutch Pharmacogenetics Working Group (DPWG), the French Network of Pharmacogenetics (Réseau national de pharmacogénétique (RNPGx) and The Canadian Pharmacogenomics Network for Drug Safety (CPNDS) are probably the most well-known and influential pharmacogenetic consortia in North America and Europe.

Among these groups, the Dutch is the one that has published more recommendations on cardiovascular drug-gene pairs. In most cases, they are also the more recent ones, having been updated in 2018. The CPNDS is the consortia with fewer recommendations in the cardiovascular area, having only issued recommendations for warfarin and CYP2C9.

With the exception of the RNpGx, the guidelines do not often address when and for which patients pharmacogenetic testing must be ordered, leaving that to doctor's criteria.

Differences in the methodology used by these groups, as well as discrepant allele terminology, classification and phenotype assignment make it even more difficult to compare and select specific recommendations to be used in clinical practice. Differences in clinical practices between countries are also conditioning, as is the case of the use of different VKAs in different countries or unequal access to direct measurement of plasma levels or drug's effect (e.g., INR monitoring).

Whenever discrepant recommendations are available, considering the country of origin's clinical practices in relation to yours is advisable. Also, considering which one is more recent can be helpful since new evidence may have arisen and is being incorporated.

The recently published ESC guideline on the role of pharmacogenomics in cardiology marks an important milestone towards clinical implementation. Although cautious in most of its recommendations, the impact the society guidelines have in setting practice standards will undoubtedly help convince many reluctant clinicians. To the best of our knowledge, no specific guidelines on pharmacogenomics have been yet issued by the AHA.

4. Conclusions

Cardiovascular drugs are amongst the most widely prescribed medicines in the world, which is why treatment optimization is fundamental to reduce associated morbidity and mortality. Tailoring treatment according to a patient's genotype has proven effective for a number of drug-gene pairs in order to reduce adverse events and increase effectiveness. However, significant differences exist between recommendations given by Pharmacogenetic Consortia and other relevant Societies. In order to effectively apply this into clinical practice, a wider consensus must be reached and official recommendations on how to adjust treatment based on a patient´s genetic profile must be issued.

Author Contributions: Conceptualization, X.G.-G. and S.S.-M.; methodology, X.G.-G. and S.S.-M.; investigation, X.G.-G. and S.S.-M.; resources, X.G.-G. and S.S.-M.; writing—original draft preparation, X.G.-G. and S.S.-M.; writing—review and editing, X.G.-G. and S.S.-M.; All authors have read and agreed to the published version of the manuscript.

Funding: This research received no external funding.

Institutional Review Board Statement: Not applicable.

Informed Consent Statement: Not applicable.

Conflicts of Interest: The authors declare no conflict of interest.

References

1. World Health Organization. Cardiovascular Diseases (CVDs). 2021. Available online: https://www.who.int/news-room/fact-sheets/detail/cardiovascular-diseases-(cvds) (accessed on 12 July 2021).
2. Roth, G.A.; Mensah, G.A.; Johnson, C.O.; Addolorato, G.; Ammirati, E.; Baddour, L.M.; Barengo, N.C.; Beaton, A.Z.; Benjamin, E.J.; Benziger, C.P.; et al. Global Burden of Cardiovascular Diseases and Risk Factors, 1990–2019: Update from the GBD 2019 Study. *J. Am. Coll. Cardiol.* **2020**, *76*, 2982–3021. [CrossRef] [PubMed]
3. Yip, V.; Hawcutt, D.B.; Pirmohamed, M.; Yip, V. Pharmacogenetic Markers of Drug Efficacy and Toxicity. *Clin. Pharmacol. Ther.* **2015**, *98*, 61–70. [CrossRef] [PubMed]
4. Roden, D.M.; McLeod, H.L.; Relling, M.V.; Williams, M.S.; Mensah, G.A.; Peterson, J.F.; Van Driest, S.L. Pharmacogenomics. *Lancet* **2019**, *394*, 521–532. [CrossRef]
5. CPIC. Clinical Pharmacogenetics Implementation Consortium (CPIC). Available online: https://cpicpgx.org/ (accessed on 12 October 2021).
6. DPWG. Dutch Pharmacogenetics Working Group (DPWG). Available online: https://www.knmp.nl/patientenzorg/medicatiebewaking/farmacogenetica/pharmacogenetics-1/pharmacogenetics (accessed on 12 October 2021).
7. SFPT. French Society of Pharmacology and Therapeutics. Available online: https://sfpt-fr.org/ (accessed on 12 October 2021).
8. CPNDS. Canadian Pharmacogenomics Network for Drug Safety. Available online: https://cpnds.ubc.ca/ (accessed on 12 October 2021).
9. SEFF. Spanish Society of Pharmacogenetics and Pharmacogenomics. Available online: https://seff.es/ (accessed on 12 October 2021).
10. Magavern, E.F.; Kaski, J.C.; Turner, R.M.; Drexel, H.; Janmohamed, A.; Scourfield, A.; Burrage, D.; Floyd, C.N.; Adeyeye, E.; Tamargo, J.; et al. The role of pharmacogenomics in contemporary cardiovascular therapy: A position statement from the European Society of Cardiology Working Group on Cardiovascular Pharmacotherapy. *Eur. Heart J. Cardiovasc. Pharmacother.* **2021**. [CrossRef] [PubMed]
11. Duarte, J.D.; Cavallari, L.H. Pharmacogenetics to guide cardiovascular drug therapy. *Nat. Rev. Cardiol.* **2021**, *18*, 649–665. [CrossRef]
12. World Health Organization. WHOCC-ATC/DDD Index. Available online: https://www.whocc.no/atc_ddd_index/ (accessed on 28 November 2020).
13. DPWG. VKORC1: Acenocoumarol (1909/1910). Available online: https://www.g-standaard.nl/risicoanalyse/B0001910.PDF (accessed on 30 September 2021).
14. Lamoureux, F.; Duflot, T. Pharmacogenetics in cardiovascular diseases: State of the art and implementation-recommendations of the French National Network of Pharmacogenetics (RNPGx). *Therapie* **2017**, *72*, 257–267. [CrossRef]
15. DPWG. SLCO1B1: Atorvastatin (4057/4058). Available online: https://www.g-standaard.nl/risicoanalyse/B0004058.PDF (accessed on 30 September 2021).
16. Scott, S.; Sangkuhl, K.; Gardner, E.E.; Stein, C.M.; Hulot, J.-S.; Johnson, J.A.; Roden, D.M.; Klein, T.E.; Shuldiner, A. Clinical Pharmacogenetics Implementation Consortium Guidelines for Cytochrome P450-2C19 (CYP2C19) Genotype and Clopidogrel Therapy. *Clin. Pharmacol. Ther.* **2011**, *90*, 328–332. [CrossRef]
17. DPWG. CYP2C19: Clopidogrel (2548/2549/2550). Available online: https://www.g-standaard.nl/risicoanalyse/B0002549.PDF (accessed on 30 September 2021).
18. DPWG. CYP2D6: Flecainide (1592/1593/1594). Available online: https://www.g-standaard.nl/risicoanalyse/B0001593.PDF (accessed on 30 September 2021).
19. DPWG. CYP2D6: Metoprolol (1554/1555/1556). Available online: https://www.g-standaard.nl/risicoanalyse/B0001554.PDF (accessed on 30 September 2021).
20. DPWG. VKORC1: Phenprocoumon (1911/1912). Available online: https://www.g-standaard.nl/risicoanalyse/B0001912.PDF (accessed on 30 September 2021).

21. DPWG. CYP2D6: Propafenone (1595/1596/1597). Available online: https://www.g-standaard.nl/risicoanalyse/B0001596.PDF (accessed on 30 September 2021).
22. Ramsey, L.B.; Johnson, S.G.; Caudle, K.E.; Haidar, C.E.; Voora, D.; Wilke, R.A.; Maxwell, W.D.; McLeod, H.L.; Krauss, R.M.; Roden, D.M.; et al. The Clinical Pharmacogenetics Implementation Consortium Guideline for SLCO1B1 and Simvastatin-Induced Myopathy: 2014 Update. *Clin. Pharmacol. Ther.* **2014**, *96*, 423–428. [CrossRef]
23. DPWG. SLCO1B1: Simvastatin (4055/4056). Available online: https://www.g-standaard.nl/risicoanalyse/B0004056.PDF (accessed on 30 September 2021).
24. Johnson, J.; Caudle, K.; Gong, L.; Whirl-Carrillo, M.; Stein, C.; Scott, S.; Lee, M.; Gage, B.; Kimmel, S.; Perera, M.; et al. Clinical Pharmacogenetics Implementation Consortium (CPIC) Guideline for Pharmacogenetics-Guided Warfarin Dosing: 2017 Update. *Clin. Pharmacol. Ther.* **2017**, *102*, 397–404. [CrossRef]
25. DPWG. CYP2C9: Warfarin (6228 t/m 6234). Available online: https://www.g-standaard.nl/risicoanalyse/B0006233.PDF (accessed on 30 September 2021).
26. Shaw, K.; Amstutz, U.; Kim, R.B.; Lesko, L.J.; Turgeon, J.; Michaud, V.; Hwang, S.; Ito, S.; Ross, C.; Carleton, B. Clinical Practice Recommendations on Genetic Testing of CYP2C9 and VKORC1 Variants in Warfarin Therapy. *Ther. Drug Monit.* **2015**, *37*, 428–436. [CrossRef]
27. DPWG. VKORC1: Warfarin (6235/6236). Available online: https://www.g-standaard.nl/risicoanalyse/B0006236.PDF (accessed on 30 September 2021).
28. DPWG. CYP2C9: Acenocoumarol (1863 to 1869). Available online: https://www.g-standaard.nl/risicoanalyse/B0001868.PDF (accessed on 30 September 2021).
29. DPWG. CYP2D6: Amiodarone (2542/2543/2544). Available online: https://www.g-standaard.nl/risicoanalyse/B0002543.PDF (accessed on 30 September 2021).
30. Theken, K.; Lee, C.; Gong, L.; Caudle, K.E.; Formea, C.M.; Gaedigk, A.; Klein, T.E.; Agundez, J.; Grosser, T. Clinical Pharmacogenetics Implementation Consortium Guideline (CPIC) for CYP2C9 and Nonsteroidal Anti-Inflammatory Drugs. *Clin. Pharmacol. Ther.* **2020**, *108*, 191–200. [CrossRef] [PubMed]
31. DPWG. CYP2D6: Atenolol (2453/2454/2455). Available online: https://www.g-standaard.nl/risicoanalyse/B0002453.PDF (accessed on 30 September 2021).
32. DPWG. CYP2D6: Bisoprolol (2456/2457/2458). Available online: https://www.g-standaard.nl/risicoanalyse/B0002457.PDF (accessed on 30 September 2021).
33. DPWG. CYP2D6: Carvedilol (2344/2345/2346). Available online: https://www.g-standaard.nl/risicoanalyse/B0002345.PDF (accessed on 30 September 2021).
34. DPWG. CYP2D6: Clonidine (2530/2531/2532). Available online: https://www.g-standaard.nl/risicoanalyse/B0002531.PDF (accessed on 30 September 2021).
35. DPWG. CYP2D6: Disopyramide (2536/2537/2538). Available online: https://www.g-standaard.nl/risicoanalyse/B0002537.PDF (accessed on 30 September 2021).
36. DPWG. SLCO1B1: Fluvastatin (4059/4060). Available online: https://www.g-standaard.nl/risicoanalyse/B0004060.PDF (accessed on 30 September 2021).
37. DPWG. CYP2C9: Phenprocoumon (1870 to 1876). Available online: https://www.g-standaard.nl/risicoanalyse/B0001876.PDF (accessed on 30 September 2021).
38. DPWG. CYP2C19: Prasugrel (2545/2546/2547). Available online: https://www.g-standaard.nl/risicoanalyse/B0002546.PDF (accessed on 30 September 2021).
39. DPWG. CYP2D6: Quinidine (2533/2534/2535). Available online: https://www.g-standaard.nl/risicoanalyse/B0002533.PDF (accessed on 30 September 2021).
40. DPWG. CYP2D6: Sotalol (2539/2540/2541). Available online: https://www.g-standaard.nl/risicoanalyse/B0002540.PDF (accessed on 30 September 2021).
41. DPWG. CYP2C19: Ticagrelor (3515 to 3517). Available online: https://www.g-standaard.nl/risicoanalyse/B0003516.PDF (accessed on 30 September 2021).
42. Kaminsky, L.S.; Zhang, Z.-Y. Human P450 metabolism of warfarin. *Pharmacol. Ther.* **1997**, *73*, 67–74. [CrossRef]
43. Takeuchi, F.; McGinnis, R.; Bourgeois, S.; Barnes, C.; Eriksson, N.; Soranzo, N.; Whittaker, P.; Ranganath, V.; Kumanduri, V.; McLaren, W.; et al. A Genome-Wide Association Study Confirms VKORC1, CYP2C9, and CYP4F2 as Principal Genetic Determinants of Warfarin Dose. *PLoS Genet.* **2009**, *5*, e1000433. [CrossRef] [PubMed]
44. Lee, C.; Goldstein, J.A.; Pieper, J.A. Cytochrome P450 2C9 polymorphisms: A comprehensive review of the in-vitro and human data. *Pharmacogenetics* **2002**, *12*, 251–263. [CrossRef] [PubMed]
45. Aithal, G.P.; Day, C.P.; Kesteven, P.J.; Daly, A.K. Association of polymorphisms in the cytochrome P450 CYP2C9 with warfarin dose requirement and risk of bleeding complications. *Lancet* **1999**, *353*, 717–719. [CrossRef]
46. Cavallari, L.H.; Langaee, T.Y.; Momary, K.M.; Shapiro, N.L.; Nutescu, E.A.; Coty, W.A.; Viana, M.A.G.; Patel, S.R.; Johnson, J.A. Genetic and Clinical Predictors of Warfarin Dose Requirements in African Americans. *Clin. Pharmacol. Ther.* **2010**, *87*, 459–464. [CrossRef] [PubMed]

47. Wang, D.; Chen, H.; Momary, K.M.; Cavallari, L.H.; Johnson, J.A.; Sadée, W. Regulatory polymorphism in vitamin K epoxide reductase complex subunit 1 (VKORC1) affects gene expression and warfarin dose requirement. *Blood* **2008**, *112*, 1013–1021. [CrossRef]
48. Li, T.; Lange, L.A.; Li, X.; Susswein, L.; Bryant, B.; Malone, R.; Lange, E.M.; Huang, T.-Y.; Stafford, D.W.; Evans, J.P. Polymorphisms in the VKORC1 gene are strongly associated with warfarin dosage requirements in patients receiving anticoagulation. *J. Med. Genet.* **2006**, *43*, 740–744. [CrossRef]
49. Caldwell, M.D.; Awad, T.; Johnson, J.A.; Gage, B.F.; Falkowski, M.; Gardina, P.; Hubbard, J.; Turpaz, Y.; Langaee, T.Y.; Eby, C.; et al. CYP4F2 genetic variant alters required warfarin dose. *Blood* **2008**, *111*, 4106–4112. [CrossRef]
50. Danese, E.; Raimondi, S.; Montagnana, M.; Tagetti, A.; Langaee, T.; Borgiani, P.; Ciccacci, C.; Carcas, A.J.; Borobia, A.M.; Tong, H.Y.; et al. Effect of CYP 4F2, VKORC 1, and CYP 2C9 in Influencing Coumarin Dose: A Single-Patient Data Meta-Analysis in More Than 15,000 Individuals. *Clin. Pharmacol. Ther.* **2019**, *105*, 1477–1491. [CrossRef]
51. Bress, A.; Patel, S.R.; Perera, M.A.; Campbell, R.T.; Kittles, R.A.; Cavallari, L.H. Effect of NQO1 and CYP4F2 genotypes on warfarin dose requirements in Hispanic–Americans and African–Americans. *Pharmacogenomics* **2012**, *13*, 1925–1935. [CrossRef]
52. Klein, T.E.; Altman, R.B.; Eriksson, N.; Gage, B.F.; Kimmel, S.E.; Lee, M.-T.M.; Limdi, N.A.; Page, D.; Roden, D.M.; Wagner, M.J.; et al. Estimation of the Warfarin Dose with Clinical and Pharmacogenetic Data. *N. Engl. J. Med.* **2009**, *360*, 753–764. [CrossRef] [PubMed]
53. Gage, B.F.; Eby, C.; Johnson, J.A.; Deych, E.; Rieder, M.J.; Ridker, P.M.; Milligan, P.E.; Grice, G.; Lenzini, P.; Rettie, A.E.; et al. Use of Pharmacogenetic and Clinical Factors to Predict the Therapeutic Dose of Warfarin. *Clin. Pharmacol. Ther.* **2008**, *84*, 326–331. [CrossRef] [PubMed]
54. Le Heuzey, J.Y.; Ammentorp, B.; Darius, H.; De Caterina, R.; Schilling, R.J.; Schmitt, J.; Zamorano, J.L.; Kirchhof, P. Differences among western European countries in anticoagulation management of atrial fibrillation. *Thromb. Haemost.* **2014**, *111*, 833–841. [CrossRef]
55. Tàssies, D.; Freire, C.; Pijoan, J.; Maragall, S.; Monteagudo, J.; Ordinas, A.; Reverter, J.C. Pharmacogenetics of acenocoumarol: Cytochrome P450 CYP2C9 polymorphisms influence dose requirements and stability of anticoagulation. *Haematologica* **2002**, *87*, 1185–1191. [PubMed]
56. Sangkuhl, K.; Klein, T.E.; Altman, R.B. Clopidogrel pathway. *Pharm. Genom.* **2010**, *20*, 463–465. [CrossRef] [PubMed]
57. Pratt, V.M.; Del Tredici, A.L.; Hachad, H.; Ji, Y.; Kalman, L.V.; Scott, S.A.; Weck, K.E. Recommendations for Clinical CYP2C19 Genotyping Allele Selection. *J. Mol. Diagn.* **2018**, *20*, 269–276. [CrossRef]
58. Wallentin, L.; Becker, R.C.; Budaj, A.; Cannon, C.P.; Emanuelsson, H.; Held, C.; Horrow, J.; Husted, S.; James, S.; Katus, H.; et al. Ticagrelor versus Clopidogrel in Patients with Acute Coronary Syndromes. *N. Engl. J. Med.* **2009**, *361*, 1045–1057. [CrossRef]
59. AEMPS. Clopidogrel (Plavix) Summary of Products characteristics. Spanish Medicines Agency. Available online: https://cima.aemps.es/cima/dochtml/ft/98069001/FT_98069001.html (accessed on 14 October 2021).
60. AEMPS. Prasugrel (Efient) Summary of Product Characteristics. Spanish Medicines Agency. Available online: https://cima.aemps.es/cima/dochtml/ft/08503013/FT_08503013.html (accessed on 14 October 2021).
61. AEMPS. Ticagrelor (Brilique) Summary of Products Characteristics. Spanish Medicines Agency. Available online: https://cima.aemps.es/cima/dochtml/ft/110655013/FT_110655013.html (accessed on 14 October 2021).
62. FDA. FDA Drug Safety Communication: Reduced Effectiveness of Plavix (Clopidogrel) in Patients Who Are Poor Metabolizers of the Drug. Available online: https://www.fda.gov/drugs/postmarket-drug-safety-information-patients-and-providers/fda-drug-safety-communication-reduced-effectiveness-plavix-clopidogrel-patients-who-are-poor (accessed on 10 October 2021).
63. FDA. Clopidogrel (Plavix) Drug label. US Food and Drug Administration. Available online: https://www.accessdata.fda.gov/scripts/cder/daf/index.cfm?event=overview.process&ApplNo=020839 (accessed on 10 October 2021).
64. Collet, J.-P.; Thiele, H.; Barbato, E.; Barthélémy, O.; Bauersachs, J.; Bhatt, D.L.; Dendale, P.; Dorobantu, M.; Edvardsen, T.; Folliguet, T.; et al. 2020 ESC Guidelines for the management of acute coronary syndromes in patients presenting without persistent ST-segment elevation. *Eur. Heart J.* **2021**, *42*, 1289–1367. [CrossRef]
65. Levine, G.N.; Bates, E.R.; Bittl, J.A.; Brindis, R.G.; Fihn, S.D.; Fleisher, L.A.; Granger, C.B.; Lange, R.A.; Mack, M.J.; Mauri, L.; et al. 2016 ACC/AHA Guideline Focused Update on Duration of Dual Antiplatelet Therapy in Patients With Coronary Artery Disease: A Report of the American College of Cardiology/American Heart Association Task Force on Clinical Practice Guidelines: An Update of the 2011 ACCF/AHA/SCAI Guideline for Percutaneous Coronary Intervention, 2011 ACCF/AHA Guideline for Coronary Artery Bypass Graft Surgery, 2012 ACC/AHA/ACP/AATS/PCNA/SCAI/STS Guideline for the Diagnosis and Management of Patients With Stable Ischemic Heart Disease, 2013 ACCF/AHA Guideline for the Management of ST-Elevation Myocardial Infarction, 2014 AHA/ACC Guideline for the Management of Patients With Non–ST-Elevation Acute Coronary Syndromes, and 2014 ACC/AHA Guideline on Perioperative Cardiovascular Evaluation and Management of Patients Undergoing Noncardiac Surgery. *Circulation* **2016**, *134*, e123–e155. [CrossRef]
66. Claassens, D.M.F.; Vos, G.J.; Bergmeijer, T.O.; Hermanides, R.S.; Van't Hof, A.W.V.; Van Der Harst, P.; Barbato, E.; Morisco, C.; Gin, R.M.T.J.; Asselbergs, F.W.; et al. A Genotype-Guided Strategy for Oral P2Y12 Inhibitors in Primary PCI. *N. Engl. J. Med.* **2019**, *381*, 1621–1631. [CrossRef] [PubMed]
67. Notarangelo, F.M.; Maglietta, G.; Bevilacqua, P.; Cereda, M.; Merlini, P.A.; Villani, G.Q.; Moruzzi, P.; Patrizi, G.; Tagliazucchi, G.M.; Crocamo, A.; et al. Pharmacogenomic Approach to Selecting Antiplatelet Therapy in Patients with Acute Coronary Syndromes. *J. Am. Coll. Cardiol.* **2018**, *71*, 1869–1877. [CrossRef]

68. Pereira, N.L.; Farkouh, M.E.; So, D.; Lennon, R.; Geller, N.; Mathew, V.; Bell, M.; Bae, J.-H.; Jeong, M.H.; Chavez, I.; et al. Effect of Genotype-Guided Oral P2Y12 Inhibitor Selection vs Conventional Clopidogrel Therapy on Ischemic Outcomes After Percutaneous Coronary Intervention. *JAMA* **2020**, *324*, 761–771. [CrossRef] [PubMed]
69. Baigent, C.; Keech, A.C.; Kearney, P.; Blackwell, L.; Buck, G.; Pollicino, C.; Kirby, A.; Sourjina, T.; Peto, R.; Collins, R.; et al. Efficacy and safety of cholesterol-lowering treatment: Prospective meta-analysis of data from 90 056 participants in 14 randomised trials of statins. *Lancet* **2005**, *366*, 1267–1278. [CrossRef] [PubMed]
70. SEARCH Collaborative Group; Link, E.; Parish, S.; Armitage, J.; Bowman, L.; Heath, S.; Matsuda, F.; Gut, I.; Lathrop, M.; Collins, R. SLCO1B1 Variants and Statin-Induced Myopathy—A Genomewide Study. *N. Engl. J. Med.* **2008**, *359*, 789–799. [CrossRef] [PubMed]
71. Shitara, Y. Clinical Importance of OATP1B1 and OATP1B3 in Drug-Drug Interactions. *Drug Metab. Pharmacokinet.* **2011**, *26*, 220–227. [CrossRef] [PubMed]
72. Kitzmiller, J.P.; Mikulik, E.B.; Dauki, A.M.; Mukherjee, C.; Luzum, J.A. Pharmacogenomics of statins: Understanding susceptibility to adverse effects. *Pharm. Pers. Med.* **2016**, *9*, 97–106. [CrossRef]
73. Kadam, P.; Ashavaid, T.F.; Ponde, C.K.; Rajani, R.M. Genetic determinants of lipid-lowering response to atorvastatin therapy in an Indian population. *J. Clin. Pharm. Ther.* **2016**, *41*, 329–333. [CrossRef]
74. Pasanen, M.K.; Neuvonen, M.; Neuvonen, P.J.; Niemi, M. SLCO1B1 polymorphism markedly affects the pharmacokinetics of simvastatin acid. *Pharm. Genom.* **2006**, *16*, 873–879. [CrossRef]
75. Linskey, D.W.; English, J.D.; Perry, D.A.; Ochs-Balcom, H.M.; Ma, C.; Isackson, P.J.; Vladutiu, G.D.; Luzum, J.A. Association of SLCO1B1 c.521T>C (rs4149056) with discontinuation of atorvastatin due to statin-associated muscle symptoms. *Pharm. Genom.* **2020**, *30*, 208–211. [CrossRef]
76. Shin, J.; Johnson, J.A. Pharmacogenetics of β-Blockers. *Pharmacother. J. Hum. Pharmacol. Drug Ther.* **2007**, *27*, 874–887. [CrossRef]
77. Bijl, M.; Visser, L.; Van Schaik, R.; Kors, J.; Witteman, J.; Hofman, A.; Vulto, A.; Van Gelder, T.; Stricker, B. Genetic Variation in the CYP2D6 Gene Is Associated with a Lower Heart Rate and Blood Pressure in β-Blocker Users. *Clin. Pharmacol. Ther.* **2008**, *85*, 45–50. [CrossRef] [PubMed]
78. Anstensrud, A.K.; Molden, E.; Haug, H.J.; Qazi, R.; Muriq, H.; Fosshaug, L.E.; Spigset, O.; Øie, E. Impact of genotype-predicted CYP2D6 metabolism on clinical effects and tolerability of metoprolol in patients after myocardial infarction–a prospective observational study. *Eur. J. Clin. Pharmacol.* **2020**, *76*, 673–683. [CrossRef] [PubMed]
79. Rau, T.; Wuttke, H.; Michels, L.; Werner, U.; Bergmann, K.; Kreft, M.; Fromm, M.; Eschenhagen, T. Impact of the CYP2D6 Genotype on the Clinical Effects of Metoprolol: A Prospective Longitudinal Study. *Clin. Pharmacol. Ther.* **2008**, *85*, 269–272. [CrossRef] [PubMed]
80. Pratt, V.M.; Scott, S.A.; Pirmohamed, M.; Esquivel, B.; Kane, M.S.; Kattman, B.L.; Malheiro, A.J. (Eds.) Metoprolol therapy and CYP2D6 genotype. In *Medical Genetics Summaries*; National Center for Biotechnology Information: Bethesda, MD, USA, 2012.
81. Pratt, V.M.; Scott, S.A.; Pirmohamed, M.; Esquivel, B.; Kane, M.S.; Kattman, B.L.; Malheiro, A.J. (Eds.) Propafenone therapy and CYP2D6 genotype. In *Medical Genetics Summaries*; National Center for Biotechnology Information: Bethesda, MD, USA, 2012.
82. Hindricks, G.; Potpara, T.; Dagres, N.; Arbelo, E.; Bax, J.J.; Blomström-Lundqvist, C.; Boriani, G.; Castella, M.; Dan, G.-A.; Dilaveris, P.E.; et al. 2020 ESC Guidelines for the diagnosis and management of atrial fibrillation developed in collaboration with the European Association for Cardio-Thoracic Surgery (EACTS): The Task Force for the diagnosis and management of atrial fibrillation of the European Society of Cardiology (ESC) Developed with the special contribution of the European Heart Rhythm Association (EHRA) of the ESC. *Eur. Heart J.* **2020**, *42*, 373–498. [CrossRef]
83. Jazwinska-Tarnawska, E.; Orzechowska-Juzwenko, K.; Niewinski, P.; Rzemislawska, Z.; Loboz-Grudzien, K.; Dmochowska-Perz, M.; Slawin, J. The influence of CYP2D6 polymorphism on the antiarrhythmic efficacy of propafenone in patients with paroxysmal atrial fibrillation during 3 months propafenone prophylactic treatment. *Int. J. Clin. Pharmacol. Ther.* **2001**, *39*, 288–292. [CrossRef]
84. Paré, G.; Eriksson, N.; Lehr, T.; Connolly, S.; Eikelboom, J.; Ezekowitz, M.D.; Axelsson, T.; Haertter, S.; Oldgren, J.; Reilly, P.; et al. Genetic Determinants of Dabigatran Plasma Levels and Their Relation to Bleeding. *Circulation* **2013**, *127*, 1404–1412. [CrossRef]
85. Joy, M.S.; Dornbrook-Lavender, K.; Blaisdell, J.; Hilliard, T.; Boyette, T.; Hu, Y.; Hogan, S.L.; Candiani, C.; Falk, R.J.; Goldstein, J.A. CYP2C9 genotype and pharmacodynamic responses to losartan in patients with primary and secondary kidney diseases. *Eur. J. Clin. Pharmacol.* **2009**, *65*, 947–953. [CrossRef]
86. Göktaş, M.T.; Pepedil, F.; Karaca, Ö.; Kalkışım, S.; Cevik, L.; Gumus, E.; Guven, G.S.; Babaoglu, M.O.; Bozkurt, A.; Yasar, U. Relationship between genetic polymorphisms of drug efflux transporter MDR1 (ABCB1) and response to losartan in hyper-tension patients. *Eur. Rev. Med. Pharmacol. Sci.* **2016**, *20*, 2460–2467.
87. Jacobsen, P.; Rossing, K.; Rossing, P.; Tarnow, L.; Mallet, C.; Poirier, O.; Cambien, F.; Parving, H.-H. Angiotensin converting enzyme gene polymorphism and ACE inhibition in diabetic nephropathy. *Kidney Int.* **1998**, *53*, 1002–1006. [CrossRef]
88. Sasaki, M.; Oki, T.; Iuchi, A.; Tabata, T.; Yamada, H.; Manabe, K.; Fukuda, K.; Abe, M.; Ito, S. Relationship between the angiotensin converting enzyme gene polymorphism and the effects of enalapril on left ventricular hypertrophy and impaired diastolic filling in essential hypertension: M-mode and pulsed Doppler echocardiographic studies. *J. Hypertens.* **1996**, *14*, 1403–1408. [CrossRef] [PubMed]
89. Cicoira, M.; Rossi, A.; Bonapace, S.; Zanolla, L.; Perrot, A.; Francis, D.P.; Golia, G.; Franceschini, L.; Osterziel, K.J.; Zardini, P. Effects of ACE gene insertion/deletion polymorphism on response to spironolactone in patients with chronic heart failure. *Am. J. Med.* **2004**, *116*, 657–661. [CrossRef] [PubMed]

90. Zubiaur, P.; Koller, D.; Saiz-Rodríguez, M.; Navares-Gómez, M.; Abad-Santos, F. Important Pharmacogenetic Information for Drugs Prescribed During the SARS-CoV-2 Infection (COVID-19). *Clin. Transl. Sci.* **2020**, *13*, 1023–1033. [CrossRef] [PubMed]
91. Choi, H.D.; Suh, J.H.; Lee, J.Y.; Bae, S.K.; Kang, H.E.; Lee, M.G.; Shin, W.G. Effects of ACE and ADD1 gene polymorphisms on blood pressure response to hydrochlorothiazide: A meta-analysis. *Int. J. Clin. Pharmacol. Ther.* **2013**, *51*, 718–724. [CrossRef]
92. Strauss, D.G.; Vicente, J.; Johannesen, L.; Blinova, K.; Mason, J.W.; Weeke, P.; Behr, E.; Roden, D.M.; Woosley, R.; Kosova, G.; et al. Common Genetic Variant Risk Score Is Associated with Drug-Induced QT Prolongation and Torsade de Pointes Risk. *Circulation* **2017**, *135*, 1300–1310. [CrossRef]

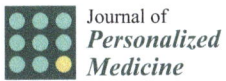

Review

Pharmacogenetics of Direct Oral Anticoagulants: A Systematic Review

Johanna Raymond [1,2], Laurent Imbert [2,3], Thibault Cousin [1], Thomas Duflot [3], Rémi Varin [1], Julien Wils [2,3] and Fabien Lamoureux [2,3,*]

1. Pharmacy Department, Rouen University Hospital, 76031 Rouen, France; johanna.raymond@chu-rouen.fr (J.R.); thibault_cousin@hotmail.fr (T.C.); remi.varin@chu-rouen.fr (R.V.)
2. Laboratory of Pharmacology, Toxicology and Pharmacogenetic, Pharmacology Department, Rouen University Hospital, 76031 Rouen, France; laurent.imbert@chu-rouen.fr (L.I.); julien.wils@chu-rouen.fr (J.W.)
3. Department of Pharmacology, Normandie University, UNIROUEN, INSERM U1096, CHU Rouen, F-76000 Rouen, France; thomas.duflot@chu-rouen.fr
* Correspondence: fabien.lamoureux@chu-rouen.fr; Tel.: +33-232-886-643

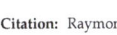

Citation: Raymond, J.; Imbert, L.; Cousin, T.; Duflot, T.; Varin, R.; Wils, J.; Lamoureux, F. Pharmacogenetics of Direct Oral Anticoagulants: A Systematic Review. *J. Pers. Med.* **2021**, *11*, 37. https://doi.org/10.3390/jpm11010037

Received: 13 November 2020
Accepted: 7 January 2021
Published: 11 January 2021

Publisher's Note: MDPI stays neutral with regard to jurisdictional claims in published maps and institutional affiliations.

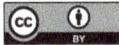

Copyright: © 2021 by the authors. Licensee MDPI, Basel, Switzerland. This article is an open access article distributed under the terms and conditions of the Creative Commons Attribution (CC BY) license (https://creativecommons.org/licenses/by/4.0/).

Abstract: Dabigatran, rivaroxaban, apixaban, edoxaban, and betrixaban are direct oral anticoagulants (DOACs). Their inter-individual variability in pharmacodynamics and pharmacokinetics (transport and metabolism) is high, and could result from genetic polymorphisms. As recommended by the French Network of Pharmacogenetics (RNPGx), the management of some treatments in cardiovascular diseases (as antiplatelet agents, oral vitamin K antagonists, and statins) can rely on genetic testing in order to improve healthcare by reducing therapeutic resistance or toxicity. This paper is a review of association studies between single nucleotide polymorphisms (SNPs) and systemic exposure variation of DOACs. Most of the results presented here have a lot to do with some SNPs of CES1 (rs2244613, rs8192935, and rs71647871) and ABCB1 (rs1128503, rs2032582, rs1045642, and rs4148738) genes, and dabigatran, rivaroxaban, and apixaban. Regarding edoxaban and betrixaban, as well as SNPs in the *CYP3A4* and *CYP3A5* genes, literature is scarce, and further studies are needed.

Keywords: direct oral anticoagulants; pharmacogenetics; adverse drug reactions; clinical implementation

1. Introduction

Dabigatran, rivaroxaban, apixaban, edoxaban, and betrixaban are direct oral anticoagulants (DOACs). Their mechanism of action is based on the direct inhibition of coagulation factors: either thrombin (factor IIa) for dabigatran, or Stuart factor (Xa) for rivaroxaban, apixaban, edoxaban, and betrixaban. DOACs are alternative treatments to oral anti-vitamin K anticoagulants (AVK: fluindione, warfarin, and acenocoumarol). However, the inter-individual variability of these treatments is significant, and can lead to hemorrhagic or thromboembolic events. This variability could be related to polymorphisms of genes coding for proteins responsible for the activation, transport, or metabolism of DOACs, such as *CES1*, *ABCB1*, *CYP3A4*, and *CYP3A5* (Table 1). Their pharmacokinetic and pharmacodynamic variability is also impacted by drug interactions when CYP450 or P-glycoprotein inducers or inhibitors are co-administered. DOACs are not subject to pharmacogenetic testing in clinical practice, unlike other cardiovascular drugs (antiplatelet agents, anti-vitamin K, and statins), for which such testing is recommended [1].

Table 1. Genes coding for proteins involved in the activation, transport, and metabolism of DOACs [2–6].

DCI	Activation	Transport	Metabolism
Dabigatran	CES1, CES2	ABCB1	UGT1A9, UGT2B7, UGT2B15
Rivaroxaban	-	ABCB1, ABCG2	CYP3A4/5, CYP2J2
Apixaban	-	ABCB1, ABCG2	CYP3A4/5, CYP1A2, CYP2J2
Edoxaban	-	ABCB1, SLCO1B1	CES1, CYP3A4/5
Betrixaban	-	ABCB1	CYP450-independent hydolysis

ABCB1: ATP-binding cassette isoforme B1; ABCG2: ATP-binding cassette isoforme G2; CES: carboxyesterase; CYP: Cytochrome P450; SLCO1B1: solute carrier organic anion transporter family, member 1B1; UGT: UDP-glucuronyltransferase.

2. Materials and Methods

A literature review was conducted using PubMed in order to identify studies evaluating the impact of CYP genetic polymorphisms on DOAC exposure, taking into account adverse events. The terms "DABIGATRAN", "RIVAROXABAN", "APIXABAN", "EDOXABAN", and "BETRIXABAN" have been crossed with "PHARMACOGENETICS", "PHARMACOGENOMICS", "POLYMORPHISM", "CYP3A4", "CYP3A5", or "ABCB1" and "BLEEDING", "HEMORRHAGE", or "THROMBOEMBOLIC EVENTS". "DABIGATRAN" and "EDOXABAN" have been also crossed with "CES".

3. Results

3.1. Dabigatran

3.1.1. Pharmacodynamics and Pharmacokinetics

Dabigatran is administered as a prodrug dabigatran etexilate. Its bioavailability is 7% [7]. It is a P-glycoprotein substrate, which implies drug interactions with potent P-glycoprotein inducers (rifampin, St. John's wort, carbamazepine, phenytoin, etc.) and P-glycoprotein inhibitors (systemic ketoconazole, itraconazole, ritonavir, cyclosporine, clarithromycin, dronedarone, amiodarone, quinidine, verapamil, ticagrelor) [3,7]. Dabigatran etexilate is activated by intestinal (CES2 isoform) and hepatocyte (CES1 isoform) carboxylesterases (CES) to form short-lived metabolites, BIBR 951 and BIBR 1087. Non-enzymatic hydrolysis also converts the prodrug to BIBR 1087. The intermediate metabolites are in turn hydrolyzed by CES1 in hepatocytes to yield active dabigatran [8,9]. The plasma protein binding of dabigatran is 35% [10]. Dabigatran is metabolized to a small extent (< 10%) by the UDP-glucuronyltransferase (UGTs) isoforms 1A9, 2B7, and 2B15, leading to the formation of four active metabolites [9]. Dabigatran is not metabolized by CYP450 and does not induce or inhibit CYP450, except at supra-therapeutic concentrations (in vitro at 100 µM: inhibition of CYP3A4 and CYP2E1) [7,10]. Dabigatran and its metabolites are eliminated mainly via the urinary route (80–90%). It has a relatively long plasma elimination half-life of 12–17 h [7].

3.1.2. Pharmacogenetics

Genetic Polymorphism of *CES1*

The *CES1* and *CES2* genes are located on chromosome 16, and contain 14 and 12 exons respectively. In humans, the CES1 protein is the most hepatically active isoform, with approximately 90% of the activity [11]; 2000 polymorphisms have been described for *CES1* [12]. The single nucleotide polymorphisms (SNPs) rs2244613 (C > A), rs8192935 (T > C), and rs71647871 (G > A) [13] have been associated with pharmacokinetic variations of dabigatran [11,14–17] (Table 2). The first two SNPs are in incomplete linkage disequilibrium ($r^2 = 0.45$) [14], and their impact on the expression or activity of CES1 has not been clearly established, unlike rs71647871, which induces a loss of CES1 function by substitution of one of the three glycines at the active site by a glutamate [12]. Overall, these three SNPs lead to a decrease in systemic exposure to dabigatran, reducing the risk of hemorrhage, without thromboembolic events being associated [12,14].

Table 2. Pharmacokinetic variations in DOACs based on genetic polymorphisms of *CES1, ABCB1, CYP3A4, CYP3A5, ABCG2,* and *SLCO1B1*.

Gene SNP Allelic Change Amino Acid Change Frequency	DABIGATRAN	RIVAROXABAN	APIXABAN	EDOXABAN	BETRIXABAN
CES1 rs2244613 intron C > A — C = 0.266 [13]	↓ [trough] by 15% per mutated allele ($p = 1.2 \times 10^{-8}$) [14] ↓ risk of bleeding ($p = 7 \times 10^{-5}$) [14] ↓ bleeding compared to warfarin for mutated alleles ($p = 0.002$) [14] Not associated with ischemic events [14] ↓ [trough] of dabigatran ($p = 0.04$) HTZ = 2% and MT = 3% [15] No effect on AUC (NS) or [peak] (NS) [16] ↓ [trough] for mutated alleles carriers (NS) [17]	NI	NI	NI	NI
CES1 rs8192935 intron T > C — T = 0.420 [13]	↓ [peak] by 12% ($p = 3.2 \times 10^{-8}$) [14] Not associated with ischemic or bleeding events [14] ↓ [trough] ($p = 0.033$) HTZ = 3% and MT «T» = 11% [15]	NI	NI	NI	NI
CES1 rs71647871 536 G > A 143 Gly > Glu A = 0.014 [13]	Loss of CES1 function: ↓ by 41% of the transformation of the prodrug and metabolites in dabigatran ($p = 0.026$ for BIBR 951) [12]	NI	NI	NI	NI
ABCB1 rs1128503 1236 C > T 412 Gly > Gly T = 0.46 [13]	Results not significant for AUC and [peak] of dabigatran Haplotype HTZ: $p = 0.61$ Haplotype MT: $p = 0.58$ [16]	Major bleeding under rivaroxaban for three MT patients [18]	No impact on [trough]/dose ratio for apixaban [19]	NI	NI
ABCB1 rs2032582 2677 G > T/A 893 Ala > Ser/Thr T = 0.42 A = 0.08 [13]	Results not significant for AUC and [peak] of dabigatran Haplotype HTZ: $p = 0.61$ Haplotype MT: $p = 0.58$ [16]	One case of rivaroxaban-induced hemorrhage with homozygous mutated genotypes 'TT' [20] No significant increase of rivaroxaban [peak] [16] Major bleeding under rivaroxaban for three MT patients [18]	No impact on [trough]/dose ratio for apixaban [19] One case of highly increased [peak] and concentration 12 h post dose in a homozygous patient (TT), along with other mutations on *ABCB1* (rs1045642, MT), *ABCG2* (rs2231142, HTZ), and *CYP3A5* (rs776746, MT) [21]	NI	NI

Table 2. Cont.

Gene SNP Allelic Change Amino Acid Change Frequency	DABIGATRAN	RIVAROXABAN	APIXABAN	EDOXABAN	BETRIXABAN
ABCB1 rs4148738 intron: A > G G = 0.38 [13]	Associated with ↑ [peak] by 12% ($p = 8.2 \times 10^{-8}$), but not associated with ischemic or bleeding events [14] No effect on [trough] and [peak] of dabigatran [17] Associated with ↑ [peak] of dabigatran [17] No impact on dabigatran pharmacokinetics [25]	Major bleeding under rivaroxaban for three MT patients [18]	Associated with ↑ [peak] of apixaban ($p = 0.048$) [26] No impact on apixaban pharmacokinetics [23]	NI	NI
CYP3A4 rs35599367 intron: C > T - T = 0.03 [13]	NI	No significant increase of rivaroxaban [peak] in mutated patients compared to wild type (haplotype of ABCB1 rs1045642 and CYP3A4 rs35599367) [22]	NI	NI	NI
CYP3A5 rs776746 intron: T > C - T = 0.29 [13]	NI	NI	Significant ↑ of ratio [trough]/dose of apixaban in HTZ or MT patients [19] One case of highly increased [peak] and concentration 12 h post dose in a MT patient, along with other mutations on ABCB1 (rs2032582 and rs1045642, MT), and ABCC2 (rs2231142, HTZ) [21] No impact on apixaban pharmacokinetics [23]	NI	NI
ABCG2 rs2231142 421 C > A 141 Gln > Lys A = 0.12 [13]	NI	NI	Significant ↑ of [trough]/dose ratio of apixaban in MT patients [19] One case of highly increased [peak] and concentration 12 h post dose in an HTZ patient, along with other mutations on ABCB1 (rs2032582 and rs1045642, MT), and CYP3A5 (rs776746, MT) [21] ↑ [peak] et [trough] of apixaban [27]	NI	NI
SLCO1B1 rs4149056 521 T > C 174 Val > Ala C = 0.13 [13]	NI	NI	NI	It seems to have no impact on the pharmacokinetics of edoxaban [24]	NI

AUC: area under curve; MT: mutated homozygous; HTZ: heterozygous; ↓: decrease; ↑: increase; [peak]: peak concentration; [trough]: trough concentration; NI: no information; NS: non significant.

Genetic Polymorphism of *ABCB1*

The *ABCB1* gene is located on chromosome 7 and contains 29 exons (4872 bp) [28]. In 2009, 1279 SNPs, including 22 silent mutations, 41 nonsense mutations and one in the start codon, were known [29]. The most common polymorphisms are rs1128503 (1236 C > T), rs2032582 (2677 G > T), rs1045642 (3435 C > T), and rs4148738 (intronic in the promoter, A > G) [13]. The first three SNPs are in partial linkage disequilibrium and form several haplotypes [30,31] (Table 3). The rs1045642 and rs4148738 are also in partial linkage disequilibrium [16]. These polymorphisms impact the pharmacokinetics of many P-glycoprotein substrate drugs, but the genotype/phenotype relationship of these variants is not clearly established [32]; only rs1045642 and rs4148738 are associated with increased peak concentration of dabigatran [14,17] (Table 2). In the systematic review and meta-analysis of Xie et al. in 2018, which included a total of 13 clinical studies involving 3144 patients, DOAC peak concentrations in wild homozygous carriers for rs1045642 and rs2032582 of *ABCB1* were lower than those of homozygous mutant carriers; the DOAC peak was also lower in wild homozygous carriers for rs1045642 [25]. However, rs4148738 did not show any impact on the pharmacokinetics of dabigatran [25].

Table 3. *ABCB1* haplotypes.

ABCB1 SNP	rs1128503	rs2032582	rs1045642	rs10276036 Intronic	rs2235033 Intronic	rs2235013 Intronic
*ABCB1*1 (Kim et al.) [30]	C	G	C	G	T	G
*ABCB1*2 (Kim et al.) [30]	T	T	T			
*ABCB1*2 (Kroetz et al.) [31]	C	G	T	G	T	G
*ABCB1*13 (Kroetz et al.) [31]	T	T	T	A	C	A

A: adenine; C: cytosine; G: guanine; T: thymine. Several definitions of the haplotype have been made according to the teams. The haplotypes *ABCB1*2 of Kim et al. and *ABCB1*13 of Kroetz et al. can be differentiated by three intronic SNPs (rs10276036, rs2235033, and rs2235013).

A study on the stability of P-glycoprotein mRNA (messenger ribonucleic acid) by Wang et al. showed an association between the presence of the 3435C > T mutation (rs1045642) and the amount of mRNA present in vitro in human liver samples [33]. Indeed, the substitution of cytosine (C) by thymine (T) would modify the secondary structure of the mRNA by a cis-regulatory mechanism, affecting its stability and thus its quantity in the liver. The two other SNPs, rs1128503 and rs2032582, also induced a secondary structure of mRNA in the model. On the other hand, during in vitro and in vivo experiments, only the 3435C > T mutation was associated with a decrease in P-glycoprotein expression and activity.

Epigenetics of *ABCB1*

The synthesis of mRNA, coding for the P-glycoprotein, is synergistically regulated by the genetic variations mentioned above, and epigenetic variations via methylation of the promoter in *ABCB1* gene [34]. Thus, homozygous patients mutated for the haplotype rs1128503-rs2032582-rs1045642 and who have a high methylation rate have the lowest amount of ABCB1 mRNA compared to homozygous mutated patients with a low methylation rate, then to wild homozygous with a high methylation rate, and finally to wild homozygous with a low methylation rate [34].

Genetic Polymorphism of *UGT1A9*, *2B7*, and *2B15*

The impact of *UGT1A9*, *2B7*, and *2B15* polymorphisms on systemic exposure to dabigatran has not been studied to date. However, we can assume that their role is likely to be minimal, since they are involved in the production of active metabolites, and in a small proportion [9].

3.2. Rivaroxaban

3.2.1. Pharmacodynamics and Pharmacokinetics

Rivaroxaban has an oral bioavailability of approximately 80% [2]. The systemic exposure is increased when rivaroxaban is administered during a meal [35]. Peak plasma concentrations occur 2–4 h after administration. The inter-individual variability of exposure is between 30 and 40%. Rivaroxaban is transported by P-glycoprotein and the breast cancer resistance protein (BCRP) encoded by the *ABCG2* gene [36]. It is highly bound to plasma proteins, in the order of 95% [37]. Two-thirds of the administered dose is metabolized, mainly by cytochrome P450 isoforms 3A4, 3A5, and 2J2, and also by mechanisms independent of CYP450. This metabolization leads to the formation of 18 different inactive metabolites, which are in turn eliminated in the urine (50%) and feces (50%). The remaining third of rivaroxaban is eliminated unchanged in the urine. The mean plasma elimination half-life is 10 h. Rivaroxaban does not induce or inhibit CYP450 [4]. Administration of potent CYP3A4/5 and P-glycoprotein enzyme inhibitors (such as ritonavir, ketoconazole, itraconazole, voriconazole, posaconazole, etc.) increases rivaroxaban plasma concentrations by an average of 2.6-fold, significantly increasing its pharmacodynamics and the risk of bleeding [4]. However, a smaller increase in plasma concentration with other potent CYP3A4/5 and/or P-glycoprotein inhibitors (such as erythromycin, clarithromycin, and fluconazole) was not considered clinically relevant; data for dronedarone are limited [4]. Coadministration of rivaroxaban with potent CYP3A and P-glycoprotein enzyme inducers (rifampin, phenytoin, carbamazepine, phenobarbital, or St. John's wort) may reduce its plasma concentration [4].

3.2.2. Pharmacogenetics

Concerning the *ABCB1* gene, Ing Lorenzini's team reported in 2016 a case of rivaroxaban-induced hemorrhage in a patient with homozygous mutated TT genotype for rs2032582 and rs1045642 [20], which is in line with the results highlighted by Xie et al. in 2018 (higher peak concentrations for these homozygous mutated genotypes, as well as AUC for rs1045642) [25]. In Gouin-Thibault's 2017 study, these two variants did not show a significant increase in rivaroxaban peak concentrations in a cohort of healthy volunteers [16]. Among three patients who experienced major bleeding associated with a residual blood concentration > 136 ng/mL in the 2018 Sennesael study, all were heterozygous for rs1128503, rs2032582, and rs4148738; two were heterozygous and one was a homozygous mutated TT for *ABCB1* rs1045642 [18]. These results are shown in Table 2.

For *CYP3A4*, it was shown in a study by Sychev et al. in 2018 that the peak and trough rivaroxaban concentrations depended on *CYP3A4* activity [38]. In addition, a number of *CYP3A4* polymorphisms are known to decrease its activity, such as *CYP3A4*22*/rs35599367 [13,39] or *CYP3A4*17*/rs4987161 [40]. In 2019, another study by Sychev et al. in 78 patients showed no significant difference in peak concentration between the mutated haplotypes *ABCB1*-rs1045642/*CYP3A4*-rs35599367 and *ABCB1*-rs4148738/*CYP3A4*-rs35599367 compared to the respective wild haplotypes [22]. These results are shown in Table 2.

3.3. Apixaban

3.3.1. Pharmacodynamics and Pharmacokinetics

Apixaban has an oral bioavailability of approximately 50% [2]. The peak plasma concentration is reached 3–4 h after administration. Intra-individual and inter-individual variabilities are approximately 20% and 30%, respectively [5]. Apixaban is transported by P-glycoprotein and BCRP. Plasma protein binding is high (87%) [37]. A quarter of the absorbed amount is converted to inactive metabolites, mainly by CYP3A4 and CYP3A5, but also by CYP1A2, CYP2C8, CYP2C9, CYP2C19, and CYP2J2 [36], and the sulfotransferases SULT1A1 and SULT1A2 (leading to O-desmethyl-apixaban sulfate), mainly SULT1A1 [41]. A proportion of 27% of apixaban is excreted in urine in an unchanged form. The remaining part of apixaban and inactive metabolites are excreted in the feces. The half-life of apixaban is approximately 12 h [5]. Concomitant administration of potent enzyme inhibitors of CYP3A4/5 and P-glycoprotein increases the blood concentration of apixaban by an average of two-fold [5]. Other active substances, weaker CYP3A4/5 and P-glycoprotein inhibitors (diltiazem, naproxen, clarithromycin, amiodarone, verapamil, quinidine), may increase apixaban plasma concentrations to a lesser extent [5]. Conversely, co-administration of apixaban with CYP3A4/5 and P-glycoprotein enzyme inducers (rifampicin, phenytoin, carbamazepine, phenobarbital, or St. John's wort) may reduce its plasma concentration [5].

3.3.2. Pharmacogenetics

In 2016, Dimatteo's team demonstrated an association between the intronic variant rs4148738 of *ABCB1* and an increase in the peak concentration of apixaban ($p < 0.05$) [26]. In 2017, Ueshima's study of a cohort of 44 Japanese patients treated for non-valvular atrial fibrillation showed a significant increase in the ratio of residual concentration/dose of apixaban with *CYP3A5*1/*3* or **3/*3* (rs776746) and *ABCG2* 421A > A (rs2231142) genotypes [13] compared to *CYP3A5*1/*1* and *ABCG2* 421C > C genotypes respectively; variants 1236C > T (rs1128503), 2677G > T (rs2032582), and 3435C > T (rs1045642) of the *ABCB1* gene had no impact on this ratio [19]. The 2018 Kruykov study in a sample of 17 Russian patients treated with apixaban, 10 mg daily, did not show a significant impact of *ABCB1* rs1045642 and rs4148738 or *CYP3A5* rs776746 on the pharmacokinetics of apixaban [23]. In 2019, Huppertz reported the case of one woman with dramatically increased apixaban plasma concentrations 3 h (peak) and 12 h after an oral dose: 1100 ng/mL and 900 ng/mL, respectively, compared to the range expected (91 to 321 ng/mL at peak and 41 to 231 ng/mL after 12 h). Four polymorphisms may have result in such increase: *ABCB1* rs2032582, rs1045642, and *CYP3A5* rs776746 were found mutated homozygous, and *ABCG2* rs2231142 was found heterozygous [21]. She also suffered from moderate renal impairment, which could also lead to increased plasma concentrations. Finally, in 2020, Gulilat's study of 358 Caucasian patients with atrial fibrillation demonstrated the relationship between the *ABCG2* 421C > A variant (resulting in impaired transporter function) and higher peak and trough blood levels of apixaban [27]. These results are shown in Table 2.

The sulfotransferase SULT1A1 has three main allelic variants: *SULT1A1*1* (wild type), *SULT1A1*2* (638 G > A), and *SULT1A1*3* (667 A > G). The effect on apixaban metabolism is very small for *SULT1A1*2* and moderate for *SULT1A1*3*, which could lead to variations in the efficacy of apixaban by variation in its metabolites [41]. To date, no studies have investigated the impact of these variants on the efficacy or toxicity of apixaban.

3.4. Edoxaban

3.4.1. Pharmacodynamics and Pharmacokinetics

The bioavailability of edoxaban is around 60% [2]. Absorption is not altered in the presence of food [35]. The peak concentration is reached within 1–2 h. Edoxaban is a substrate for P-glycoprotein. It is 55% bound to plasma proteins [37], and is metabolized by CES1 and CYP3A4/5 to three active metabolites in a small proportion (about 10%), of which M4 is a substrate of the OATP1B1 (organic anion transporter protein 1B1) transporter encoded by the *SLCO1B1* (solute carrier organic anion transporter family, member 1B1) gene [36]. The urinary excretion of edoxaban is 35% remaining of the unchanged fraction, and metabolites are excreted in the feces. Its half-life is 10–14 h [6]. Potent enzyme inhibitors of P-glycoprotein increase systemic exposure to edoxaban by a factor of 1.5 to 2 [6].

3.4.2. Pharmacogenetics

Edoxaban is metabolized mainly by CES1, but very little by CYP3A4/3A5, and is transported by P-glycoprotein. Variations in systemic exposure could be related to the *CES1* and *ABCB1* polymorphisms [42]. To date, only one study has investigated the rs1045642 (3435 C > T) variants of *ABCB1* and rs4149056 (521 T > C) of *SLCO1B1* [13]. These variants do not seem to impact the pharmacokinetics of edoxaban [24] (Table 2).

3.5. Betrixaban

3.5.1. Pharmacodynamics and Pharmacokinetics

Betrixaban has an oral bioavailability of approximately 34%. The peak plasma concentration appears within 3–4 h after administration [43,44]. The mean plasma elimination half-life is 20 h, with a terminal half-life of 37 h. Administration with food is recommended to reduce plasma concentration variability [43]. Plasma protein binding is 60% [43,44]. Betrixaban is transported by P-glycoprotein [43], and concomitant use of P-glycoprotein inhibitors results in a 2.5- to five-fold increase in plasma peak concentrations, and a two- to three-fold increase in AUC, depending on the inhibitors [44]. Betrixaban is transformed into two inactive major metabolites by a CYP-independent hydrolysis [44]. Unlike the other factor Xa inhibitors, betrixaban has a minimal (less than 1%) hepatic metabolism by CYP450 (CYP1A1, 1A2, 2B6, 2C9, 2C19, 2D6, and 3A4), which reduces drug–drug interactions [44]. The active drug is excreted unchanged through the biliary system, then the feces for 85% and in urine for 8 to 11% [43,44].

3.5.2. Pharmacogenetics

To date, there is no data on genetic polymorphisms and betrixaban pharmacokinetics and pharmacodynamics. However, one would expect that *ABCB1* polymorphisms could impact plasma concentrations of betrixaban.

3.6. Plasma Concentrations and Adverse Events

To the best of our knowledge and to date, there is little data about the relationship between DOAC's pharmacokinetics and pharmacodynamics. However, two studies are of interest about dabigatran and edoxaban.

Regarding the risk of major bleeding in patients on dabigatran therapy, Reilly previously showed that this risk increased with dabigatran exposure ($p < 0.0001$) [45]. The median trough concentration and post-dose concentration were, respectively, 55% (116 versus 75.3 ng/mL) and 36% higher in patients with major bleeding compared to those without bleeding. Age was also an important covariate ($p < 0.0001$) [45]. No difference was shown in the median plasma concentration between patients with ischemic stroke or systemic embolism and patients who did not experience these events [45].

Ruff et al., based on ENGAGE AF-TIMI 48 trial data, have described the dose–concentration relationship and impact on anti-FXa activity for edoxaban [46]. The reduction from an oral dose of 60 mg to 30 mg and from 30 mg to 15 mg decreased mean exposure by 29% (34.6 versus 48.5 ng/mL) and 35% (16 versus 24.5 ng/mL), respectively, as well as mean anti-FXa activity by 25% and 20%, respectively [46]. Regarding the link between plasma concentrations and adverse events, this trial showed that with increasing edoxaban concentration, a gradual linear decrease in the risk of stroke or systemic embolic events occurred by contrast with the steeper increase in the risk of major bleeding [46]. Overall, the risk of major bleeding exceeded the risk of stroke or systemic embolic events, and the therapeutic window for edoxaban appeared narrower for major bleeding than thromboembolism [46]. Globally, the risk of major bleeding seems to be correlated with increasing plasma levels of direct oral anticoagulants. The risk of stroke or systemic embolic events fluctuates less with concentration variation.

4. Discussion and Conclusions: Implementation in Clinical Practice Guidelines

To date, there is no recommendation with a high level of evidence regarding the search for polymorphisms of the *CES1*, *ABCB1*, *CYP3A4*, *CYP3A5*, and *ABCG2* genes as part of therapeutic optimization for patients undergoing DOAC treatment. The methodological evaluation of studies of the association between genetic polymorphisms and cardiovascular drugs using the AGREE (Appraisal of Guidelines, Research, and Evaluation) method demonstrated the good methodological quality of the search for rs2244613 *CES1* polymorphism in patients treated with dabigatran in the same way as the search for *CYP2C19* and clopidogrel, or *CYP2C9* and warfarin polymorphisms. This finding supported the use in clinical practice of this polymorphism of interest in dabigatran-treated patients [47]. In addition, according to the PharmGKB database (www.pharmgkb.org), the earch for rs2244613 and rs8192935 *CES1* polymorphisms is indicated at Evidence Level 3 (low) for dabigatran, and for the rs776746 *CYP3A5* and rs2231142 *ABCG2* polymorphisms for apixaban. However, this level of evidence is insufficient to allow implementation of pharmacogenetic testing in clinical practice. This low level of evidence is due to the lack of reproducibility of results between studies [48]. The DAPHNE clinical study involving a cohort of 350 patients on rivaroxaban and apixaban is currently being conducted by Victoria Rollason's team (University Hospitals of Geneva); it aims to analyze the impact of certain polymorphisms of the *CYP3A4*, *CYP3A5*, *CYP3A7*, and *ABCB1* genes, as well as the phenotyping of the proteins encoded by these genes on the pharmacokinetics of these two DOACs [49]. The results of this trial will be useful to clarify the use of pharmacogenetic testing during DOAC treatment. Randomized controlled trials, similar to those undertaken for *CYP2C9* and *VKORC1* genotyping prior to anti-vitamin K treatment [50,51] or *CYP2C19* genotyping prior to clopidogrel treatment [52], will demonstrate the clinical utility of a priori genotyping of patients before introduction of direct oral anticoagulants [53,54]. In clinical practice, pharmacogenetic testing could help prescribers in choosing the most appropriate DOAC treatment according to each patient's characteristics with the lowest risk of plasma concentration variability, thus optimizing an individual patient's risk of bleeding and thromboembolic events. Therapeutic drug monitoring (TDM) could then be use as a complement to individualize oral doses in order to obtain optimal plasma levels. Lastly, there is no clear evidence between hemorrhage risk increase and a particular genetic polymorphism.

Author Contributions: F.L. proposed the subject of the study. J.R. conducted the literature review and wrote the manuscript. F.L., R.V., L.I., J.W., T.C. and T.D. provided advice on data analysis. All authors contributed to the review and approval of this final version. All authors have read and agreed to the published version of the manuscript.

Funding: This research received no external funding.

Institutional Review Board Statement: Not applicable.

Informed Consent Statement: Not applicable.

Data Availability Statement: Data sharing is not applicable to this article.

Conflicts of Interest: The authors declare no conflict of interest.

References

1. Picard, N.; Boyer, J.C.; Etienne-Grimaldi, M.C.; Barin-Le Guellec, C.; Thomas, F.; Loriot, M.A.; French National Network of Pharmacogenetics (RNPGx). Pharmacogenetics-based personalized therapy: Levels of evidence and recommendations from the French Network of Pharmacogenetics (RNPGX). *Therapie* **2017**, *72*, 185–192. [CrossRef] [PubMed]
2. Bertoletti, L.; Ollier, E.; Duvillard, C.; Delavenne, X.; Beyens, M.N.; De Magalhaes, E.; Bellet, F.; Basset, T.; Mismetti, P.; Laporte, S. Direct oral anticoagulants: Current indications and unmet needs in the treatment of venous thromboembolism. *Pharmacol. Res.* **2017**, *118*, 33–42. [CrossRef] [PubMed]
3. Pradaxa: Summary of Product Characteristics. Available online: https://www.ema.europa.eu/en/documents/product-information/pradaxa-epar-product-information_en.pdf (accessed on 27 August 2020).
4. Xarelto: Summary of Product Characteristics. Available online: https://www.ema.europa.eu/en/documents/product-information/xarelto-epar-product-information_en.pdf (accessed on 27 August 2020).
5. Eliquis: Summary of Product Characteristics. Available online: https://www.ema.europa.eu/en/documents/product-information/eliquis-epar-product-information_en.pdf (accessed on 27 August 2020).
6. Lixiana: Summary of Product Characteristics. Available online: https://www.ema.europa.eu/en/documents/product-information/lixiana-epar-product-information_en.pdf (accessed on 27 August 2020).

7. Ufer, M. Comparative efficacy and safety of the novel oral anticoagulants dabigatran, rivaroxaban and apixaban in preclinical and clinical development. *Thromb. Haemost.* **2010**, *103*, 572–585. [CrossRef] [PubMed]
8. Ganetsky, M.; Babu, K.M.; Salhanick, S.D.; Brown, R.S.; Boyer, E.W. Dabigatran: Review of pharmacology and management of bleeding complications of this novel oral anticoagulant. *J. Med. Toxicol.* **2011**, *7*, 281–287. [CrossRef]
9. Ishiguro, N.; Kishimoto, W.; Volz, A.; Ludwig-Schwellinger, E.; Ebner, T.; Schaefer, O. Impact of endogenous esterase activity on in vitro p-glycoprotein profiling of dabigatran etexilate in Caco-2 monolayers. *Drug Metab. Dispos.* **2014**, *42*, 250–256. [CrossRef]
10. Blech, S.; Ebner, T.; Ludwig-Schwellinger, E.; Stangier, J.; Roth, W. The metabolism and disposition of the oral direct thrombin inhibitor, dabigatran, in humans. *Drug Metab. Dispos.* **2008**, *36*, 386–399. [CrossRef]
11. Merali, Z.; Ross, S.; Paré, G. The pharmacogenetics of carboxylesterases: CES1 and CES2 genetic variants and their clinical effect. *Drug Metabol. Drug Interact.* **2014**, *29*, 143–151. [CrossRef]
12. Shi, J.; Wang, X.; Nguyen, J.H.; Bleske, B.E.; Liang, Y.; Liu, L.; Zhu, H.J. Dabigatran etexilate activation is affected by the CES1 genetic polymorphism G143E (rs71647871) and gender. *Biochem. Pharmacol.* **2016**, *119*, 76–84. [CrossRef]
13. Sherry, S.T.; Ward, M.H.; Kholodov, M.; Baker, J.; Phan, L.; Smigielski, E.M.; Sirotkin, K. dbSNP: The NCBI database of genetic variation. *Nucleic Acids Res.* **2001**, *29*, 308–311. [CrossRef]
14. Paré, G.; Eriksson, N.; Lehr, T.; Connolly, S.; Eikelboom, J.; Ezekowitz, M.D.; Axelsson, T.; Haertter, S.; Oldgren, J.; Reilly, P.; et al. Genetic determinants of dabigatran plasma levels and their relation to bleeding. *Circulation* **2013**, *127*, 1404–1412. [CrossRef]
15. Dimatteo, C.; D'Andrea, G.; Vecchione, G.; Paoletti, O.; Cappucci, F.; Tiscia, G.L.; Buono, M.; Grandone, E.; Testa, S.; Margaglione, M. Pharmacogenetics of dabigatran etexilate interindividual variability. *Thromb. Res.* **2016**, *144*, 1–5. [CrossRef] [PubMed]
16. Gouin-Thibault, I.; Delavenne, X.; Blanchard, A.; Siguret, V.; Salem, J.E.; Narjoz, C.; Gaussem, P.; Beaune, P.; Funck-Brentano, C.; Azizi, M.; et al. Interindividual variability in dabigatran and rivaroxaban exposure: Contribution of ABCB1 genetic polymorphisms and interaction with clarithromycin. *J. Thromb. Haemost.* **2017**, *15*, 273–283. [CrossRef] [PubMed]
17. Sychev, D.A.; Levanov, A.N.; Shelekhova, T.V.; Bochkov, P.O.; Denisenko, N.P.; Ryzhikova, K.A.; Mirzaev, K.B.; Grishina, E.A.; Gavrilov, M.A.; Ramenskaya, G.V.; et al. The impact of ABCB1 (rs1045642 and rs4148738) and CES1 (rs2244613) gene polymorphisms on dabigatran equilibrium peak concentration in patients after total knee arthroplasty. *Pharmgenomics Pers. Med.* **2018**, *11*, 127–137. [CrossRef] [PubMed]
18. Sennesael, A.L.; Larock, A.S.; Douxfils, J.; Elens, L.; Stillemans, G.; Wiesen, M.; Taubert, M.; Dogné, J.M.; Spinewine, A.; Mullier, F. Rivaroxaban plasma levels in patients admitted for bleeding events: Insights from a prospective study. *Thromb. J.* **2018**, *16*, 28. [CrossRef]
19. Ueshima, S.; Hira, D.; Fujii, R.; Kimura, Y.; Tomitsuka, C.; Yamane, T.; Ozawa, T.; Itoh, H.; Horie, M.; Terada, T.; et al. Impact of ABCB1, ABCG2, and CYP3A5 polymorphisms on plasma trough concentrations of apixaban in Japanese patients with atrial fibrillation. *Pharm. Genom.* **2017**, *27*, 329–336. [CrossRef]
20. Ing Lorenzini, K.; Daali, Y.; Fontana, P.; Desmeules, J.; Samer, C. Rivaroxaban-Induced Hemorrhage Associated with ABCB1 Genetic Defect. *Front. Pharmacol.* **2016**, *7*, 494. [CrossRef]
21. Huppertz, A.; Grond-Ginsbach, C.; Dumschat, C.; Foerster, K.I.; Burhenne, J.; Weiss, J.; Czock, D.; Purrucker, J.C.; Rizos, T.; Haefeli, W.E. Unexpected excessive apixaban exposure: Case report of a patient with polymorphisms of multiple apixaban elimination pathways. *BMC Pharmacol. Toxicol.* **2019**, *20*, 53. [CrossRef]
22. Sychev, D.; Minnigulov, R.; Bochkov, P.; Ryzhikova, K.; Yudina, I.; Lychagin, A.; Morozova, T. Effect of CYP3A4, CYP3A5, ABCB1 gene polymorphisms on rivaroxaban pharmacokinetics in patients undergoing total hip and knee replacement surgery. *High Blood Press Cardiovasc. Prev.* **2019**, *26*, 413–420. [CrossRef]
23. Kryukov, A.V.; Sychev, D.A.; Andreev, D.A.; Ryzhikova, K.A.; Grishina, E.A.; Ryabova, A.V.; Loskutnikov, M.A.; Smirnov, V.V.; Konova, O.D.; Matsneva, I.A.; et al. Influence of ABCB1 and CYP3A5 gene polymorphisms on pharmacokinetics of apixaban in patients with atrial fibrillation and acute stroke. *Pharmgenomics Pers. Med.* **2018**, *11*, 43–49. [CrossRef]
24. Vandell, A.G.; Lee, J.; Shi, M.; Rubets, I.; Brown, K.S.; Walker, J.R. An integrated pharmacokinetic/pharmacogenomic analysis of ABCB1 and SLCO1B1 polymorphisms on edoxaban exposure. *Pharm. J.* **2018**, *18*, 153–159. [CrossRef]
25. Xie, Q.; Xiang, Q.; Mu, G.; Ma, L.; Chen, S.; Zhou, S.; Hu, K.; Zhang, Z.; Cui, Y.; Jiang, J. Effect of ABCB1 Genotypes on the Pharmacokinetics and Clinical Outcomes of New Oral Anticoagulants: A Systematic Review and Meta-analysis. *Curr. Pharm. Des.* **2018**, *24*, 3558–3565. [CrossRef] [PubMed]
26. Dimatteo, C.; D'Andrea, G.; Vecchione, G.; Paoletti, O.; Tiscia, G.; Santacroce, R.; Correale, M.; Brunetti, N.; Grandone, E.; Testa, S.; et al. ABCB1 SNP rs4148738 modulation of apixaban interindividual variability. *Thromb. Res.* **2016**, *145*, 24–26. [CrossRef] [PubMed]
27. Gulilat, M.; Keller, D.; Linton, B.; Pananos, A.D.; Lizotte, D.; Dresser, G.K.; Alfonsi, J.; Tirona, R.G.; Kim, R.B.; Schwarz, U.I. Drug interactions and pharmacogenetic factors contribute to variation in apixaban concentration in atrial fibrillation patients in routine care. *J. Thromb. Thrombolysis* **2020**, *49*, 294–303. [CrossRef] [PubMed]
28. Bodor, M.; Kelly, E.J.; Ho, R.J. Characterization of the human MDR1 gene. *AAPS J.* **2005**, *7*, E1–E5. [CrossRef] [PubMed]
29. Hodges, L.M.; Markova, S.M.; Chinn, L.W.; Gow, J.M.; Kroetz, D.L.; Klein, T.E.; Altman, R.B. Very important pharmacogene summary: ABCB1 (MDR1, P-glycoprotein). *Pharm. Genom.* **2011**, *21*, 152–161. [CrossRef] [PubMed]
30. Kim, R.B.; Leake, B.F.; Choo, E.F.; Dresser, G.K.; Kubba, S.V.; Schwarz, U.I.; Taylor, A.; Xie, H.G.; McKinsey, J.; Zhou, S.; et al. Identification of functionally variant MDR1 alleles among European Americans and African Americans. *Clin. Pharmacol. Ther.* **2001**, *70*, 189–199. [CrossRef] [PubMed]

31. Kroetz, D.L.; Pauli-Magnus, C.; Hodges, L.M.; Huang, C.C.; Kawamoto, M.; Johns, S.J.; Stryke, D.; Ferrin, T.E.; DeYoung, J.; Taylor, T.; et al. Sequence diversity and haplotype structure in the human ABCB1 (MDR1, multidrug resistance transporter) gene. *Pharmacogenetics* **2003**, *13*, 481–494. [CrossRef]
32. Leschziner, G.D.; Andrew, T.; Pirmohamed, M.; Johnson, M.R. ABCB1 genotype and PGP expression, function and therapeutic drug response: A critical review and recommendations for future research. *Pharm. J.* **2007**, *7*, 154–179. [CrossRef]
33. Wang, D.; Johnson, A.D.; Papp, A.C.; Kroetz, D.L.; Sadée, W. Multidrug resistance polypeptide 1 (MDR1, ABCB1) variant 3435C>T affects mRNA stability. *Pharm. Genom.* **2005**, *15*, 693–704. [CrossRef]
34. Wu, L.X.; Zhao, H.B.; Wen, C.J.; Li, Y.; Shao, Y.Y.; Yang, Z.; Zhou, H.H. Combined influence of genetic polymorphism and DNA methylation on ABCB1 expression and function in healthy chinese males. *Eur. J. Drug Metab. Pharm.* **2016**, *42*, 627–634. [CrossRef]
35. Stampfuss, J.; Kubitza, D.; Becka, M.; Mueck, W. The effect of food on the absorption and pharmacokinetics of rivaroxaban. *Int. J. Clin. Pharmacol. Ther.* **2013**, *51*, 549–561. [CrossRef] [PubMed]
36. O'connor, C.T.; Kiernan, T.J.; Yan, B.P. The genetic basis of antiplatelet and anticoagulant therapy: A pharmacogenetic review of newer antiplatelets (clopidogrel, prasugrel and ticagrelor) and anticoagulants (dabigatran, rivaroxaban, apixaban and édoxaban). *Expert Opin. Drug Metab. Toxicol.* **2017**, *13*, 725–739. [CrossRef] [PubMed]
37. Harder, S. Pharmacokinetic and pharmacodynamic evaluation of rivaroxaban: Considerations for the treatment of venous thromboembolism. *Thromb. J.* **2014**, *12*, 22. [CrossRef] [PubMed]
38. Sychev, D.A.; Vardanyan, A.; Rozhkov, A.; Hachatryan, E.; Badanyan, A.; Smirnov, V.; Ananichuk, A.; Denisenko, N. CYP3A Activity and Rivaroxaban Serum Concentrations in Russian Patients with Deep Vein Thrombosis. *Genet. Test. Mol. Biomark.* **2018**, *22*, 51–54. [CrossRef] [PubMed]
39. Wang, D.; Guo, Y.; Wrighton, S.A.; Cooke, G.E.; Sadee, W. Intronic polymorphism in CYP3A4 affects hepatic expression and response to statin drugs. *Pharm. J.* **2011**, *11*, 274–286. [CrossRef] [PubMed]
40. Dai, D.; Tang, J.; Rose, R.; Hodgson, E.; Bienstock, R.J.; Mohrenweiser, H.W.; Goldstein, J.A. Identification of variants of CYP3A4 and characterization of their abilities to metabolize testosterone and chlorpyrifos. *J. Pharmacol. Exp. Ther.* **2001**, *299*, 825–831.
41. Kanuri, S.H.; Kreutz, R.P. Pharmacogenomics of novel direct oral anticoagulants: Newly identified genes and genetic variants. *J. Pers. Med.* **2019**, *9*, 7. [CrossRef]
42. Ašić, A.; Marjanović, D.; Mirat, J.; Primorac, D. Pharmacogenetics of novel oral anticoagulants: A review of identified gene variants & future perspectives. *PerMed* **2018**, *15*, 209–221. [CrossRef]
43. Palladino, M.; Merli, G.; Thomson, L. Evaluation of the oral direct factor Xa inhibitor–Betrixaban. *Expert Opin. Investig. Drugs.* **2013**, *22*, 1465–1472. [CrossRef]
44. Betrixaban: Highlights of Prescribing Information. Available online: https://www.accessdata.fda.gov/drugsatfda_docs/label/2017/208383s000lbl.pdf (accessed on 21 December 2020).
45. Reilly, P.A.; Lehr, T.; Haertter, S.; Connolly, S.J.; Yusuf, S.; Eikelboom, J.W.; Ezekowitz, M.D.; Nehmiz, G.; Wang, S.; Wallentin, L.; et al. The effect of dabigatran plasma concentrations and patient characteristics on the frequency of ischemic stroke and major bleeding in atrial fibrillation patients: The RE-LY Trial (Randomized Evaluation of Long-Term Anticoagulation Therapy). *J. Am. Coll. Cardiol.* **2014**, *63*, 321–328. [CrossRef]
46. Ruff, C.T.; Giugliano, R.P.; Braunwald, E.; Morrow, D.A.; Murphy, S.A.; Kuder, J.F.; Deenadayalu, N.; Jarolim, P.; Betcher, J.; Shi, M.; et al. Association between edoxaban dose, concentration, anti-Factor Xa activity, and outcomes: An analysis of data from the randomised, double-blind ENGAGE AF-TIMI 48 trial. *Lancet* **2015**, *385*, 2288–2295. [CrossRef]
47. Kaufman, A.L.; Spitz, J.; Jacobs, M.; Sorrentino, M.; Yuen, S.; Danahey, K.; Saner, D.; Klein, T.E.; Altman, R.B.; Ratain, M.J.; et al. Evidence for Clinical Implementation of Pharmacogenomics in Cardiac Drugs. *Mayo Clin. Proc.* **2015**, *90*, 716–729. [CrossRef] [PubMed]
48. Whirl-Carrillo, M.; McDonagh, E.M.; Hebert, J.M.; Gong, L.; Sangkuhl, K.; Thorn, C.F.; Altman, R.B.; Klein, T.E. Pharmacogenomics knowledge for personalized medicine. *Clin. Pharmacol. Ther.* **2012**, *92*, 414–417. [CrossRef] [PubMed]
49. DAPHNE Study: Direct Anticoagulant PHarmacogeNEtic. Available online: https://clinicaltrials.gov/ct2/show/NCT03112525 (accessed on 27 August 2020).
50. Kimmel, S.E.; French, B.; Kasner, S.E.; Johnson, J.A.; Anderson, J.L.; Gage, B.F.; Rosenberg, Y.D.; Eby, C.S.; Madigan, R.A.; McBane, R.B.; et al. A pharmacogenetic versus a clinical algorithm for warfarin dosing. *N. Engl. J. Med.* **2013**, *369*, 2283–2293. [CrossRef]
51. Pirmohamed, M.; Burnside, G.; Eriksson, N.; Jorgensen, A.L.; Toh, C.H.; Nicholson, T. A randomized trial of genotype-guided dosing of warfarin. *N. Engl. J. Med.* **2013**, *369*, 2294–2303. [CrossRef]
52. Claassens, D.M.F.; Vos, G.J.A.; Bergmeijer, T.O.; Hermanides, R.S.; van't Hof, A.W.J.; van der Harst, P.; Barbato, E.; Morisco, C.; Tjon Joe Gin, R.M.; Asselbergs, F.W.; et al. A genotype-guided strategy for oral P2Y12 inhibitors in primary PCI. *N. Engl. J. Med.* **2019**, *381*, 1621–1631. [CrossRef]
53. Roden, D.M. Clopidogrel pharmacogenetics-why the wait? *N. Engl. J. Med.* **2019**, *381*, 1677–1678. [CrossRef]
54. Ragia, G.; Manolopoulos, V.G. Pharmacogenomics of anticoagulation therapy: The last 10 years. *Pharmacogenomics* **2019**, *20*, 1113–1117. [CrossRef]

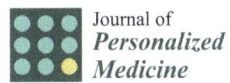

Article

A Novel Nomenclature for Repeat Motifs in the Thymidylate Synthase Enhancer Region and Its Relevance for Pharmacogenetic Studies

Dominic Schaerer [1,2,†], Tanja K. Froehlich [1,†], Seid Hamzic [1,2], Steven M. Offer [3], Robert B. Diasio [3], Markus Joerger [4]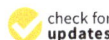, Ursula Amstutz [1] and Carlo R. Largiadèr [1,*]

1. University Institute of Clinical Chemistry, Inselspital, Bern University Hospital, University of Bern, 3010 Bern, Switzerland; Dominic.schaerer@extern.insel.ch (D.S.); tanja.froehlich@insel.ch (T.K.F.); se.hamzic@gmail.com (S.H.); ursula.amstutz@insel.ch (U.A.)
2. Graduate School for Cellular and Biomedical Sciences, University of Bern, 3012 Bern, Switzerland
3. Department of Molecular Pharmacology and Experimental Therapeutics, Mayo Clinic, Rochester, MN 55905, USA; offer.steven1@mayo.edu (S.M.O.); diasio.robert@mayo.edu (R.B.D.)
4. Department of Medical Oncology, Cantonal Hospital St. Gallen, 9007 St. Gallen, Switzerland; markus.joerger@kssg.ch
* Correspondence: carlo.largiader@insel.ch; Tel.: +41-31-632-9545
† These authors contributed equally to this work.

Received: 21 September 2020; Accepted: 16 October 2020; Published: 19 October 2020

Abstract: Inhibition of thymidylate synthase (TS) is the primary mode of action for 5-fluorouracil (5FU) chemotherapy. TS expression is modulated by a variable number of tandem repeats in the TS enhancer region (TSER) located upstream of the TS gene (*TYMS*). Variability in the TSER has been suggested to contribute to 5FU-induced adverse events. However, the precise genetic associations remain largely undefined due to high polymorphism and ambiguity in defining genotypes. To assess toxicity associations, we sequenced the TSER in 629 cancer patients treated with 5FU. Of the 13 alleles identified, few could be unambiguously named using current TSER-nomenclature. We devised a concise and unambiguous systematic naming approach for TSER-alleles that encompasses all known variants. After applying this comprehensive naming system to our data, we demonstrated that the number of upstream stimulatory factor (USF1-)binding sites in the TSER was significantly associated with gastrointestinal toxicity in 5FU treatment.

Keywords: 5-fluorouracil; capecitabine; fluoropyrimidine; thymidylate synthase; thymidylate synthase enhancer region; upstream stimulatory factor 1; adverse drug reactions

---

1. Introduction

As the only de novo source of thymidylate, thymidylate synthase (TS) has a major role in DNA replication through catalyzing the conversion of deoxyuridine-monophosphate to deoxythymidine-monophosphate (dTMP), a precursor of deoxythymidine-triphosphate. Thymidylate synthase gene (TYMS) expression levels are low in resting phase cells and high in proliferating cells [1]. Inhibition of TS in proliferating cells leads to severe DNA damage, eventually resulting in cell death [2] and, thus, represents an enticing therapeutic target in cancer. The antimetabolite 5-fluorouracil (5FU) and its oral prodrug capecitabine (Cp) are among the most commonly used chemotherapeutic agents for the treatment of solid carcinomas [3], systemically affecting proliferating cells. Fluorodeoxyuridine-monophosphate, a metabolite of 5FU, forms a stable ternary complex with TS and the co-factor 5,10-methylene tetrahydrofolate, resulting in inhibition of dTMP synthesis. The subsequent imbalance of the nucleotide pool leads to DNA damage and apoptosis [2]. Although

TS is the major target of 5FU, and its systemic inhibition leads to serious toxicity, no TYMS variants have been shown to be clinically relevant predictive markers of 5FU toxicity.

TYMS is located on chromosome 18p11.32, has a length of ~16 kb, and consists of seven exons. It does not contain typical eukaryotic promoter DNA motifs, such as a TATA or CAAT box. However, other regulating motifs in its 5′-UTR have been identified [4]. A 28bp variable number of tandem repeats (rs45445694) in the TYMS enhancer region (TSER) has been reported to affect transcription [5] with two repeats being less efficient than three [6]. A vast majority of the population carries alleles with either two or three repeats in this region [7]; however, individuals with as many as nine TSER-repeats have been described [8,9]. Those repeats are commonly named according to the corresponding number of repeats, e.g., TSER-2R or simply 2R for the two repeats, 3R for three, etc. [7,10,11]. This nomenclature is referred to here as "repeat number" (RN-) nomenclature. Furthermore, a G > C SNP (rs2853542) at position 12 of the second repeat of the triple repeat allele has been suggested to reduce transcription by abolishing an upstream stimulatory factor (USF1)-binding site [12,13]. SNP status is commonly depicted by listing the nucleotide directly following the repeat (e.g., 3RG or 3RC [8,14,15]). In addition, a rare G > C SNP (rs183205964) has been described in the TSER-2R allele, carrying a G > C base change at the 12th nucleotide of the first 28bp-repeat, which is commonly depicted as 2RG or 2RC [14,15]. This nomenclature, which also takes the SNP into account (e.g., 2RC, 3RG, etc.), is referred to herein as "repeat number, binding site, SNP" (RNBS-) nomenclature. A functional study showed that the 2RC allele has the lowest transcriptional activity of all known TSER-alleles [16]. Studies of TYMS and the TSER as potential markers for tumor progression, overall survival, and 5FU-induced toxicity have yielded inconclusive and, often, conflicting results, likely due to varying considerations for TSER-repeat number and SNP status, as well as ambiguity in allele definitions [6,12,15–25].

A recently published meta-analysis [10] reported that the polymorphism c.742-227G>A (rs2612091) within the Enolase Superfamily Member 1 gene (ENOSF1) was associated with the development of severe hand-foot syndrome (HFS) in 5FU/Cp-treated patients. The ENOSF1 and TYMS genes partially overlap on chromosome 18 and are transcribed in opposite directions. In-vitro studies suggested that ENOSF1 might regulate TYMS at the protein and RNA levels [26]. In addition to the polymorphism in ENOSF1, the TSER-2R variant was also associated with an increased risk of HFS in the same study. However, consistent with other studies, only 2R and 3R alleles were distinguished and considered in analyses, and SNP status was not taken into account [7,11]. Therefore, for the present study, we investigated the complex enhancer structure of TYMS in a large Caucasian cohort and assessed the effect of genetic variation in this region on the development of 5FU-related toxicity.

The TSER was sequenced in 629 patients of primarily Caucasian ancestry that were treated with the fluoropyrimidine-based chemotherapy containing either 5FU or Cp. In total, 13 unique TSER-sequence variants were discovered. Using RN-and RNBS-nomenclature, we were not able to classify all detected variants unambiguously. Therefore, we devised an improved naming strategy that permits systematic classification of all discovered sequence variants in the TSER. Furthermore, associations between the identified repeat structures and severe fluoropyrimidine-related toxicity were also investigated. The focus of the present study was specifically on early-onset toxicities where the clinical relevance of predictive genetic markers is likely to be highest.

2. Materials and Methods

2.1. Patient Samples

This study included 515 patients from a previously described cohort [27] and 114 additional patients recruited between February 2013 and December 2014 at the same centers using the same inclusion criteria. Except for nine subjects, all patients self-declared their ancestry as Caucasian. Of the 629 total patients, 614 were prospectively recruited and 15 were retrospective cases (toxicity grade 2–5). All patients were treated with 5FU- or Cp-based chemotherapy (Table 1). Blood samples were collected and adverse events for 13 hematologic, gastrointestinal, infection, and dermatologic categories were recorded during the first two chemotherapy cycles. Adverse events were classified according to the Common Terminology Criteria for Adverse Events (CTCAE) v3.0 [28]. All subjects gave their informed consent for inclusion before they participated in the study. The study was conducted in accordance with the Declaration of Helsinki, and the protocol was approved by the Ethics Committees of the Cantons of Bern, Switzerland (131/07; 150/2015) and St. Gallen, Switzerland (09/104/2B).

Table 1. Clinical, demographic, and toxicity data. The cohort consisted of 629 participants. FOLFOX: chemotherapy regimen based on a combination of LV, 5FU (5-fluorouracil), and oxaliplatin; FOLFIRI: chemotherapy regimen based on a combination of LV, 5FU, and irinotecan; Cp: capecitabine; CPL: cis-or carboplatin; D: docetaxel; E: epirubicin; LV: leucovorin.

	Grade 3–5		Grade 0–2		Total
	N	%	N	%	N
Total					
Total cohort	106	17	523	83	629
Collection					
Prospectively	92	15	522	85	614
Retrospectively	14	93	1	7	15
Sex					
Female	55	22	192	78	247
Male	51	13	331	87	382
Ancestry					
Caucasian	104	17	516	83	620
Arab	0	0	3	100	3
African	1	50	1	50	2
Asian	0	0	2	100	2
Unknown	1	50	1	50	2
Treatment					
FOLFOX, FOLFIRI	22	10	192	90	214
5FU +/−LV	12	11	100	89	112
5FU, CPL +/−D,E	36	30	86	70	122
Other 5FU regimen	10	28	26	72	36
Cp	26	18	119	82	145
Toxicity category					
Hematologic toxicity	58	9	571	91	629
Gastrointestinal toxicity	55	9	574	91	629
Infection	24	4	605	96	629
Dermatologic toxicity	15	2	614	98	629

2.2. PCR and Sequence Analysis

Genomic DNA was extracted from EDTA blood samples using the BioRobot EZ1 (Qiagen, Hilden, Germany) and the EZ1 DNA blood 350 L Kit (Qiagen). PCR reactions were performed using the GC-rich PCR System (Roche Applied Science, Basel, Switzerland) on GeneAmp 9700 Thermal Cyclers (Applied Biosystems, Foster City, CA, USA). Detailed information for primers and PCR products are shown in Figure 1A. PCR conditions consisted of a denaturation step of 3 min at 96 °C, followed by 45 cycles of 30 s at 96 °C, 30 s at 60 °C and 45 s at 72 °C, and a final extension step of 10 min at 72 °C. In five patients the genotype could not be inferred unambiguously. Therefore, the amplification products were separated by gel electrophoresis followed by a purification of the corresponding bands with the QIAquick Gel Extraction Kit (Qiagen). The purified fragments were amplified again with the GC-rich PCR System. Amplification products were sequenced using the Big Dye Terminator v3.1 Cycle Sequencing kit (Applied Biosystems, Foster City, CA, USA) and an ABI Prism 3130× L Genetic Analyzer (Applied Biosystems, Foster City, CA, USA). Forward and reverse sequence analysis, including SNP calling and repeat structure detection, were performed using Sequencher 4.10.1 (Gene Codes Corporation, Ann Arbor, MI, USA) with heterozygous base calling. Heterozygous genotypes were called using the IUPAC nucleotide ambiguity code provided by Sequencher, as each heterozygous allele combination generates a specific nucleotide ambiguity code pattern.

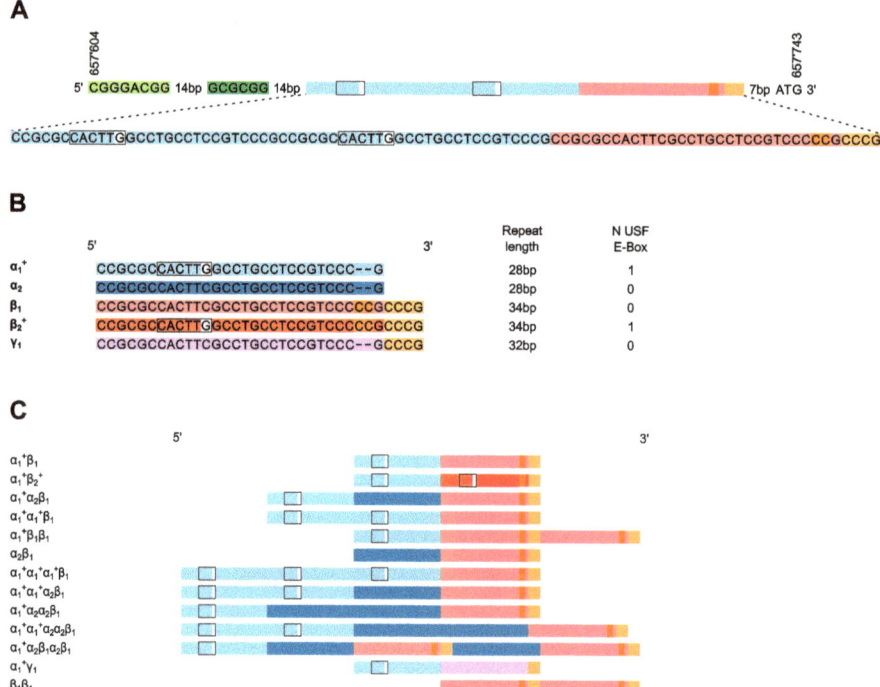

Figure 1. The reference and observed structures of the *TYMS* TSER-region. (A) The reference structure of the TSER (NC_000018.10:657'604.657'743) consists of three imperfect repeats. Upstream of the repeats, an inverted repeat is indicated in light and dark green. The region was PCR-amplified using the forward primer 5'-GTG-GCT-CCT-GCG-TTT-CCC-CC-3' (position 657543; 200bp upstream of the start codon in the NC_000018.10 reference) and the reverse primer 5'-GCT-CCG-AGC-CGG-CCA-CAG-GCA-TG-3' (including the start codon at the 3'-end indicated in bold) (B) Shown here are five variants of the imperfect tandem repeats together with the length of each repeat that were observed in 1258 sequenced *TYMS*-promoter region alleles. The presence of the USF1-binding E-box is indicated as a box for each of the five repeats. (C) Shown here are the 13 different TSER-alleles observed in 629 sequenced patients with the corresponding new nomenclature.

2.3. Statistical Analyses

The cohort was tested for deviations from Hardy-Weinberg-Equilibrium (HWE) with respect to TSER using the Genepop package of R (v3.6.3) [29]. Differences in allele frequencies between populations were assessed using Fisher's exact tests. Univariable and multivariable logistic regression analyses for the assessment of genetic associations of TSER-repeat number and of binding site number with 5FU toxicity (two toxicity groups: grade 0–2, 3–5) as well as the Fisher's exact test were performed using the R package Stats [30]. Multivariable regression models were adjusted for sex, age, concomitant cis-or carboplatin (CPL) administration, and *DPYD*-risk variant carrier status. Co-administration of cis- or carboplatin was previously shown to be associated with increased early-onset toxicity in this cohort, whereas no effect was observed for other concomitant chemotherapeutics (e.g., oxaliplatin, anthracyclines), or for 5FU versus capecitabine [27]. *DPYD*-risk variants were defined for this study as the minor alleles for rs3918290, rs67376798, rs55886062, and rs75017182, all of which have been demonstrated to significantly increase risk for 5FU-induced toxicity [31]. Association tests between 5FU-toxicity and TSER-repeat numbers were performed using additive genetic models for the TSER-repeat number variable; patients carrying alleles with more than three TSER-repeat elements were excluded from these specific analyses. In all analyses, p-values < 0.05 were considered significant.

3. Results

3.1. Polymorphisms in the TSER

Sequencing analysis of the TSER, which encompassed the inverted repeat located upstream of the variable number of tandem repeats through the ATG-initiation codon (Figure 1A), was performed in 629 patients. Thirteen unique TSER-variants were identified among the 1258 sequenced alleles (Table 2). All TSER-genotypes were found to be in HWE. No variation was detected in the upstream inverted repeat region (NC_000018.10:657'604.657'645) or in the region between the TSER and the ATG-initiation codon.

Several sequence variants within the TSER-repeats could not be distinguished by fragment-length analyses. Therefore, those alleles could not be classified unambiguously according to the commonly used RN-nomenclature of TSER-polymorphisms that is based on scoring the apparent number of tandem repeats (Figure 1B, Table 2). Specifically, all TSER-alleles were composed of varying combinations of five different variants of the imperfect tandem-repeat elements. Several combinations of these variants could not be classified even with the more specific RNBS-nomenclature, and the unambiguous classification of variant combinations using reference SNPs was not possible. Therefore, we devised a new nomenclature to designate a 28bp-, a 34bp-, and a 32bp-variant of the repeat element using combinations of the Greek letters α, β, and γ, respectively. Compared to the α-variant, the β-and γ-variants are characterized by six and four additional bases, respectively, at the 3'-end of the repeat element. Subscript numbers are used to differentiate different alleles within a repeat. Additionally, the presence of a putative USF1-binding site within a repeat (created by the G allele at position 12 in α- or β-repeats) is denoted with a superscript plus sign (Figure 1B). While USF1-binding site presence would also be indicated by specific subscript numbers, the inclusion of the plus superscript notation enables rapid assessment of the number of sites in a given allele.

It is noted that this nomenclature is highly extensible. Any newly identified repeat with a length other than 28 bp, 32 bp, or 34 bp can be labelled with subsequent Greek letters. Similarly, the already known repeat structures can be extended as new sequence variants are discovered by increasing the subscript number. If the new variant contains a USF1-binding site, the plus superscript designation would also apply.

For all TSER-alleles observed in this study, the most 3'-repeat element was a β- or γ-variant. The β-elements almost exclusively contained a C at position 12 and were designated β_1. In the majority of TSER-alleles, the 3'-terminal β-element was preceded by one or multiple α-elements (Figure 1C). However, rare TSER-alleles containing multiple β-elements were observed. One example of such a multiple β-element-containing allele was also observed previously in a Japanese cohort [8], in which it was referred to as 3Rc-ins. The sequence structure of this 3Rc-ins allele is consistent with a duplication of the β_1-repeat region, indicating that the haploid genotype would be denoted as $\alpha_1\beta_1\beta_1$. One allele carrying a G at position 12 in the β-repeat and one allele with a deletion of CC at position 28 in the β-repeat were observed. These variants were designated β_2 and γ_1, respectively. Besides the single β_2 and γ_1 alleles, no alleles without a β_1 repeat were observed in the remaining 1256 alleles. Seven alleles with two repeats and no USF-binding site were observed. The new nomenclature allowed us to depict the highly variable repeat patterns (Figure 1C) in a concise and unambiguous way that simultaneously denotes the number of repeats, the type and the order of repeat elements, and the presence of USF-binding sites ($\alpha_1^+ + \beta_2^+$). For example, the allele previously named as 3RG consists of two identical 28bp-repeats followed by a 34bp-repeat, which has a C instead of a G at position 12. With the proposed nomenclature the 3RG-allele is designated $\alpha_1^+\alpha_1^+\beta_1$ and consists of two α_1^+-and one β_1-subunits, indicating that the allele contains two potential USF1-binding sites

Table 2. Frequencies of TSER (TYMS enhancer region)-polymorphisms. Each of the 13 alleles in our cohort (N = 629) plus one allele ($\alpha_1^+\alpha_1^+\alpha_1^+\alpha_2\beta_1$) only detected in the Japanese cohort (N = 263) previously reported by Kim et al. [8] is listed using the "New", the "repeat number" (RN-), and the "repeat number, binding site, SNP" (RNBS-) nomenclature (columns 1, 2, and 3; *: allelic designations given by Kim et al. [8]; na: no name could be assigned using this nomenclature). For each allele, the number (N) of USF1 (upstream stimulatory factor)-binding sites (column 4), the number (N) of alleles (column 5), and the allele frequency (f%) (column 6) within the cohort is shown. For comparison, column 7 shows the frequency of the common alleles in a Japanese cohort. Column 8 lists the p-values from Fisher's exact test for population allele frequency differences between the study cohort and the population from Kim et al. [8].

New Nomenclature	Repeat Number (RN-) Nomenclature	Repeat Number, Binding Site, SNP (RNBS-) Nomenclature	USF1-Binding Sites N	Allele N	Allele f%	Kim et al. f%	p-Value
$a_1^+b_1$	2R	2RG	1	561	44.6	12.4	<0.0001
$a_1^+a_2b_1$	3R	3RC	1	360	28.6	42.0	<0.0001
$a_1^+a_1^+b_1$	3R	3RG	2	308	24.5	42.1	<0.0001
$a_1^+b_1b_1$	3R	3RC-ins *	1	12	1.0	0.2	ns
a_2b_1	2R	2RC	0	6	0.5	-	-
$a_1^+a_1^+a_1^+b_1$	4R	na	3	4	0.3	-	-
$a_1^+b_2$	2R	2RG	2	1	0.1	-	-
$a_1^+a_1^+a_2b_1$	4R	4RC *	2	1	0.1	0.2	ns
$a_1^+a_2b_1$	4R	na	1	1	0.1	-	-
$a_1^+a_1^+a_2a_2b_1$	5R	na	2	1	0.1	-	-
$a_1^+a_2b_1a_2b_1$	5R	na	1	1	0.1	-	-
$a_1^+\gamma_1$	2R	2RG	1	1	0.1	-	-
b_1b_1	2R	2RC	0	1	0.1	-	-
$a_1^+a_1^+a_1^+a_2b_1$	5R	5RC *	3	0	0.0	2.1	<0.0001

Because different TSER-repeat numbers were observed in different ethnic groups [9,32], we compared the polymorphism frequencies of our large cohort with a Japanese cohort [8] to assess ethnic differences at the repeat-structure level. Indeed, we observed that frequencies of $\alpha_1^+\beta_1$, $\alpha_1^+\alpha_2\beta_1$ and $\alpha_1^+\alpha_1^+\beta_1$ TSER-variants differed substantially between Caucasian and Japanese populations (Table 2), with $\alpha_1^+\beta_1$ being more frequent in Caucasians and $\alpha_1^+\alpha_2\beta_1$ and $\alpha_1^+\alpha_1^+\beta_1$ being more frequent in the Japanese population. Interestingly, the frequency of the G > C polymorphism containing α_2-repeat as a second repeat in alleles with three repeat elements was similar compared to the frequency of α_1^+ in this position. This was true in both populations. Approximately half of the three-repeat element-alleles contained α_2 as the second repeat. The $\alpha_1^+\alpha_1^+\alpha_1^+\alpha_2\beta_1$-allele was only observed in the Japanese cohort, whereas the similar $\alpha_1^+\alpha_1^+\alpha_2\alpha_2\beta_1$-allele was only detected in the Caucasian cohort.

3.2. Distribution of the Number of USF1-Binding Sites Between Different TSER-Repeat Genotypes

The transcription factor USF1 has been shown to bind to the consensus recognition domains in the TSER to activate *TYMS* transcription [13]. Therefore, for further correlative studies we also classified the alleles based on the number of USF1-binding sites. The USF1-binding sites number in the most commonly detected TSER-repeat genotypes was assessed (Figure 2). Patients homozygous for the 2R-genotype almost exclusively carried two USF1-binding sites. Three 2R/2R patients carried only one USF1-binding site in the TSER; one patient carried three USF1-binding sites. In heterozygous 2R/3R-carriers, the most frequent number of binding sites was also two. Among patients with a homozygous 3R-genotype, three binding sites were observed most frequently. In total, eight patients carried alleles with more than three repeat elements and could therefore not be assigned to any of the three genotype combinations (2R/2R, 2R/3R, 3R/3R). These participants carried between two and five USF1-binding sites in TSERs.

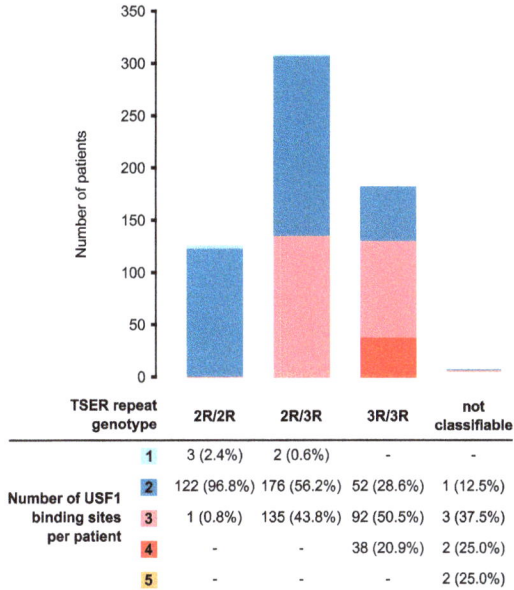

Figure 2. Number of USF1-binding sites per TSER-repeat genotype. Patients were classified according to the number of repeat elements. The number of USF1-binding sites per patient was subsequently determined. Eight patients carried alleles with more than three repeat elements and could therefore not be assigned to a 2R-3R genotype.

3.3. Association Analyses of TYMS TSER-Variants with Severe 5FU Toxicity

The association of the TSER-repeat polymorphisms with toxicity was assessed using univariable and multivariable logistic regression analyses with two different models of allele classification. Model I was based on the number of USF-binding sites per patient extracted from the new nomenclature and which allowed the inclusion of all TSER-genotypes. Model II was based on RN-nomenclature and excluded patients carrying alleles with more than three repeat elements.

In the univariable analysis, the number of USF1-binding sites was associated with the risk of developing early-onset gastrointestinal toxicity (OR 1.66, $p = 0.043$; Table 3). After adjustment for sex, age, carboplatin treatment, and *DPYD*-risk variant carrier status, the risk of severe gastrointestinal toxicity remained significantly higher in patients with fewer USF1-binding sites in TSER (OR 1.74, $p = 0.034$). The association between gastrointestinal toxicity and the number of USF1-binding sites was also significant in a subgroup analysis containing only patients with 2R and 3R genotypes ($n = 621$; data not shown). As shown in Figure 3A, the frequency of gastrointestinal toxicity decreased gradually from 20% in patients carrying one USF1-binding site to 0% in patients with five binding sites. Associations did not reach significance when assessing other toxicity classes or overall toxicity.

Table 3. Toxicity association with number of USF1-binding sites. Associations were assessed in the full cohort ($n = 629$). *p*-values from logistic regression models; [1] adjusted for cis-and carboplatin co-administration, sex, age, and *DPYD*-risk variants. Significant *p*-values are shown in bold.

Outcome	Univariable			Multivariable [1]		
	OR	95% CI	*p*-Value	OR	95% CI	*p*-Value
Overall toxicity	1.04	0.76–1.46	0.793	1.08	0.77–1.54	0.670
Hematologic toxicity	0.73	0.49–1.10	0.122	0.73	0.48–1.13	0.148
Gastrointestinal toxicity	1.66	1.04–2.77	**0.043**	1.74	1.06–2.99	**0.034**
Infection	1.1	0.59–2.20	0.769	1.14	0.57–2.43	0.723
Dermatologic toxicity	1.29	0.58–3.27	0.558	1.28	0.57–3.25	0.576

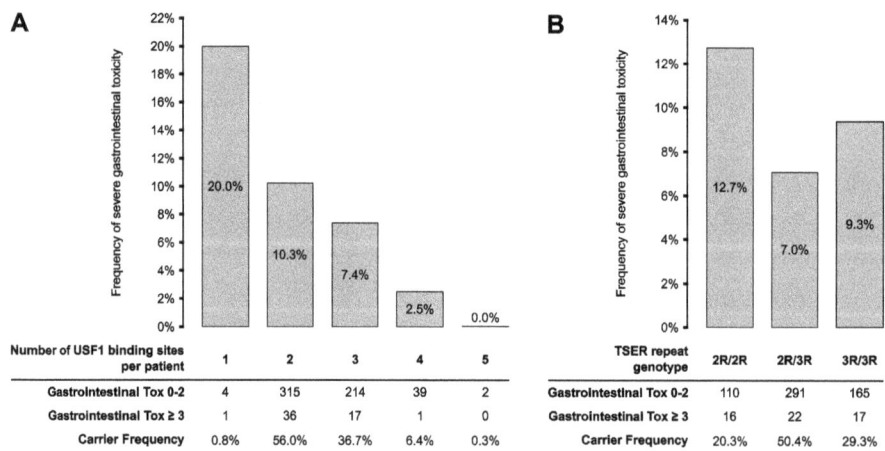

Figure 3. Frequency of severe gastrointestinal toxicity according to number of USF1-binding sites and TSER-repeat genotypes. Gastrointestinal toxicity frequencies were stratified according to (**A**) the number of USF1-binding sites in the full cohort of 629 patients and (**B**) TSER-repeat genotype in a subcohort of 607 patients carrying only 2R or 3R polymorphisms.

The number of TSER-repeats alone (i.e., in analyses that did not evaluate the number of USF1-binding sites) was not significantly associated with gastrointestinal toxicity (univariable: OR 1.28, $p = 0.424$; multivariable: OR 1.21, $p = 0.348$; Table 4). However, the frequency of severe gastrointestinal toxicity was higher in homozygous 2R patients compared to the other two genotypes (Figure 3B), consistent with the lower number of USF1-bindings sites in these patients. Of 182 patients homozygous for 3R, 9.3% experienced toxicity grade ≥3 vs. 12.7% of 126 patients homozygous for 2R. Other toxicities were also not associated with the number of TSER-repeats in univariable or multivariable analyses.

Table 4. Toxicity association with number of TSER-repeats. Associations were assessed in the 621 patients carrying only two or three repeat-element alleles. *p*-values from logistic regression models; [1] adjusted for cis-and carboplatin co-administration, sex, age, and *DPYD*-risk variants.

Outcome	Univariable			Multivariable [1]		
	OR	95% CI	*p*-Value	OR	95% CI	*p*-Value
Overall toxicity	0.96	0.71–1.30	0.814	0.98	0.71–1.34	0.887
Hematological toxicity	0.73	0.49–1.08	0.119	0.75	0.49–1.13	0.174
Gastrointestinal toxicity	1.18	0.79–1.75	0.424	1.21	0.81–1.82	0.348
Infection	0.93	0.51–1.66	0.803	1.06	0.58–1.93	0.845
Dermatological toxicity	1.05	0.50–2.19	0.895	0.97	0.45–2.04	0.929

4. Discussion

In the present study, we performed a sequence-based analysis of the TSER-region in a cohort of 629 5FU-treated patients that self-declared as "Caucasian". Thirteen unique TSER-sequence variants were observed (Table 2), of which not all could be assigned unambiguous genotypes using the current RN or RNBS nomenclatures. Based on available information, we hypothesized that the number of intact USF1-binding sites, which is dependent upon both the number of repeats and the variant status within each repeat, is a contributor to 5FU toxicity risk. To address this hypothesis, we developed a novel approach to assigning allele designations in the TSER that incorporates this information. These genotypes were then assessed in correlative studies. We demonstrated that this improved naming system can unambiguously assign allele names to all known TSER-sequences. Using this information, we subsequently demonstrated that the number of USF1-binding sites within the TSER, not the repeat status itself, was significantly associated with gastrointestinal toxicity in 5FU/Cp treatment.

The RN-nomenclature was previously introduced to classify TSER-fragment-length polymorphisms by gel-electrophoresis [12]. Later studies added *HaeIII* digestion to detect the G > C SNP at position 12 of the repeats, giving rise to RNBS-nomenclature [19]. Neither naming system can accommodate sequence-level information. The novel nomenclature system introduced herein overcomes those limitations by distinguishing 28, 34, and 32 base pair repeat motifs as α, β, and γ, respectively, and by designating sequence variants within each repeat using subscript numbers (Figure 1B). Using this new method, all previously reported [8,33] repeat combinations, their structural order, and variant status can be designated in a concise and unambiguous manner.

USF1 is a transcription factor that usually binds symmetrical E-box sequences (5′-CACGTG-3′) and for *TYMS* TSER, it was shown that the factor can also bind to the sequence 5′-CACTTG-3′ [13]. With the TSER, the number of USF1-binding sites varies depending on the number of repeat sequences (Figure 2) and the genotype (G/C) at position 12 in the repeat, with the C allele abolishing the consensus-binding site. The TSER-nomenclature we present in this manuscript clearly denotes the presence of a USF1-binding site within each repeat, overcoming another limitation of RN/RNBS-nomenclature. For example, a 4R-allele has been previously reported [9], the repeat-motif composition of which is not overtly clear using the RN-nomenclature. In the present study, we observed three alleles ($\alpha_1^+\alpha_1^+\alpha_1^+\beta_1$, $\alpha_1^+\alpha_1^+\alpha_2\beta_1$, $\alpha_1^+\alpha_2\alpha_2\beta_1$) that would be classified as 4R; however, the number of USF1-binding sites, as well as the SNP composition, varies in each.

The number of USF1-binding sites per patient in our cohort varied between one and five. Our data demonstrate a significant inverse correlation between gastrointestinal toxicity and the number of TSER USF1-binding sites. This finding is consistent with another recent study that found ≤1 TSER USF1-binding site per patient to be associated with an increased risk of overall severe toxicity to 5FU [15]. In that study, gastrointestinal toxicity was also more common in patients with ≤1 binding site;

however, statistical significance was not achieved [15]. Another study reported a similar non-significant trend for this apparent protective effect against 5FU-induced toxicity [34]. These observations can be explained by increased *TYMS* transcriptional activity in patients with more USF1-binding sites. It is noted that in a small cohort of 29 colorectal cancer patients, transcriptional activity was not shown to be conclusively associated with the number of USF1-binding sites [16]. Therefore, additional adequately powered in vivo and in vitro studies are needed to precisely define the role of USF1-driven transcription of *TYMS* in 5FU toxicity.

Notable differences in TSER-genotype frequencies have been reported for populations with different racial/ethnic compositions, providing further impetus for a robust naming system that can accommodate diverse genotypes. Whereas our cohort displayed similar TSER-repeat frequencies as in other large Caucasian cohorts [34,35], the frequencies of $\alpha_1^+\beta_1$, $\alpha_1^+\alpha_2\beta_1$, $\alpha_1^+\alpha_1^+\beta_1$, and $\alpha_1^+\alpha_1^+\alpha_1^+\alpha_2\beta_1$ differed substantially from a previously reported Japanese population [8]. Eight TSER-variants were identified in our cohort that were not present in the Japanese cohort (Table 2). Further comparisons with other ethnic groups could provide additional insight into toxicity risk predictors; however, other studies, including a study of African individuals [9], only reported the number of repeats, limiting potential analyses. As a first application of the proposed nomenclature, our results highlight the importance of considering USF1-binding sites, as the analysis based on the RN-nomenclature failed to identify a toxicity association.

Several large meta-analyses [7,10,11] have reported that either the 2R/2R-genotype or the 2R-allele were associated with a higher toxicity risk. In a cohort of Cp-treated patients, 2R-carriers were predominantly associated with increased risk for diarrhea [7]. In partial agreement with this finding, our study found higher levels of severe gastrointestinal toxicity in homozygous 2R-allele carriers; however, this finding was not statistically significant. Collectively, the correlations between toxicity and 2R that have been reported by previous studies remains consistent with our results because 2R-repeats are more likely to carry a reduced number of USF1-binding sites compared to larger repeat expansions (e.g., 3R; Figure 2). Our data suggest that expanded considerations that encompass USF1-binding sites may offer greater predictive value.

One limitation to our study was that the cohort was not large enough to fully investigate rare TSER-variants for toxicity associations. Anecdotal evidence suggests that 5FU-treated patients with rare TSER-genotype combinations, for example without any USF1-binding site, might have a strongly increased risk of severe adverse events [15]. However, the limited sample size in the present report was inadequate to address this question; future expanded studies are planned where we can fully utilize all information encoded by the new nomenclature. In contrast to Hamzic et al. [10], we did not observe an association between the 2R-allele and HFS. Notably, our cohort consisted mainly of 5FU-treated patients, and HFS is considered an adverse event specific to Cp, not 5FU [36]. The limited number of Cp-treated patients, coupled with the low overall occurrence of severe HFS in our cohort, provided inadequate statistical power to assess this association. An additional trial conducted in North America did not find TSER-repeat number to be associated with toxicity [18]. While the exact reason for this discrepancy with our results cannot be inferred, the focus on irinotecan-based therapies in that trial and the masking effects of uninvestigated *DPYD*-risk variants may have contributed.

5. Conclusions

In conclusion, we propose a simple nomenclature for TSER-alleles that encodes multiple levels of information pertaining to repeats, variants, and USF1-binding sites. This concise and unambiguous naming system can accommodate rare and novel sequence variants and, therefore, enables expanded analyses of TSER in association studies. After applying this comprehensive naming system to sequencing data gathered in a Caucasian cohort encompassing 629 5FU-treated cancer patients, we demonstrated that the number of upstream stimulatory factor (USF1-)binding sites in the TSER was significantly associated with gastrointestinal toxicity in 5FU treatment.

Author Contributions: Conceptualization, D.S., T.K.F., S.H., S.M.O., R.B.D., U.A. and C.R.L.; methodology, T.K.F.; software, T.K.F.; validation, D.S. and T.K.F.; formal analysis, D.S. and T.K.F.; investigation, D.S. and T.K.F.; resources, T.K.F., M.J. and C.R.L.; data curation, D.S. and T.K.F.; writing—original draft preparation, D.S., T.K.F. and C.R.L.; writing—review and editing, D.S., T.K.F., S.H., S.M.O., R.B.D., M.J., U.A. and C.R.L.; visualization, D.S. and T.K.F.; supervision, C.R.L; project administration, C.R.L.; funding acquisition, C.R.L. All authors have read and agreed to the published version of the manuscript.

Funding: This research was funded by Swiss National Science Foundation, grant number 163205.

Acknowledgments: We thank all investigators from participating oncology centers and G.A., G.M., D.S.-E., M.A., A.A. and D.S. for their laboratory work.

Conflicts of Interest: The authors declare no conflict of interest.

References

1. Navalgund, L.G.; Rossana, C.; Muench, A.J.; Johnson, L.F.; Gollakota, L.; Rossana, C.; Muench, A.J.; Johnson, L.F. Cell cycle regulation of thymidylate synthetase gene expression in cultured mouse fibroblasts. *J. Biol. Chem.* **1980**, *255*, 7386–7390. [PubMed]
2. Longley, D.B.; Harkin, D.P.; Johnston, P.G. 5-Fluorouracil: Mechanisms of action and clinical strategies. *Nat. Rev. Cancer* **2003**, *3*, 330–338. [CrossRef] [PubMed]
3. Meyerhardt, J.A.; Mayer, R.J. Systemic therapy for colorectal cancer. *N. Engl. J. Med.* **2005**, *352*, 476–487. [CrossRef] [PubMed]
4. Horie, N.; Takeishi, K. Identification of functional elements in the promoter region of the human gene for thymidylate synthase and nuclear factors that regulate the expression of the gene. *J. Biol. Chem.* **1997**, *272*, 18375–18381. [CrossRef]
5. Kaneda, S.; Nalbantoglu, J.; Takeishi, K.; Shimizu, K.; Gotoh, O.; Seno, T.; Ayusawa, D. Structural and functional analysis of the human thymidylate synthase gene. *J. Biol. Chem.* **1990**, *265*, 20277–20284.
6. Horie, N.; Takeishi, K.; Aiba, H.; Oguro, K.; Hojo, H. Functional analysis and DNA polymorphism of the tandemly repeated sequences in the 5'-Terminal Regulatory Region of the human gene for thymidylate synthase. *Cell Struct. Funct.* **1995**, *20*, 191–197. [CrossRef]
7. Rosmarin, D.; Palles, C.; Church, D.; Domingo, E.; Jones, A.; Johnstone, E.; Wang, H.; Love, S.; Julier, P.; Scudder, C.; et al. Genetic markers of toxicity from capecitabine and other fluorouracil-based regimens: Investigation in the QUASAR2 study, systematic review, and meta-analysis. *J. Clin. Oncol.* **2014**, *32*, 1031–1039. [CrossRef]
8. Kim, S.R.; Ozawa, S.; Saito, Y.; Kurose, K.; Kaniwa, N.; Kamatani, N.; Hamaguchi, T.; Shirao, K.; Muto, M.; Ohtsu, A.; et al. Fourteen novel genetic variations and haplotype structures of the TYMS gene encoding human thymidylate synthase (TS). *Drug Metab. Pharmacokinet.* **2006**, *21*, 509–516. [CrossRef]
9. Marsh, S.; Ameyaw, M.M.; Githang'a, J.; Indalo, A.; Ofori-Adjei, D.; McLeod, H.L. Novel thymidylate synthase enhancer region alleles in African populations. *Hum. Mutat.* **2000**, *16*, 528. [CrossRef]
10. Hamzic, S.; Kummer, D.; Froehlich, T.K.; Joerger, M.; Aebi, S.; Palles, C.; Thomlinson, I.; Meulendijks, D.; Schellens, J.H.M.; García-González, X.; et al. Evaluating the role of ENOSF1 and TYMS variants as predictors in fluoropyrimidine-related toxicities: An IPD meta-analysis. *Pharmacol. Res.* **2020**, *152*, 104594. [CrossRef]
11. Jennings, B.A.; Kwok, C.S.; Willis, G.; Matthews, V.; Wawruch, P.; Loke, Y.K. Functional polymorphisms of folate metabolism and response to chemotherapy for colorectal cancer, a systematic review and meta-analysis. *Pharmacogenet. Genom.* **2012**, *22*, 290–304. [CrossRef] [PubMed]
12. Kawakami, K.; Watanabe, G. Identification and functional analysis of single nucleotide polymorphism in the tandem repeat sequence of thymidylate synthase gene. *Cancer Res.* **2003**, *63*, 6004–6007. [PubMed]
13. Mandola, M.V.; Stoehlmacher, J.; Muller-Weeks, S.; Cesarone, G.; Yu, M.C.; Lenz, H.-J.J.; Ladner, R.D. A novel single nucleotide polymorphism within the 5' tandem repeat polymorphism of the thymidylate synthase gene abolishes USF-1 binding and alters transcriptional activity. *Cancer Res.* **2003**, *63*, 2898–2904. [PubMed]
14. Gusella, M.; Bolzonella, C.; Crepaldi, G.; Ferrazzi, E.; Padrini, R. A novel G/C single-nucleotide polymorphism in the double 28-bp repeat thymidylate synthase allele. *Pharmacogenomics J.* **2006**, *6*, 421–424. [CrossRef] [PubMed]
15. Meulendijks, D.; Jacobs, B.A.W.; Aliev, A.; Pluim, D.; Van Werkhoven, E.; Deenen, M.J.; Beijnen, J.H.; Cats, A.; Schellens, J.H.M. Increased risk of severe fluoropyrimidine-associated toxicity in patients carrying a G to

C substitution in the first 28-bp tandem repeat of the thymidylate synthase 2R allele. *Int. J. Cancer* **2016**, *138*, 245–253. [CrossRef]
16. De Bock, C.E.; Garg, M.B.; Scott, N.; Sakoff, J.A.; Scorgie, F.E.; Ackland, S.P.; Lincz, L.F. Association of thymidylate synthase enhancer region polymorphisms with thymidylate synthase activity in vivo. *Pharmacogenomics J.* **2011**, *11*, 307–314. [CrossRef] [PubMed]
17. Ruzzo, A.; Graziano, F.; Loupakis, F.; Rulli, E.; Canestrari, E.; Santini, D.; Catalano, V.; Ficarelli, R.; Maltese, P.; Bisonni, R.; et al. Pharmacogenetic profiling in patients with advanced colorectal cancer treated with first-line FOLFOX-4 chemotherapy. *J. Clin. Oncol.* **2007**, *25*, 1247–1254. [CrossRef] [PubMed]
18. McLeod, H.L.; Sargent, D.J.; Marsh, S.; Green, E.M.; King, C.R.; Fuchs, C.S.; Ramanathan, R.K.; Williamson, S.K.; Findlay, B.P.; Thibodeau, S.N.; et al. Pharmacogenetic predictors of adverse events and response to chemotherapy in metastatic colorectal cancer: Results from North American gastrointestinal intergroup trial N9741. *J. Clin. Oncol.* **2010**, *28*, 3227–3233. [CrossRef]
19. Lecomte, T.; Ferraz, J.M.; Zinzindohoué, F.; Loriot, M.A.; Tregouet, D.A.; Landi, B.; Berger, A.; Cugnenc, P.H.; Jian, R.; Beaune, P.; et al. Thymidylate synthase gene polymorphism predicts toxicity in colorectal cancer patients receiving 5-fluorouracil-based chemotherapy. *Clin. Cancer Res.* **2004**, *10*, 5880–5888. [CrossRef]
20. Nief, N.; Le Morvan, V.; Robert, J. Involvement of gene polymorphisms of thymidylate synthase in gene expression, protein activity and anticancer drug cytotoxicity using the NCI-60 panel. *Eur. J. Cancer* **2007**, *43*, 955–962. [CrossRef]
21. Marcuello, E.; Altés, A.; Del Rio, E.; César, A.; Menoyo, A.; Baiget, M. Single nucleotide polymorphism in the 5′ tandem repeat sequences of Thymidylate synthase gene predicts for response to fluorouracil-based chemotherapy in advanced colorectal cancer patients. *Int. J. Cancer* **2004**, *112*, 733–737. [CrossRef] [PubMed]
22. Sharma, R.; Hoskins, J.M.; Rivory, L.P.; Zucknick, M.; London, R.; Liddle, C.; Clarke, S.J. Thymidylate synthase and methylenetetrahydrofolate reductase gene polymorphisms and toxicity to capecitabine in advanced colorectal cancer patients. *Clin. Cancer Res.* **2008**, *14*, 817–825. [CrossRef]
23. Jakobsen, A.; Nielsen, J.N.; Gyldenkerne, N.; Lindeberg, J. Thymidylate synthase and methylenetetrahydrofolate reductase gene polymorphism in normal tissue as predictors of fluorouracil sensitivity. *J. Clin. Oncol.* **2005**, *23*, 1365–1369. [CrossRef] [PubMed]
24. Pullarkat, S.T.; Stoehlmacher, J.; Ghaderi, V.; Xiong, Y.-P.; Ingles, S.A.; Sherrod, A.; Warren, R.; Tsao-Wei, D.; Groshen, S.; Lenz, H.-J.J. Thymidylate synthase gene polymorphism determines response and toxicity of 5-FU chemotherapy. *Pharmacogenomics J.* **2001**, *1*, 65–70. [CrossRef] [PubMed]
25. Joerger, M.; Huitema, A.D.R.R.; Boot, H.; Cats, A.; Doodeman, V.D.; Smits, P.H.M.M.; Vainchtein, L.; Rosing, H.; Meijerman, I.; Zueger, M.; et al. Germline TYMS genotype is highly predictive in patients with metastatic gastrointestinal malignancies receiving capecitabine-based chemotherapy. *Cancer Chemother. Pharmacol.* **2015**, *75*, 763–772. [CrossRef]
26. Wu, Q.; Dolnick, B.J. Detection of thymidylate synthase modulators by a novel screening assay. *Mol. Pharmacol.* **2003**, *63*, 167–173. [CrossRef]
27. Froehlich, T.K.; Amstutz, U.; Aebi, S.; Joerger, M.; Largiadèr, C.R. Clinical importance of risk variants in the dihydropyrimidine dehydrogenase gene for the prediction of early-onset fluoropyrimidine toxicity. *Int. J. Cancer* **2015**, *136*, 730–739. [CrossRef]
28. NCI USNCI Cancer Therapy Evaluation Program: Common Terminology Criteria for Adverse Events (CTCAE) v3.0. Available online: https://ctep.cancer.gov/protocoldevelopment/electronic_applications/docs/CTCAE_v5_Quick_Reference_8.5x11.pdf (accessed on 4 February 2020).
29. Rousset, F. Genepop'007: A complete re-implementation of the genepop software for Windows and Linux. *Mol. Ecol. Res.* **2008**, *8*, 103–106. [CrossRef]
30. R Core Team R: *A Language and Environment for Statistical Computing*; R Foundation for Statistical Computing: Vienna, Austria, 2019.
31. Amstutz, U.; Henricks, L.M.; Offer, S.M.; Barbarino, J.; Schellens, J.H.M.; Swen, J.J.; Klein, T.E.; McLeod, H.L.; Caudle, K.E.; Diasio, R.B.; et al. Clinical pharmacogenetics implementation consortium (CPIC) guideline for dihydropyrimidine dehydrogenase genotype and fluoropyrimidine dosing: 2017 update. *Clin. Pharmacol. Ther.* **2018**, *103*, 210–216. [CrossRef]
32. Marsh, S.; Collie-Duguid, E.S.R.; Li, T.; Liu, X.; McLeod, H.L. Ethnic variation in the thymidylate synthase enhancer region polymorphism among Caucasian and Asian populations. *Genomics* **1999**, *58*, 310–312. [CrossRef]

33. Luo, H.R.; Lü, X.M.; Yao, Y.G.; Horie, N.; Takeishi, K.; Jorde, L.B.; Zhang, Y.P. Length polymorphism of thymidylate synthase regulatory region in Chinese populations and evolution of the novel alleles. *Biochem. Genet.* **2002**, *40*, 41–51. [CrossRef] [PubMed]
34. Loganayagam, A.; Arenas Hernandez, M.; Corrigan, A.; Fairbanks, L.; Lewis, C.M.; Harper, P.; Maisey, N.; Ross, P.; Sanderson, J.D.; Marinaki, A.M. Pharmacogenetic variants in the DPYD, TYMS, CDA and MTHFR genes are clinically significant predictors of fluoropyrimidine toxicity. *Br. J. Cancer* **2013**, *108*, 2505–2515. [CrossRef] [PubMed]
35. Schwab, M.; Zanger, U.M.; Marx, C.; Schaeffeler, E.; Klein, K.; Dippon, J.; Kerb, R.; Blievernicht, J.; Fischer, J.; Hofmann, U.; et al. Role of genetic and nongenetic factors for fluorouracil treatment-related severe toxicity: A prospective clinical trial by the German 5-FU toxicity study group. *J. Clin. Oncol.* **2008**, *26*, 2131–2138. [CrossRef]
36. Petrelli, F.; Cabiddu, M.; Barni, S. 5-Fluorouracil or capecitabine in the treatment of advanced colorectal cancer: A pooled-analysis of randomized trials. *Med. Oncol.* **2012**, *29*, 1020–1029. [CrossRef]

Publisher's Note: MDPI stays neutral with regard to jurisdictional claims in published maps and institutional affiliations.

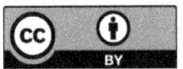

© 2020 by the authors. Licensee MDPI, Basel, Switzerland. This article is an open access article distributed under the terms and conditions of the Creative Commons Attribution (CC BY) license (http://creativecommons.org/licenses/by/4.0/).

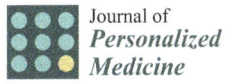

Review

The Road so Far in Colorectal Cancer Pharmacogenomics: Are We Closer to Individualised Treatment?

Ana Rita Simões [1,2,†], **Ceres Fernández-Rozadilla** [1,2,*,†], **Olalla Maroñas** [1] and **Ángel Carracedo** [1,2,3,4]

1. Grupo de Medicina Xenómica, Universidade de Santiago de Compostela (USC), 15706 Santiago de Compostela, Spain; anarita.santos.simoes@rai.usc.es (A.R.S.); olalla.maronas@usc.es (O.M.); angel.carracedo@usc.es (Á.C.)
2. Instituto de Investigación Sanitaria de Santiago (IDIS), 15706 Santiago de Compostela, Spain
3. Fundación Pública Galega de Medicina Xenómica; SERGAS, 15706 Santiago de Compostela, Spain
4. Consorcio Centro de Investigación Biomédica en Red de Enfermedades Raras—CIBERER, 28029 Madrid, Spain
* Correspondence: ceres.fernandez.rozadilla@gmail.com
† These authors contributed equally to this work.

Received: 13 October 2020; Accepted: 17 November 2020; Published: 19 November 2020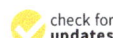

Abstract: In recent decades, survival rates in colorectal cancer have improved greatly due to pharmacological treatment. However, many patients end up developing adverse drug reactions that can be severe or even life threatening, and that affect their quality of life. These remain a limitation, as they may force dose reduction or treatment discontinuation, diminishing treatment efficacy. From candidate gene approaches to genome-wide analysis, pharmacogenomic knowledge has advanced greatly, yet there is still huge and unexploited potential in the use of novel technologies such as next-generation sequencing strategies. This review summarises the road of colorectal cancer pharmacogenomics so far, presents considerations and directions to be taken for further works and discusses the path towards implementation into clinical practice.

Keywords: colorectal cancer; adverse drug reactions; pharmacogenomics; personalised medicine; toxicity

1. Introduction

Colorectal cancer (CRC) is the second leading cause of cancer-related death and the third most commonly diagnosed cancer [1]. Surgical resection is the preferable treatment independently of stage, but chemotherapy is widely used too across stages. There are different chemotherapeutic schemes for CRC treatment (Table 1).

Table 1. Guidelines for colorectal cancer (CRC) treatment.

CRC Stage	Treatment	
	Surgery	Pharmacological Treatment
I	Wide surgical resection and anastomosis	No adjuvant chemotherapy recommended
II	Wide surgical resection and anastomosis	Adjuvant chemotherapy for high-risk could be considered

Table 1. Cont.

CRC Stage	Treatment	
	Surgery	Pharmacological Treatment
III	Wide surgical resection and anastomosis	Adjuvant administration of oxaliplatin plus 5-FU or capecitabine
IV	The majority of patients have metastases that initially are not suitable for potentially curative resection. Revaluate after chemotherapy	Cytotoxic agents: 1st line: 5-FU or capecitabine alone or in combination either with oxaliplatin or irinotecan 2nd line: if refractory to irinotecan-based treatment, FOLFOX is recommended; and if refractory to oxaliplatin-based treatment, FOLFIRI is recommended
		Biological targeted agents: 1st line: monoclonal antibodies against VEGF (bevacizumab, aflibercept) and/or EGFR (cetuximab, panitumumab), if *RAS* mutation excluded Multi-kinase inhibitor: regorafenib

FOLFOX: folinic acid (leucovorin-LV) + fluorouracil + oxaliplatin; FOLFIRI: leucovorin + fluorouracil + irinotecan; VEGF: vascular endothelial growth factor; EGFR: epidermal growth factor receptor.

Usually, the first line of treatment is based on fluoropyrimidines: 5-fluorouracil (5-FU) or its oral prodrug capecitabine, either alone or in different combinations with other agents, the most common being leucovorin, oxaliplatin (named FOLFOX or XELOX -if capecitabine is used instead of 5FU) or irinotecan (FOLFIRI) [2–5]. Besides these cytotoxic agents, metastatic CRC (mCRC) treatment may in addition include biological targeted agents to improve patient outcome, such as monoclonal antibodies against vascular endothelial growth factor (VEGF) (bevacizumab), or against epidermal growth factor receptor (EGFR) (cetuximab and panitumumab) (Table 1) [4].

There are two essential factors to be taken into account when considering efficacy and appropriateness of a treatment: response and toxicity. Response is often evaluated based on overall survival, progression-free survival or response evaluation criteria in solid tumors (RECIST), in the case of unresectable CRC [6]. On the other hand, patients subject to chemotherapy are prone to develop adverse drug reactions (ADRs) that might be severe or even fatal, and have a considerable impact on healthcare and burden. These ADRs can affect the patients' quality of life (even in the long term) and may hinder treatment, due to necessary delays or dose reduction. A study with more than four thousand mCRC patients receiving FOLFOX, FOLFIRI or XELOX saw that 90% of patients had one ADR, and 66% of patients had >1 ADR during the first line of treatment [7]. These toxic events also come with an increased economic burden to resolve them, with haematological toxicities being the most costly to resolve, followed by respiratory, endocrine/metabolic, central nervous system and cardiovascular ones.

Since both response and toxicity events have heterogeneous distributions amongst patients, it has been hypothesised that these ADRs may be caused by underlying genetic variants. Moreover, because chemotherapy agents have only been used since the 1950s, any genomic variants having large effects on toxicity responses have not had time to be washed away by negative selection [8,9]. Moreover, because cancer is usually related to later stages of life and does not affect fitness, purifying selection against these variants is not in place. Therefore, it is feasible that genetic variants having moderate-to-large effects (detectable by classical association studies) could be responsible for the observed variability.

Pharmacogenetics is a science that aims to learn about the inherited inter-variability in response and ADRs after drug exposure. First-generation studies were focused on the analysis of genes with an a priori relationship to drug effect, i.e., those involved mainly in the adsorption, distribution, metabolism and excretion (ADME) of chemotherapeutic agents. Later, these studies started to apply global approaches without a previous functional hypothesis, like genome-wide association studies (GWAS). The Pharmacogenomics Knowledgebase (PharmGKB [10]) is a free database that aggregates, curates, integrates and disseminates the knowledge obtained from these studies regarding the impact of human genetic variation on drug response and toxicity. Other important sources of pharmacogenomic information have also launched from the efforts of The Clinical Pharmacogenetics Implementation Consortium (CPIC), which aims to create, curate and post free detailed gene/drug clinical practice guidelines (https://cpicpgx.org/ (accessed on 29 October 2020)).

In this review, we summarise the available data on CRC pharmacogenomics to date and go beyond the typically discussed candidate gene approaches, to cover genome-wide studies and next-generation sequencing. We also reflect on the necessity of comprehensive works including molecular studies to assess variant functionality, and discuss the limitations towards clinical implementation in the light of cost-effectiveness to health systems. Last but not least, we discuss considerations for further studies towards a routine implementation of personalised medicine strategies in clinical practice.

2. Chemotherapeutic Agents in CRC Treatment

Chemotherapy based on fluoropyrimidines, specifically 5-FU, has been used for over thirty years now, and is still the backbone of CRC treatment (Figure 1) [11]. However, there have been reports that show that up to 94% of patients treated with this drug end up developing ADRs, some of which may be severe or life threatening (Table 2) [12]. For instance, some studies have shown that around 40–56% of patients treated with 5-FU develop severe neutropenia, and 10–15% present grade 3–4 diarrhoea [13]. Patients receiving capecitabine have a similar incidence of ADRs, although with less severe neutropenia, but present hand–foot syndrome (HFS) at a high incidence (54%) instead (Table 2) [14].

Table 2. The most common toxicity profile of CRC treatments.

Treatment	Significant ADRs (According to FDA Labels) *	ADR Incidence (% Patients)	Ref.
5-Fluororacil	Diarrhoea, neutropenia, mucositis, nausea/vomiting, stomatitis, asthenia, leukopenia, anaemia.	94%	[12]
Capecitabine	Hand-and-foot syndrome, diarrhoea, nausea/vomiting, abdominal pain, fatigue, hyperbilirubinemia.	96%	[12]
Oxaliplatin	Peripheral sensory neuropathy, neutropenia, thrombocytopenia, anaemia, nausea/vomiting, increase in transaminases and alkaline phosphatase, diarrhoea, fatigue, stomatitis.	>92%	[15]
Irinotecan	Nausea/vomiting, diarrhoea, neutropenia, alopecia, abdominal pain, constipation, anorexia, leukopenia, anaemia, asthenia, fever, body weight decreasing.	100%	[16]
Cetuximab	Cutaneous adverse reactions, headache, diarrhoea, infection.	>87%	[17]
Panitumumab	Skin rash, paronychia, fatigue, nausea, diarrhoea.	>90%	[18]
Bevacizumab	Haemorrhage, hypertension, headache, rhinitis, proteinuria, taste alteration, dry skin, lacrimation disorder, back pain, exfoliative dermatitis.	>60%	[19]

* According to Food and Drug Administration (FDA) label section: Warnings and Precautions, Contraindications, and Boxed Warning Sections of Labelling for Human Prescription Drug and Biological Products.

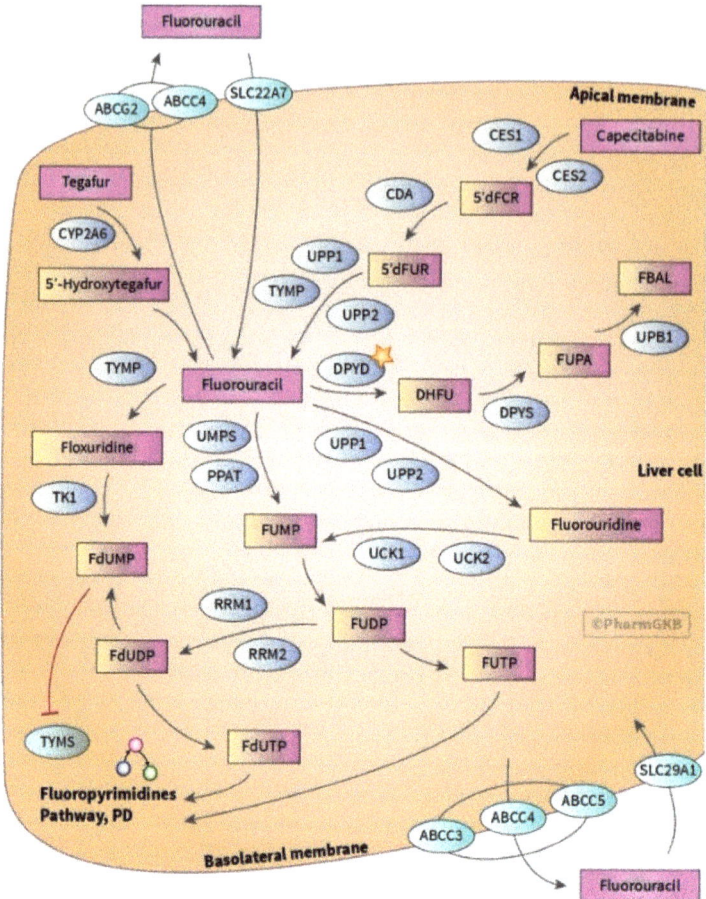

Figure 1. Graphic scheme of the genes involved in the adsorption, distribution, metabolism and excretion (ADME) of fluoropyrimidines [20]. Capecitabine passes through the gut wall and is metabolised into 5-deoxyfluorocytidine (5'dFCR) and 5'-deoxy-5-fluorouridine (5'dFUR) by carboxyl esterases (CES) and cytidine deaminase (CDA), respectively, and activated into 5-FU by thymidine phosphorylase (TP). - 5-FU is metabolised mostly in the liver by dihydropyrimidine dehydrogenase (DPD) (<80%) into dihydrofluorouracil (DHFU). The secondary elimination pathway is through urinary excretion or catabolism in extrahepatic tissues [21]. Its mechanism of action involves the methylenetetrahydrofolate reductase (MTHFR)—converting 5,10-methylentetrahydrofolate (5,10-MTHF) into 5-MTHF, which is required for purine and thymidine synthesis, and thymidylate synthase (TS) enzymes—forming a complex with 5,10-MTHF and deoxyuridine monophosphate (dUMP), which in the end disrupts DNA replication and repair. Used with PharmGKB and Stanford University permission (available at https://www.pharmgkb.org/pathway/PA150653776 (accessed on 24 September 2020)).

Platinum-based drugs, mainly oxaliplatin, are cytotoxic agents that prevent neoplastic proliferation, by forming DNA–platinum adducts, which block replication and transcription and induce apoptosis (Figure 2) (Table 1) [22]. The main oxaliplatin dose-limiting toxicity is neuropathy, occurring in about >90% of treated patients (Table 2) [15].

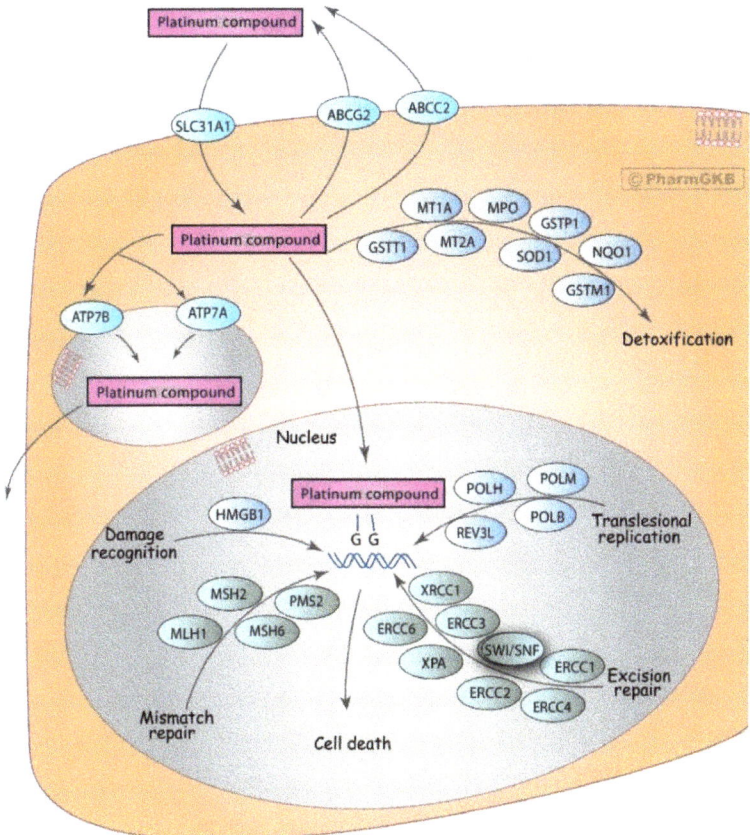

Figure 2. Graphic scheme of the genes involved in the ADME of platinum compounds, including oxaliplatin [23]. The glutathione S-transferases (GSTs), a multigene family of enzymes, undertake oxaliplatin detoxification. The solute carriers (SLCs) and adenosine-triphosphate binding cassette (ABC) transporters are responsible for oxaliplatin uptake and efflux in the liver, respectively, and so impact on drug bioavailability and toxicity profile. Further, the nucleotide excision repair (NER) and base excision repair (BER) pathways, which include the ERCC1 and ERCC2, and XRCC1 proteins, respectively, repair the damages cause by this drug. Used with PharmGKB and Stanford University permission (available at https://www.pharmgkb.org/pathway/PA150642262 (accessed on 24 September 2020)).

Irinotecan (CPT-11) is another cytotoxic agent used in the treatment of CRC in combination with 5-FU (FOLFIRI) (Table 1). FOLFIRI treatments result in better response rates and longer progression-free survival and overall survival of mCRC patients (Figure 3) [2,24]. CPT-11 is a semi-synthetic soluble analogue of the natural alkaloid camptothecin [25,26]. Some clinical trials report an ADR incidence for this drug of up to 100% of patients, where common ADRs include diarrhoea, neutropenia and alopecia (Table 2) [16].

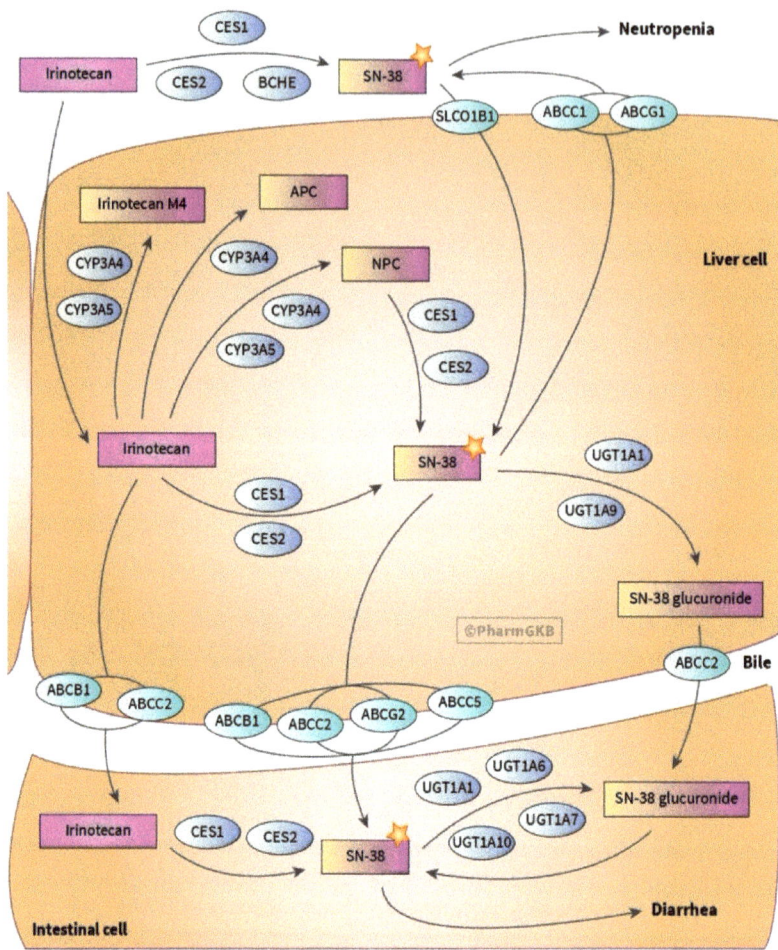

Figure 3. Graphic scheme of the genes involved in the ADME of irinotecan [10]. Irinotecan is converted into SN-38 by CES, which inhibits topoisomerase I, an enzyme essential for DNA replication and then into inactive SN-38G by UGTs. Further, it can suffer oxidation into 7-ethyl-10-[4-N-(5-aminopentanoic acid)-1-piperidino] carbonyloxycamptothecin (APC), M4 and 7-ethyl-10-[4-(1-piperidino)-1-amino] carbonyloxycamptothecin (NPC) by CYP3A4 and CYP3A5. NPC can be reactivated by CES into SN-38. Irinotecan and its metabolites' uptake and efflux are conducted by SLCs and ABC transporters, respectively. Used with PharmGKB and Stanford University permission (available at https://www.pharmgkb.org/pathway/PA2001 (accessed on 24 September 2020)).

In case of unresectable CRC, patients may also be given biological targeted agents. Cetuximab and panitumumab bind specifically to the human EGFR protein, which is constitutively expressed in normal epithelial tissues and overexpressed in some cancers like CRC. Some of the pioneer pharmacogenetics studies on treatment efficacy found, however, that because *RAS* mutations can constitutively activate the response pathway downstream from EGFR, anti-EGFR therapy efficacy is limited to patients' wild type for *KRAS* and *NRAS* [4]. These belong to signalling pathways downstream of EGFR, and mutations in these genes may cause EGFR-independent pathway activation, leading to resistance to anti-EGFR treatments [27]. More than 87% of patients receiving cetuximab develop an ADR and are commonly (>25%) prone to develop cutaneous reactions, headache, diarrhoea and infection, whereas patients receiving panitumumab (>20%) will probably have cutaneous reactions, fatigue, nausea and diarrhoea [17,18,25,26]. On the other hand, bevacizumab binding to VEGF blocks the interactions with its receptors on the endothelial cell surface. This interaction allows cell proliferation and angiogenesis, and thus bevacizumab reduces microvascular growth and inhibits metastatic progression. Over 60% of patients receiving bevacizumab develop ADRs, where the most common are hypertension, proteinuria, mucosal bleeding and wound healing problems [4,19].

3. Pharmacogenetics: Candidate Gene Studies

As we mentioned before, pharmacogenetic studies arose in the context of studying the genetic factors that contribute to ADRs. Initial efforts utilised candidate gene approaches to inspect mainly genetic variation in genes that might have a great influence on the drug pharmacokinetics and pharmacodynamics, and that can alter drug concentration levels, leading to toxicity.

3.1. Dihydropyrimidine Dehydrogenase (DPYD)

DPD, encoded by the *DPYD* gene, is responsible for the vast majority of 5-FU hepatic metabolism and is responsible for the first step and rate-limiting factor in the 5-FU catabolic pathway (Figure 1). Several single nucleotide polymorphisms (SNPs) have so far been identified in this gene in association with different toxicities [28]. The most studied *DPYD* variant is rs3918290 (*DPYD**2A, IVS14+1G>A), which causes exon 14 skipping and results in a truncated and catalytically inactive protein [29,30]. A study by Toffoli et al. on 603 patients treated with 5-FU-based chemotherapy reported the association of rs3918290 (OR = 8.5, $p = 0.008$), rs67376798 (OR = 7.8, $p = 0.012$) and rs55886062 (OR = 6.0, $p = 0.131$) with general toxicity (Table 3) [28].

Table 3. Summary of CRC pharmacogenomics.

Drug	Gene	SNP (rsID)	Change	Alternative Nomenclature	Frequency of Risk Allele [a]	Associated ADR	OR (95% CI)	Evidence Level [b]	Ref.
Fluoropyrimidines	DPYD	rs55886062	NM_000110.3:c.1679T>G; NP_000101.2:p.Ile560Ser	DPYD*13	3×10^{-4} (C)	Global toxicity	6.0 (0.6–61)	1A	[28]
		rs3918290	NM_000110.4:c.1905+1G>A (Splice donor)	DPYD*2A	0.007 (T)	Global toxicity	8.5 (1.8–40.9)	1A	[29]
		rs67376798	NM_000110.3:c.2846A>T; NP_000101.2:p.Asp949Val		0.003 (A)	Global toxicity	7.8 (1.6–39.2)	1A	[31]
		rs115232898	NM_000110.3:c.557A>G; NP_000101.2:p.Tyr186Cys		0.002 (Afr: 0.023) (C)	Neutropenia, mucositis, alopecia	-	1A	[32]
		rs75017182	NM_000110.4:c.1129-5923C>G (Intronic)		0.013 (C)	Global toxicity	6.8 (2.0–23)	1A	[33]
		rs56038477	NM_000110.3:c.1236G>A; NP_000101.2:p.Glu412=		0.014 (T)	Gastrointestinal; haematological	2.0 (1.5–2.8) 2.8 (1.2–3.7)	3	[34]
		rs72549303 [c]	NM_000110.4:c.1898del; NP_000101.2:p.Pro633fs	DPYD*3	NA	NA	NA	1A	[31]
		rs72549309 [c]	NM_000110.4:c.295_298TCAT [1]; NP_000101.2:p.Phe100fs	DPYD*7	6×10^{-5} (delATGA)	NA	NA	1A	[31]
		rs1801266 [c]	NM_000110.4:c.703C>T; NP_000101.2:p.Arg235Trp	DPYD*8	3×10^{-5} (A)	NA	NA	1A	[31]
		rs1801268 [c]	NM_000110.4:c.2983G>T; NP_000101.2:p.Val995Phe	DPYD*10	NA	NA	NA	1A	[31]
		rs78060119	NM_000110.3:c.1156G>T; NP_000101.2:p.Glu386Ter	DPYD*12	8×10^{-6} (A)	Leucopenia, thrombocytopenia, mucositis	NA	1A	[35]
		rs2297595	NM_000110.3:c.496A>G; NP_000101.2:p.Met166Val		0.085 (C)	Global toxicity	5.9 (1.3–27.2)	3	[36]
		rs1801265	NM_000110.3:c.85T>C; NP_000101.2:p.Cys29Arg	DPYD*9A	0.228 (G)	Diarrhoea	0.8 (0.7–1)	3	[37]
		rs1801267 [c]	NM_000110.4:c.2657G>A; NP_000101.2:p.Arg886His	DPYD*9B	1×10^{-4} (T)	NA	NA	NA	[38]

Table 3. Cont.

Drug	Gene	SNP (rsID)	Change	Alternative Nomenclature	Frequency of Risk Allele [a]	Associated ADR	OR (95% CI)	Evidence Level [b]	Ref.
		rs1801159	NM_000110.3:c.1627A>G; NP_000101.2:p.Ile543Val	DPYD*5	0.198 (C)	Diarrhoea	4.9 (-)	3	[39]
		rs1801158	NM_000110.3:c.1601G>A; NP_000101.2:p.Ser534Asn	DPYD*4	0.015 (T)	Global toxicity	1.7 (1.1–2.6)	3	[37]
		rs17376848	NM_000110.3:c.1896T>C; NP_000101.2:p.Phe632=		0.051 (G)	Global toxicity	14.5 (1.4–155.2)	3	[36]
		rs1801160	NM_000110.3:c.2194G>A; NP_000101.2:p.Val732Ile	DPYD*6	0.048 (T)	Global toxicity	2.1 (1.5–3.0)	3	[40]
		rs12022243	NM_000110.4:c.1906-14763G>A (Intronic)		0.181 (T)	Global toxicity	1.7 (1.5–1.9)	3	[41]
		rs12119882	NM_000110.4:c.680+2545T>C (Intronic)		0.075 (G)	Hyperbilirubinemia	4.9 (1.2–20.8)	3	[42]
		rs76387818	Intergenic		0.019 (A)	Global toxicity	4.1 (3.5–4.6)	3	[41]
		rs12132152	Intergenic		0.020 (A)	HFS;global toxicity	6.1 (5.5–6.8); 1.6 (1.4–1.8)	3	[41]
		rs183205964	NM_001071.4:c.-86= (5' UTR)		3×10^{-5} (C)	Global toxicity	3.0 (1.1–8.4)	3	[43]
		rs2853741	NM_001071.4:c. (Upstream transcript)		0.322 (T)	Diarrhoea	0.3 (0.1–0.7)	3	[42]
		rs699517	NM_017512.7:c.*1289= (3' UTR)		0.379 (T)	Nausea/vomiting;asthenia	7.9 (1.5–41.6); 0.3 (0.1–0.8)	3	[42]
	TYMS	rs45445694	NM_001071.4:c. (5' UTR)		0.007 (2R2R)	Global toxicity	1.7 (-)	3	[44]
		rs2853542	NM_001071.4:c.-58= (5' UTR)			Global toxicity; HFS	1.5 (1.2–1.8); 1.4 (1.2–1.8)	NA	[45]
		rs11280056	NM_017512.7:c.*853_*861= (3' UTR)			Global toxicity	1.7 (1.2–2.2)	NA	[45]
	ENOSF1	rs2612091	NM_017512.7:c.742-227G>C (Intronic)		0.373 (C)	Global toxicity	1.6 (1.4–1.8)	3	[41]

Table 3. Cont.

Drug	Gene	SNP (rsID)	Change	Alternative Nomenclature	Frequency of Risk Allele [a]	Associated ADR	OR (95% CI)	Evidence Level [b]	Ref.
	UMPS	rs2279199	NM_000373.4:c. (Genic upstream transcript)		0.556 (T)	Nausea/vomiting	0.2 (0.1–1.0)	3	[42]
		rs4678145	NM_000373.4:c.156+607G>C (Intronic)		0.096 (C)	Asthenia	4.5 (1.6–13.2)	3	[42]
		rs1801019 d	NM_000373.4:c.638G>C; NP_000364.1:p.Gly213Ala		0.169 (C)	Global toxicity	17.6 (1.6–195.9)	3	[46]
	MTHFR	rs1801131	NM_001330358.1:c.1409A>C; NP_001317287.1:p.Glu470Ala		0.289 (G)	HFS	10.0 (3.8–27.8)	3	[47]
		rs1801133	NM_001330358.1:c.788C>T; NP_001317287.1:p.Ala263Val		0.315 (A)	Neutropenia	2.3 (1.2–4.6)	3	[48]
	TYMP	rs11479	NM_001113755.3:c.1412C>T; NP_001244917.1:p.Ser471Leu		0.094 (A)	Global toxicity	2.7 (1.2–5.9)	3	[49]
	MIR27A	rs895819	NR_029501.1:n.40A>G (Non-coding transcript)		0.335 (C)	Global toxicity	1.6 (1.1–2.2)	3	[50]
	ABCC1	rs7194667	NM_032583.4:c.1609-491A>C (Intronic)		0.063 (G)	Leucopenia	3.31 (1.3–8.7)	3	[51]
	ABCB1	rs1045642	NM_001348945.1:c.3645T>C; NP_001335874.1:p.Ile1215=	ABCB1*6	0.504 (G)	HFS	NA	3	[52]
		rs2032582	NM_001348945.1:c.2887T>G; NP_001335874.1:p.Ser963Ala	ABCB1*7	0.637 (C)	HFS	NA	3	[52]
		rs1128503	NM_001348945.1:c.1446T>C; NP_001335874.1:p.Gly482=	ABCB1*8	0.614 (G)	Neutropenia	NA	3	[52]
	SLC22A7	rs2270860	NM_006672.3:c.1269C>T; NP_006663.2:p.Ser423=		0.368 (T)	Global toxicity	17.1 (1.7–170.3)	3	[42]
		rs4149178	NM_006672.3:c.1586+206A>G (Intronic)		0.795 (A)	Diarrhoea	0.3 (0.1–0.9)	3	[42]

Table 3. Cont.

Drug	Gene	SNP (rsID)	Change	Alternative Nomenclature	Frequency of Risk Allele [a]	Associated ADR	OR (95% CI)	Evidence Level [b]	Ref.
		rs2072671	NM_001785.3:c.79A>C; NP_001776.1:p.Lys27Gln		0.279 (C)	Global toxicity	1.8 (1.1–3.0)	3	[53]
		rs1048977	NM_001785.3: c.435C>T; NP_001776.1:p.Thr145=		0.307 (T)	Hyperbilirubinemia	8.6 (1.1–70.3)	3	[42]
	CDA	rs602950	NM_001785.3:c. (Upstream transcript)		0.224 (G)	Diarrhoea	2.3 (1.3–4.2)	3	[47]
		rs3215400	NM_001785.3:c.-33_-31= (5′ UTR)		0.555 (delC)	HFS	0.5 (0.3–1.0)	3	[54]
		rs532545	NM_001785.3:c. (Upstream transcript)		0.220 (T)	Diarrhoea	2.3 (1.3–4.2)	NA	[47]
		rs3217164	NM_001025195.2:c.693+129del (Intronic)		0.607 (G)	Global toxicity	4.1 (1.8–9.0)	3	[55]
	CES1	rs2244614	NM_001025195.2:c.1171-41C>T (Intronic)		0.482 (G)	Global toxicity	4.7 (1.9–12.0)	3	[55]
		rs2244613	NM_001025195.2:c.1171-33C>T (Intronic)		0.232 (G)	Global toxicity	6.4 (1.5–27.7)	3	[55]
		rs7187684	NR_003276.2:n. (Intronic)		0.278 (T)	Global toxicity	6.5 (1.5–28.0)	3	[55]
	CES1P1	rs11861118	NR_003276.2:n. (Upstream transcript)		0.161 (G)	Global toxicity	6.5 (1.5–28.0)	3	[55]
	Intergenic	rs9936750	Intergenic		0.161 C	Global toxicity	4.6 (1.5–13.9)	3	[56]
	Intergenic	rs10876844	Intergenic		0.439 (A)	Diarrhoea	6.5 (1.6–27.2)	NA	[57]

Table 3. Cont.

Drug	Gene	SNP (rsID)	Change	Alternative Nomenclature	Frequency of Risk Allele [a]	Associated ADR	OR (95% CI)	Evidence Level [b]	Ref.
Oxaliplatin	ABCC2	rs717620	NM_000392.5:c.-24= (5' UTR)		0.171 (T)	Neuropathy	14.4 (1.6–127.0)	3	[58]
		rs3740066	NM_000392.5:c.3972C> TNP_000383.2:p.Ile1324=			Neuropathy	3.0 (1.2–7.7)	NA	[58]
		rs1885301	NM_000392.5:c. (Upstream Transcript)		0.413 (A)	Neuropathy	3.1 (1.4–6.9)	NA	[58]
		rs4148396	NM_000392.5:c.3258+56T>C (Intronic)		0.347 (T)	Neuropathy	4.7 (1.6–13.7)	NA	[58]
	ABCG2	rs3114018	NM_004827.3:c.-19-3415T>G (Intronic)		0.516 (A)	Neuropathy	2.7 (1.0–4.4)	NA	[59]
	GSTP1	rs1695	NM_000852.3:c.313A>G; NP_000843.1:p.Ile105Val	GSTP1*B	0.339 (G)	Dying	3.0 (1.2–7.6)	3	[60]
	GSTM1	Null genotype	-	GSTM1*0		Neutropenia	2.0 (1.1–3.7)	NA	[61]
	GSTT1	Null genotype	-			Neutropenia	2.0 (1.1–3.7)	NA	[61]
	ERCC1	rs11615	NM_202001.3:c.354T>C; NP_001356337.1:p.Asn118=		0.498 (A)	Neutropenia	4.6 (1.2–17.4)	3	[48]
	ERCC2	rs13181	NM_000400.3:c.2251A>C; NP_000391.1:p.Lys751Gln		0.323 (G)	Haematological	2.2 (1.3–3.8)	3	[62]
		rs238406	NM_000400.4:c.468A>C NP_000391.1:p.Arg156=		0.645 (C)	Thrombocytopenia	NA	NA	[63]
	PARD3B	rs17626122	NM_001302769.2:c.3261-6168T>C (Intronic)		0.550 (T)	Global toxicity	3.4 (1.9–6.8)	3	[57]
	Intergenic	rs7325568	Intergenic		0.409 (T)	Haematological	1.8 (1.3–2.4)	3	[57]

Table 3. Cont.

Drug	Gene	SNP (rsID)	Change	Alternative Nomenclature	Frequency of Risk Allele [a]	Associated ADR	OR (95% CI)	Evidence Level [b]	Ref.
Irinotecan	UGT1A1	rs3064744	NM_000463.3:c. (Upstream transcript)	UGT1A1*28	0.347 (dupTA) (EAS:0.122)	Global toxicity	7.2 (2.5–22.3)	2A	[64]
		rs4148323 [c]	NM_000463.2:c.211G>A; NP_000454.1:p.Gly71Arg	UGT1A1*6	0.014 (EAS: 0.144) (A)	NA	NA	2A	[65]
		rs11563250	NM_001367507.1:c. (Genic upstream transcript)		0.893 (A)	Neutropenia	0.3 (0.2–0.6)	3	[66]
		rs4124874	NM_001072.3:c.862-10021T>G (Intronic)	UGT1A1*60	0.452 (T)	Neutropenia	NA	3	[67]
		rs10929302	NM_019075.2:c.856-9898G>A (Intronic)	UGT1A1*93	0.299 (A)	Global toxicity	8.4 (1.9–37.2)	3	[68]
		rs11692021	NM_021027.3:c.855+9770T>C (Intronic)		0.349 (C)	Global toxicity	2.0 (1.1–3.6)	3	[69]
	UGT1A9	rs3832043 [e]	NM_021027.3:c. (Upstream Transcript)		0.609 (delT)	Diarrhoea	6.3 (1.3–31.7)	3	[70]
	UGT1A6	rs2070959	NM_001072.4:c.541A>G (Intronic)		0.689 (A)	Global toxicity	2.1 (1.1–3.9)	3	[69]
	ABCG1	rs225440	NM_016818.3:c.286+7029C>T (Intronic)		0.428 (T)	Neutropenia	3.1 (1.1–8.6)	3	[71]
		rs425215	NM_016818.3:c.974-898C>G (Intronic)		0.623 (G)	Gastrointestinal	11.4 (1.7–78.4)	NA	[72]
	ABCB1	rs12720066	NM_001348945.1:c.2529+971T>G (Intronic)		0.035 (C)	Neutropenia	NA	3	[73]
	ABCC1	rs17501331	NM_004996.4:c.49-12232A>G (Intronic)		0.928 (A)	Neutropenia	NA	3	[73]
		rs3743527	NM_004996.4:c.*543= (3' UTR)		0.774 (C)	Neutropenia	NA	3	[73]

Table 3. Cont.

Drug	Gene	SNP (rsID)	Change	Alternative Nomenclature	Frequency of Risk Allele [a]	Associated ADR	OR (95% CI)	Evidence Level [b]	Ref.
	ABCC5	rs2292997	NM_005688.4:c.129+7980C>T (Intronic)		0.126 (A)	Neutropenia	3.2 (1.3–7.9)	3	[71]
		rs10937158	NM_005688.4:c.130-1268A>T (Intronic)		0.612 (C)	Diarrhoea	0.4 (0.2–0.8)	3	[71]
		rs3749438	NM_005688.4:c.591+374C>T (Intronic)		0.324 (A)	Diarrhoea	5.9 (1.3–26.3)	3	[71]
		rs562	NM_005688.4:c.*1243= (3′ UTR)		0.515 (C)	Gastrointestinal	32.0 (2.8–370.8)	NA	[72]
	ABCG2	rs7699188	NM_004827.3:c. (Genic upstream transcript)		0.227 (A)	Global toxicity; non-haematological	7.3 (1.5–34.5); 15.2 (2.5–78.2)	3	[74]
	SLCO1B1	rs2306283	NM_006446.5:c.388A>G NP_006437.3:p.Asn130Asp	SLCO1B1*1b	0.529 (G)	Gastrointestinal	2.3 (0.4–15.1)	NA	[72]
	TOP1	rs6072262	NM_003286.4:c.279+61G>A (Intronic)		0.144 (A)	Neutropenia	NA	3	[75]
	TGFBR2	rs3087465	NM_001024847.2:c. (2KB upstream)		0.659 (G)	Diarrhoea	3.7 (1.0–13.3)	3	[76]
	TGFB1	rs1800469	NM_000660.7:c. (Upstream transcript)		0.701 (G)	Diarrhoea	4.4 (1.0–18.9)	3	[76]
	KCNQ5	rs9351963	NM_019842.4:c.490-17798A>C (Intronic)		0.178 (C)	Diarrhoea	3.3 (1.8–5.6)	3	[77]
	Intergenic	rs10486003	Intergenic		0.913 (C)	Neuropathy	0.3 (0.2–0.5)	NA	[78]
	Intergenic	rs2338	Intergenic		0.275 (A)	Neuropathy	2.3 (1.6–3.3)	NA	[78]
	Intergenic	rs830884	Intergenic		0.92 (T)	Neuropathy	0.3 (0.2–0.5)	NA	[78]
	ACYP2	rs843748	NM_001320586.2:c.405-28913G>A (Intronic)		0.379 (A)	Neuropathy	2.4 (1.6–3.7)	NA	[78]
	DLEU7	rs797519	NC_000013.11:g.50656996G>C (Intronic)		0.548 (G)	Neuropathy	0.5 (045–0.7)	NA	[78]
	FARS2	rs17140129	NM_001318872.2.c.-22+36771A>G (Intronic)		0.158 (G)	Neuropathy	3.3 (1.8–6.4)	NA	[78]

Table 3. Cont.

Drug	Gene	SNP (rsID)	Change	Alternative Nomenclature	Frequency of Risk Allele [a]	Associated ADR	OR (95% CI)	Evidence Level [b]	Ref.
Cetuximab	EGFR	rs712830	NM_005228.5:c.-191= (5' UTR)		0.894 (C)	Global toxicity	6.1 (1.6–23.8)	3	[79]
		rs2227983	NM_005228.5:c.1562G>A NP_005219.2:p.Arg521Lys		0.768 (G)	Skin toxicity	3.2 (1.3–8.3)	3	[80]
		rs11568315	NM_005228.5:c.88+1195AC[10] (Intronic)		$3.9 \times 10{-4}$ (CA > 35)	Skin toxicity	2.9 (1.0–8.9)	NA	[81]
	RPS7	rs10203413	NC_000002.12:g.3581588G>A (Regulatory region)		0.776 (G)	Skin toxicity	0.1 (0.1–0.4)	NA	[82]
	ZNF827	rs12646351	NC_000002.12:g.3581588G>A (Intronic)		0.815 (G)	Skin toxicity	0.04 (0.01–0.3)	NA	[82]
		rs17806780	NM_001306215.2:c.2383+11920A>T (Intronic)		0.818 (T)	Skin toxicity	0.04 (0.01–0.4)	NA	[82]
	EPHA5	rs7692430	NM_004439.8:c.2237-1876A>G (Intronic)		0.156 (G)	Skin toxicity	4.6 (2.5–8.5)	NA	[82]
Bevacizumab	VEGF	rs3025039	NM_001171623.1:c.*237= (3' UTR)		0.134 (T)	Hypertension	0.2 (0.03–0.8)	NA	[83]
		rs2010963	NM_001171623.1:c.-634= (5' UTR)		0.698 (G)	Hypertension	NA	NA	[84]
		rs833061	NM_001025366.3:c. (Upstream transcript)		0.452 (C)	Hypertension	0.2 (0.03–0.8)	NA	[85]
		rs699947	NM_001025366.3:c. (Upstream transcript)		0.414 (A)	Hypertension	0.1 (0.01–0.6)	NA	[85]

a: The risk alleles frequencies were consulted on gnomAD. b: Measure of confidence in the association, according to PharmGKB [10]. c: Associated with changes in enzymatic activity, but with a particular adverse drug reaction (ADR). d: Described for tegafur, a prodrug of 5-FU. e: Described for non-small-cell lung carcinoma. NA: not available. Note: In case of multiple studies, we have chosen a publication used by PharmGKB to support the level of evidence of the referred variant, and the corresponding OR and p-value.

A further meta-analysis including 7365 patients from eight different studies confirmed the association between *DPYD* rs55886062 (*DDYD*13*) and *DPYD* rs56038477 with gastrointestinal (OR = 5.72, p = 0.015; 2.04, p < 0.0001, respectively) and haematological toxicities (OR = 9.76, p = 0.00014; and 2.07, p = 0.013, respectively), and also between *DPYD* rs3918290 and rs67376798 with overall toxicity (OR = 20.5, p < 0.0001; and 3.02, p < 0.0001, respectively) [34].

3.2. Thymidylate Synthetase (TYMS)

TS, encoded by the *TYMS* gene, is the main target of fluoropyrimidines and low levels of expression may influence toxicity [86,87]. The two most studied SNPs in *TYMS* are rs2853542 (5′VNTR 2R/3R) and rs11280056 (3′UTR 6bp ins-del). This gene has been widely studied, but with no conclusive results so far. Some studies have reported a correlation between rs2853542 and 5-FU/capecitabine toxicity, where the haplotype 2R/ins 6-bp was found to be significantly associated with severe toxicity [45,87], but other works could not replicate this association [61]. This might be explained by a work of Rosmarin et al. in 2015, which reported an association of an intronic variant located in the overlapping *ENOSF1* gene capable of explaining the toxicity attributed to the two previous *TYMS* polymorphisms. They discovered that SNP rs2612091 and *TYMS* 5′VNTR and 3′UTR are in moderate linkage disequilibrium (LD) (r^2 = 0.40 and 0.32, respectively), but after testing for dependency, they concluded that it was the rs2612091 G allele alone that increased the risk of toxicity (p = 0.0021). Although it has been proposed that the ENOSF1 protein could influence TYMS activity, the interaction between these two genes is not yet well understood [41]. Interestingly, genetic variation in *TYMS* has also been related to response to pyrimidine treatments, with higher levels of TS implicating worse response and poorer overall survival [88,89].

3.3. Methylenetetrahydrofolate Reductase (MTHFR)

MTHFR is the other major enzyme involved in 5-FU metabolism. Polymorphisms in this gene (namely rs1801133 and rs1801131) might impact enzyme activity, causing an accumulation of 5,10-MTHF, which increases toxicity [90]. Indeed, a study involving 292 stage II/III colon cancer patients found that the rs1801133 TT genotype was associated with neutropenia (OR = 2.32, p = 0.014) [48]. Another study involving 118 mCRC patients found that the same genotype was associated with diarrhoea (p = 0.02) [91]. However, other studies have not been able to find any association between polymorphisms in this gene and toxicity events [61,62,92,93].

3.4. Carboxyl Esterases (CES) and Cytidine Deaminase (CDA)

CES2 is the first enzyme in the conversion of capecitabine to 5-FU, followed by a second step catalysed by CDA (Figure 1). There have been some attempts to prove the association of polymorphisms on these two genes with ADRs, but there are still no concrete positive results. Ribelles et al. studied 136 patients and showed a trend (p = 0.07) between HFS and *CDA* SNP rs3215400 [54]. A study including 239 patients found an association of *CDA* rs2072671 with a high risk of overall toxicity (OR= 1.84, p = 0.029) [53]. Another work including 430 patients linked the *CDA* rs602950 and *CDA* rs532545 variants with diarrhoea (OR = 2.3, p = 0.0055, and 2.3, p = 0.0082, respectively) [47]. There have also been some smaller studies on *CES* polymorphisms and their association with capecitabine toxicity [45,54,94]. CES proteins are also important in the catabolic pathway of irinotecan (Figure 3) [95]. *CES1* rs2244613 was found to be associated with diarrhoea and patients with low *CES2* expression are more prone to develop neutropenia or diarrhoea [95–98].

3.5. DNA Repair Genes

DNA repair pathways have been extensively studied in pharmacogenomic studies [99]. A meta-analysis of more than 1000 CRC patients receiving oxaliplatin found a single significant association of the *ERCC1* rs11615 C allele with a higher risk of having haematological toxicity in Asian populations (HR = 1.97, p < 0.05) [100]. Boige et al. could not, however, replicate this association, perhaps due to population differences, but did associate the *ERCC2* rs13181 C allele with a higher risk of severe haematological toxicity caused by FOLFOX (OR = 2.16, p = 0.01) [62]. A recent study on 596 CRC patients found that *ERCC1* rs11615 was significantly associated with stomatitis (p = 0.03) and nausea (p = 0.04), and that *ERCC2* rs13181 and rs238406 were associated with thrombocytopenia (p = 0.004 and p = 0.03, respectively) [63]. On the other hand, a study of 517 patients with stage II/III colon cancer concluded that polymorphisms in *ERCC1* and *XRCC1* did not have a clinically significant association with adverse effects [61]. Further smaller studies could neither confirm the relationship between these variants and toxicity [91,101].

3.6. Glutathione S-Transferases (GSTs)

GST enzymes are proteins from a multigene family, and specifically, GSTP1, GSTM1 and GSTT1 are involved in oxaliplatin detoxification (Figure 2). The most studied variations are *GSTP1* rs1695 and the complete deletion of the *GSTT1* and *GSTM1* genes. McLeod et al. tested these on 300 patients receiving FOLFOX in an advanced CRC setting. Patients bearing the *GSTM1* null genotype had a 1.7-fold increased risk of having severe neutropenia (p = 0.016), whereas homozygous patients for the rs1695 T allele had higher probability of discontinuing FOLFOX treatment due to neurotoxicity (p = 0.01) [102]. In contrast to these findings, Boige et al. did not find any significant association between these same SNPs and severe neurotoxicity on a study enrolling 349 patients [62]. Ruzzo et al. studied 517 patients and suggested a weak association between the *GST-T1/M1* null/null genotype and severe neutropenia (OR = 1.99, p = 0.032) [61], whereas Cecchin et al. analysed 154 patients receiving FOLFOX but could not replicate any markers of neurotoxicity. Interestingly, they suggested that variants other than genetics, such as the biological state of patients or disease stage, may also influence the detoxification pathway, and could therefore be responsible for the FOLFOX-related neurotoxicity [58].

3.7. Adenosine-Triphosphate Binding Cassette (ABC) Transporters

Genes within the ABC transporter family are responsible for the efflux of a variety of drugs and their metabolites, including oxaliplatin and irinotecan. However, there is a lot of controversy on the relationship of polymorphisms on *ABC* genes and chemotherapy-related toxicity. For 206 patients receiving FOLFOX, Custodio et al. reported that the *ABCG2* rs3114018 AA genotype had a significantly higher risk of neuropathy (OR = 2.67, p = 0.059) [59]. In a study including 144 patients, Cecchin et al. reported positive associations with neurotoxicity for SNPs in *ABCC2*: rs3740066 (OR = 2.99, p = 0.0231), rs1885301 (OR = 3.06, p = 0.0072), rs4148396 (OR = 4.69, p = 0.0048) and rs717620 (OR = 14.39, p = 0.0164), which are in high LD with one another. Others studies have been less successful in linking genetic variants in this gene with neurotoxicity or other toxicities [58,61,103].

In relation to irinotecan-based regimens, Salvador-Martín et al. showed that SNPs rs1128503, rs2032582 and rs1045642 in *ABCB1*, which are in LD, were associated with haematological and overall toxicity [92]. Others proposed the association of solely *ABCB1* rs1128503 (OR = 2.02, p = 0.401) with global toxicity, or of *ABCB1* rs1045642 with early toxicity (OR = 3.79, p = 0.098) (not strictly significant), while others did not find any association at all [74,93,95,96]. There have also been some reports on other *ABC transporter* genes, with conflicting results. For instance, a study on 26 mCRC patients showed that patients with the CC genotype in *ABCC5* rs562 or the GG genotype in *ABCG1* rs425215 presented higher gastrointestinal toxicity (p < 0.02) [72]. A study including 250 patients with mCRC linked the *ABCG2* rs7699188 variant with severe global toxicity (OR = 7.26, p = 0.013) [74].

3.8. Uridine Disphosphate Glucuronosyltransferases (UGTs)

UGT1A1 is the main enzyme responsible for SN-38 inactivation, followed by UGT1A7 and UGT1A9. Several groups have studied the influence of *UGT* polymorphisms on toxicity development. One of the most studied polymorphisms in *UGT1A1* is a change in the number of TA repeats $(TA)_n TAA$ in the promoter region. The wild-type allele for this polymorphism is $(TA)_6 TAA$, with $(TA)_7 TAA$

(rs3064744, *UGT1A1*28*) being frequent in Caucasians, but not in Asian populations (≈30% and ≈10%, respectively). However, rs4148323 (*UGT1A1*6*) is more frequent in Asian populations comparing with Caucasians (≈14% and ≈1%, respectively). Ando and colleagues reported that patients carrying the *UGT1A1*28* genotype were at significantly higher risk of having irinotecan-related severe toxicity (OR = 7.23, $p < 0.001$) [64]. Innocenti et al. also stated that patients with *UGT1A1*28* had more events of severe neutropenia (OR = 9.3, $p = 0.001$) [67]. Others have also showed a correlation between *UGT1A1*28* and neutropenia, diarrhoea and vomiting ($p < 0.01$) [104–107]. Additionally, as for *TYMS*, it has been proven that the *UGT1A1* genotype also affects maximum tolerated dose and therefore response [108,109].

3.9. Solute Carriers (SLCs)

Reduction or elimination of the function of SLC genes due to genetic variation can lead to a decrease in SN-38 uptake, with further accumulation in plasma, ultimately leading to toxicity [97]. rs2306283 (*SLCO1B1*1b*) has been shown to cause severe gastrointestinal toxicity, particularly diarrhoea and neutropenia [72,110,111]. A discovery study on 167 mCRC patients receiving irinotecan also revealed a protective effect of the *SLCO1B1* rs2291076 T allele against neutropenia but associated the rs2306283 GG genotype with significantly higher neutropenia events. These results were, however, not replicated in a posterior study of 250 mCRC patients [71].

3.10. Cytochrome p Gene Family (CYP)

CYP3A4 and CYP3A5 are responsible for the oxidation of irinotecan into the inactive metabolites APC, M4 and NPC. Some researchers have studied the possible association of polymorphisms on these genes and chemo-related toxicity but have not found any positive correlation [68,96,112], probably because over 80% of variants in *CYP* genes coding regions are very rare and the sample sizes of these studies were not large enough [113]. It has also been suggested that their enzymatic function might be altered by non-genetic factors such as diet, concomitant medications, altered liver function or patient's performance status [114].

3.11. Epidermal Growth Factor Receptor (EGFR)

Skin toxicity is the major ADR related to anti-EGFR agents. Parmar et al. studied 109 cancer patients and concluded that skin toxicity was linked to the *EGFR* rs2227983 GG genotype (OR = 3.24, $p = 0.014$) [80]. Dahan et al. studied 58 patients treated with third-line cetuximab and irinotecan, and reported a trend between the presence of rs11568315 (CA repeats ≤ 35) and skin toxicity (OR = 2.91, $p = 0.058$) [81]. Sunakawa et al. studied 77 patients treated with cetuximab in combination with oxaliplatin and also correlated rs11568315 (CA repeats ≤ 19) with skin toxicity [115]. A study on 52 patients treated with cetuximab and FOLFIRI found that *EGFR* rs712830 was significantly associated with severe global toxicity (OR = 6.13, $p = 0.010$), but not specifically with skin toxicity. rs712829, rs11568315 (CA repeats cut-off = 17) and rs4444903 were, however, not associated with any toxicity [79]. Another study on 46 mCRC patients receiving XELOX-bevacizumab with or without cetuximab also found no evidence for the association of either rs4444903 or rs11568315 (CA repeats cut-off = 20) with skin toxicity [116].

3.12. Vascular Endothelial Growth Factor (VEGF)

Hypertension is the major toxicity derived from anti-VEGF agent treatment. Studies on the relationship of *VEGF* polymorphisms and bevacizumab-related toxicity have also been controversial. For instance, a study on 89 patients reported a positive link between rs3025039 and hypertension (OR = 0.15, $p = 0.022$), but a meta-analysis of over 1000 cancer patients did not validate this finding [83,117]. Moreover, some researchers have reported that patients with the rs833061 TT, rs2010963 CC or rs699947 CC genotypes were less prone to hypertension caused by bevacizumab

($p < 0.03$) [84,85], but Etienne-Grimaldi et al. saw that patients harbouring the rs2010963 CC genotype alone had more toxicity than patients with other genotypes ($p = 0.01$) [118].

3.13. Immunotherapy and Toxicity

Immunotherapy has arisen in the past few years as a promising therapeutic option in many cancers, and has particular relevance in the case of tumours with microsatellite instability (MSI) [119]. Hence, the FDA approved, in 2018, the use of ipilimumab and nivolumab (anti-CTLA-4 and anti-PD1 monoclonal antibodies, respectively) for the treatment of metastatic CRC patients previously treated with standard chemotherapy [120]. In 2020, pembrolizumab (anti–PD-1) was also approved as a first-line treatment of patients with unresectable, MSI-high or mismatch repair-deficient metastatic CRC [121]. Although there have been some studies suggesting the influence of genetic variants on the development of toxicity due to these treatments in other cancer types, to date there is no sufficient data on CRC [122–124]. Surely novel data on this will shortly become available for pharmacogenomic studies as more patients undergo immunotherapy treatment.

4. Pharmacogenomic Approaches

4.1. Genome-Wide Association Studies (GWAS)

Despite the large effect sizes for toxicity variants discovered by candidate gene approaches, chemotherapy-related toxicity is likely complex and multigenic. Therefore, other discovery strategies may be more suitable to inspect genomic variation in a more comprehensive manner. This has been made possible by the increasing availability of higher-throughput technologies at increasingly affordable prices, which has allowed pharmacogenetics to go genomic. In these upcoming sections, we will describe the more recent approaches that have further expanded the knowledge on pharmacogenomics in recent years (Table 4).

Table 4. Advantages and disadvantages of different pharmacogenomics approaches.

Approach	Advantages	Disadvantages
Candidate genes	<ul><li>offers biological plausibility</li><li>associates variants with known functional consequences and direct clinical implication</li></ul>	<ul><li>bias toward certain genes/pathways (usually, ADME genes) based on prior information of relevance to phenotype, which may be incomplete</li><li>unable to discover novel genes/pathways</li><li>the selected SNPs may not represent the full variation of the studied genes</li><li>limited to protein-coding regions</li></ul>
SNP arrays (GWAS)	<ul><li>unbiased by a priori functional knowledge</li><li>potential discovery of other relevant genes/pathways</li><li>potential to identify variation in regulatory regions such as promoters or enhancers</li><li>high-throughput</li></ul>	<ul><li>need to be adequately powered to detect moderate-effect variants</li><li>require large sample sizes</li><li>multiple testing correction needs to be applied</li><li>variants might be intergenic; harder to interpret</li><li>inspects common populational variation (potential loss of rarer variants)</li><li>not suitable for CNV studies</li></ul>
SNP arrays (targeted fine-mapping approaches)	<ul><li>denser coverage</li><li>cheaper</li><li>may be population-specific</li></ul>	<ul><li>design bias</li><li>may require a priori knowledge of region to study (i.e., as defined by GWAS, for example).</li></ul>

Table 4. Cont.

Approach	Advantages	Disadvantages
NGS (targeted panels, WES, WGS)	• possibility of densely resequencing an entire gene (targeted genes) • allows a more comprehensive and unbiased identification of novel genetic biomarkers • allows the identification of relevant rare variants and CNV • rapid evolution of NGS technologies	• large number of false positives and VUS • need for validation by Sanger or other genotyping methods • higher turnaround time and costs (although decreasing) • need for high data storage capacity • need for deeper bioinformatic knowledge
Functional assays	• give mechanistic perspective on how variants exert their effect • validate the findings at the molecular level, giving further validity to the statistical association results • potentially applicable to a specific desired tissue	• assay design may be difficult, particularly in the case of intergenic variants • results must be replicated in clinical studies

GWAS make use of LD inheritance patterns to inspect common genetic variation across the entire genome. The main two advantages of GWAS over candidate gene studies are that they are unbiased by a priori functional knowledge on the variants (which may help in the discovery of other toxicity relevant pathways) and also have the potential to identify variation in regulatory regions such as promoters or enhancers, which have been largely unexplored by candidate gene approaches.

Several GWAS have been performed to inspect chemotherapy-related toxicity in CRC. In the QUASAR2 trial, Rosmarin et al. analysed over 1000 stage II/III CRC patients receiving capecitabine with or without bevacizumab to identify 1456 variants on 25 candidate genes (Table 3) [41]. Fernandez-Rozadilla et al. used 1012 patients in a two-stage study in patients treated with 5-FU and FOLFOX [57] to find a moderate association for the rs10876844 variant and diarrhoea in patients treated with 5-FU. Won et al. also completed a GWAS on 343 Korean patients receiving oxaliplatin-based regimens to identify possible genetic markers associated with chronic oxaliplatin-induced peripheral neurotoxicity (OXCPN) [78]. They found some evidence for an association that was intronic or within 100 Kb of genes related to various neuronal activities. Two subsequent and independent studies by Oguri et al. and Terrazzino et al. tried to validate these findings, but a single association between the FARS2 rs17140129 G allele and OXCPN (OR = 6.5, p = 0.034) was found [125,126]. Lastly, the CAIRO2 trial included 282 advanced or metastatic CRC individuals treated with XELOX plus bevacizumab and cetuximab. They found some novel SNPs to be moderately associated with toxicity (Table 3) [82].

In general, although GWAS present several advantages over candidate gene strategies, there are also some important limitations, some of which could be overcome post hoc. Firstly, there is a lack of replication due to discrepancies in variant frequencies amongst the different populations used between studies, as seen when comparing the works from Won et al. and Terrazzino et al. mentioned above (Asian vs. Caucasian populations, respectively). Further, most of the associated variants are intergenic, which makes it harder to interpret the results directly and design appropriate validatory functional assays. Moreover, because we are evaluating thousands to millions of variants at a time, statistical power is a concern, and adequate study sample sizes are needed [127]. As an illustration, for a GWAS with a sample size of 200 patients, assessing variants with minor allele frequency (MAF) ≥ 5%, and a statistical threshold of 80% power, the OR that we would be able to discover is OR ≈ 2, which reflects a moderate effect.

GWAS are limited to inspecting common variation (i.e., generally over 5% MAF), but it is likely that toxicity variants may be of rarer prevalence [128,129]. Some approaches have been developed to overcome this limitation. For instance, targeted SNP panels can be designed to fine-map regions of interest spanning a large section of the gene or specific to a desired population. As an example, a commercially available array has been designed to include both common and low-frequency variation as well as Mendelian and functional alleles specific to Spanish genomes, which allows for better genotyping of the Spanish population when comparing with the generic global arrays [130]. Moreover, albeit possible, GWAS strategies are not usually suitable for CNV studies, because they demand that the CNV be in high LD with a genotyped SNP [57].

Despite these limitations, GWAS still hold great potential for discovery, given appropriate study conditions. Surely, there are still pathways contributing to toxicity development to be discovered, as proven by the contribution of *RPS7* to cetuximab-related toxicity. This gene is normally overexpressed in dermal papilla cells, which makes it reasonable that genetic variants could be associated with skin toxicity [82].

4.2. Next-Generation Sequencing (NGS)

NGS, either whole-exome (WES) or whole-genome sequencing (WGS), allows for a more comprehensive identification of novel genetic biomarkers in this regard, and several studies have reported the added value of NGS to identify relevant rare pharmacogenetic variants that would not be detected by other conventional methods (Table 4) [131–136].

In 2014, Mizzi et al. compared the data from 482 healthy individuals (data from Genomes Data and the Wellderly Study) obtained either with WGS or SNP array genotyping that included 1936 known pharmacogenomic variants within 231 ADMET genes (Table 5) [131]. Focusing on these genes, the WGS revealed an average of 17,733 variants vs. 249.5 found with the SNP array. In silico analysis with the PROVEAN and SIFT algorithms, which are in silico functional predictors, showed some missense variants likely to be deleterious. Specifically, they found that 254 of the 332 variants in *UGT1A1* were novel, of which 31 were functional and 26 had a frequency of <1%. In general, the WGS approach allowed the identification of a significantly higher number of variants compared to the SNP array, which might impact the pharmacological processes.

Table 5. Summary of relevant next-generation sequencing (NGS) results.

N	Cohort	Method	Genes	Results	Ref.
482	Genomes Data, Wellderly Study	WGS or SNP array genotyping	231 pharmacogenes	≈17,733 (WGS) vs. 249.5 (SNP array) *UGT1A1* (WGS): 254 of 332 variants were novel, 31 functional and 26 with frequency < 1%.	[131]
>6500	1KG phase 3; ESP	WES and WGS	146 pharmacogenes	19,328 SNV, 62.9% exonic 6225 and 6258 variants in *ABC* transporter (22 genes) and SLC genes (49), respectively, 253 variants in *UGTs* (16) and *GTSs* (14) 92.9% rare, 82.7% very rare 56.2% missenses ≈30–40% of the functional variability in pharmacogenes	[133]
141,456	gnomAD v2.1 [a]	WES and WGS	*SLC* genes	204,287 SNVs and indels, 56.9% missenses, 2.5% frameshifts, 1.7% stop-gains and 1.5% variations in canonical splice sites Each individual had ≈29.7 putatively functional *SLC* variants, 18% of functional variability due to rare variants	[136]

Table 5. Cont.

N	Cohort	Method	Genes	Results	Ref.
100	QUASAR	Amplicon sequencing	DPYD and TYMS coding regions	Novel rare independent DPYD variant (c.1651G>A; p.Ala551Thr)—classified as strongly damaging	[41]
62,402	1 KG phase 3; ExAC [b]	WES and WGS	208 pharmacogenes	201 (97%) genes had 5589 novel CNVs, 47% deletions and 54% duplications Novel deletions responsible for >5% of loss-of-function alleles in 87, 25, 49, 48, 59 and 51 genes in non-Finnish Europeans, Finnish, East Asians, South Asians, Africans and admixed Americans, respectively	[134]

1 KG: 1000 Genomes Project; ESP: Exome Sequencing Project; a: non-Finnish Europeans, Finns, Africans, East Asians, South Asians, Latinos, Ashkenazi Jews and other populations; ExAC: Exome Aggregation Consortium; b: included six major populations: non-Finnish Europeans, Finns, Africans, South Asians, East Asians and admixed Americans.

Another study analysed sequencing data for 146 genes related to pharmacological traits from over 6500 individuals (data from the 1000 Genomes Project (1KGP) and Exome Sequencing Project (ESP)) (Table 5) [133]. They detected 19,328 single nucleotide variants (SNVs), 62.9% of which were exonic; for example, 6225 and 6258 variants in *ABC transporter* (22 genes) and *SLC* genes (49) respectively, and 253 variants in *UGTs* (16) and *GTSs* (14). Most of these variants were indeed rare (MAF < 1%; 92.9%) or very rare (MAF < 0.1%; 82.7%)—meaning that they would not be detected by conventional methods—and the majority were missenses (56.2%). The functional impact from rare variants was different across the genes, yet they concluded that rare variants contribute on average 30–40% of the functional variability in the studied pharmacogenes.

Schaller et al. analysed WES and WGS data from 141,456 individuals (data from gnomAD v2.1) and assessed the genetic variability of *SLC* genes (Table 5) [136]. They detected 204,287 SNVs and indels, of which 56.9% were missenses, and several were loss-of-function variants, such as 2.5% frameshifts, 1.7% stop-gains and 1.5% variations in canonical splice sites. They concluded that each individual presents, on average, 29.7 putatively functional *SLC* variants, with rare variants contributing 18% of this functional variability.

Following on from the results obtained from their initial GWAS, Rosmarin et al. sequenced the complete *DPYD* and *TYMS* coding regions and identified a further novel rare independent *DPYD* variant (c.1651G>A; p.Ala551Thr). This change was present in a single patient that had presented with grade 4 neutropenia and thrombocytopenia, and was predicted to be "strongly damaging" by in silico predictors (Table 4) [41].

NGS approaches can not only be useful to identify rarer variants but can be an important asset to reveal copy number variations (CNVs). The case in point is the work by Santos et al. that included CNV available data from 2504 whole genomes and 59,898 exomes (data from 1KGP and Exome Aggregation Consortium (ExAC)) and focused on 208 ADME genes (Table 5) [134]. Within these, 201 (97%) genes had a total of 5589 novel CNVs, where 47% were deletions and 54% were duplications. These novel deletions were responsible for >5% of loss-of-function alleles in a considerable number of genes (87, 25, 49, 48, 59 and 51 genes in non-Finnish Europeans, Finnish, East Asians, South Asians, Africans and admixed Americans, respectively). This demonstrates the impact that CNV might have on ADME genes, and hence the development of ADRs.

As the conventional screening methods only include common variants, a high number of variants are missed, thus explaining the need for unbiased and more comprehensive approaches. These interesting works emphasise the potential of NGS to detect novel rarer variants or CNV, not only in ADME genes, but in other pathways, which might help to explain the pharmacogenetic variability possibly associated with toxicity caused by chemotherapy.

5. Functional Assays

Functional assays on candidate variants are essential to ultimately clarify the mechanisms by which the genetic variants exert their effect on ADR development. Pharmacokinetic (PK) studies have been the most used approach to assess the functional impact of toxicity SNPs (Table 4). They have been used for many years now to evaluate enzymatic activity in patients carrying the desired variants, as they measure the level of drug and its metabolites that influence drug bioavailability and could hence lead to the toxicity profile.

By far, the most studied gene in PK studies has been *DPYD*, and there is an agreement that the DPD protein plays a crucial role in 5-FU metabolism. There are several methods to determine DPD deficiency [30,137]: testing for DPD activity in peripheral blood mononuclear cells, the uracil breath test, the uracil test dose and endogenous DHU/U ratio, or high-performance liquid chromatography (HPLC).

A study including 30 patients heterozygous for the *DPYD* rs3918290 variant analysed 5-FU plasma concentrations by HPLC and found that the mean maximum enzymatic 5-FU conversion capacity value was 40% lower in these patients (Table 6) [138].

Table 6. Pharmacokinetic studies on fluoropyrimidines and irinotecan.

Genes	Significant Variants	N	Pharmacokinetic Results	Ref.
		Fluoropyrimidines		
DPYD	rs3918290	1 case (heterozygous for IVS14+1G>A) vs. 6 controls (CRC)	inactivation of one *DPYD* allele: strong ↓CL_{5-FU}: severe toxicity	[139]
DPYD	rs1801265 rs115232898 rs55886062	175 CRC patients	rs55886062: lowest activity ($p = 0.014$) rs115232898: 46% ↓activity ($p = 0.026$) rs1801265: 27% ↑activity ($p = 0.013$)	[140]
DPYD	rs3918290 rs67376798 rs55886062	487 advanced carcinoma patients	rs3918290, rs67376798, or rs55886062: ↓CL_{5-FU} ($p < 0.001$)	[141]
DPYD	rs3918290	30 patients (heterozygous for IVS14+1G>A) and 18 controls	rs3918290: 40% ↓Vmax ($p < 0.001$)	[142]
DPYD	rs1801159	112 gastric or colon cancer patients	rs1801159: ↓k ($p = 0.022$) and nausea/vomiting ($p = 0.005$)	[143]
DPYD	rs55886062 rs1801265 rs1801158	Expression vector	rs1801158: 36% ↑activity ($p = 3.4 \times 10^{-7}$) rs1801265: 13% ↑activity ($p = 0.0013$) rs55886062: 75% ↓activity ($p = 5.2 \times 10^{-9}$)	[29]
DPYD	rs141044036 rs72549308 rs1801268 rs145773863 rs55674432 rs72547601 rs137999090 rs59086055 rs1801266 rs111858276 rs183385770 rs72549307 rs138616379 rs72549304 rs112766203 rs183105782 rs143986398 rs115232898 rs2297595	Expression vector	rs141044036, rs72549308, rs1801268, rs145773863, rs55674432, rs137999090, rs72547601, rs59086055: <12.5% activity ($p < 3.5 \times 10^{-4}$) rs1801266, rs72549307, rs111858276, rs138616379, rs183385770, rs72549304: 12.5–25% activity ($p < 0.0021$) rs112766203, rs143986398, rs183105782, rs115232898: >25% ↓activity ($p < 0.05$) rs2297595: 120% ↑activity ($p = 0.025$)	[31]
ABC	rs2271862	48 CRC patients	*ABCA2* rs2271862: ↑CL_{5-FU}	[144]

Table 6. *Cont.*

Genes	Significant Variants	N	Pharmacokinetic Results	Ref.
ABCB1￼ ABCC1￼ ABCG2￼ UGT1A1	rs12720066￼ rs6498588￼ rs10929302	85 advanced cancer patients	ABCB1 rs12720066 ($p = 6.24 \times 10^{-4}$) and rs6498588 ($p = 9.50 \times 10^{-4}$), and UGT1A1 rs10929302 ($p = 9.00 \times 10^{-5}$): ↑AUC$_{SN-38}$ ↑AUC$_{SN-38}$: G ≥ 3 neutropenia ($p = 0.0001$)	[73]
ABCG2￼ SLCO1B1￼ ABCB1￼ ABCC1￼ ABCC2￼ UGT1A1￼ UGT1A9￼ UGT1A7￼ CES￼ CYP3A4￼ CYP3A5￼ HNF1A	rs717620￼ rs1169288￼ rs4149056￼ rs35605￼ rs1092302￼ rs3740066	85 advanced cancer patients	ABCC2 rs717620 ($p = 0.002$), HNF1A rs1169288 ($p = 0.007$), SLCO1B1 rs4149056 ($p = 0.015$): ↑AUC$_{CPT-11}$ ABCC1 rs35605 ($p = 0.031$), UGT1A1 rs1092302 ($p = 0.007$): ↑AUC$_{SN-38}$ ABCC2 rs3740066: ↑AUC$_{SN-38G}$ and ↑AUC$_{APC}$ ($p = 0.012$) ABCC1 rs35605 ($p = 0.023$), rs3064744 ($p < 0.0001$): ↓GR	[111]
UGT1A1	rs3064744	250 mCRC patients	↓GR ($p = 0.01$) and ↑BI ($p = 0.003$): G ≥ 3 toxicity rs3064744: ↓GR ($p = 0.01$) and ↑BI ($p = 0.007$)	[145]
UGT1A1￼ UGT1A7￼ UGT1A9	rs4124874￼ rs10929302￼ UGT1A7*3	Subset of 71 patients	UGT1A1 rs4124874 and rs10929302: ↑BI ($p = 0.03$ and $p = 0.04$, respectively) UGT1A7*3: ↓GR ($p = 0.02$) and ↑BI ($p = 0.007$)	[146]
HNF1A	rs2244608	Subset of 49 patients	rs2244608: ↑AUC$_{SN-38}$ ($p = 0.032$), ↑BI ($p = 0.021$) and ↓GR ($p = 0.035$)	[147]
ABCC2	rs2273697￼ rs17216114￼ rs1885301￼ rs2804402￼ rs717620￼ rs3740066	31 mCRC patients	rs2273697: ↓AUC$_{CPT-11}$ ($p = 0.011$) rs17216114: ↓AUC$_{SN-38}$ rs1885301, rs2804402, rs717620 and rs3740066: ↑AUN$_{SN-38}$ ($p < 0.03$)	[148]
ABCB1￼ ABCC1￼ ABCC2￼ ABCG2￼ CES1￼ CES2￼ CYP3A4￼ CYP3A5￼ UGT1A￼ XRCC1	rs1128503	65 solid tumour patients	ABCB1 rs1128503: ↑AUC$_{CPT-11}$ ($p = 0.038$), AUC$_{SN-38}$ ($p = 0.031$) and ↓CL$_{SN-38}$ ($p = 0.015$)	[96]
UGT1A1	rs3064744	20 solid tumour patients	rs3064744 ↓GR ($p = 0.001$) and ↑BI ($p = 0.001$) AUC$_{SN-38}$: neutropenia ($p < 0.0001$)	[105]
UGT1A1￼ UGT1A9	rs3064744	94 solid tumour patients	rs3064744: ↓GR ($p = 0.022$)	[149]
UGT1A1	rs4148323￼ rs4124874￼ rs3064744	85 solid tumour patients	rs4148323: ↓GR ($p = 0.0372$) rs4124874: ↑BI ($p = 0.0048$) rs3064744: ↑BI ($p = 0.0007$)	[150]
ABCC2￼ UGT1A1	ABCC2*2￼ rs306474	167 solid tumour patients	ABCC2*2: ↓CL$_{CPT-11}$ ($p = 0.020$) rs3064744: ↓CL$_{SN-38}$ ($p < 0.001$), GR and BI ($p = 0.014$)	[151]
UGT1A1	rs3064744	62 solid tumour patients	rs3064744: ↓CL$_{SN-38}$ ($p < 0.01$) ↑SN-38 exposure: G2–3 diarrhoea ($p = 0.03$)	[152]
UGT1A1	rs3064744	65 solid tumour or lymphoma patients	rs3064744: ↑BI ($p = 0.0003$) and ↓GR ($p = 0.03$) ↑BI: G4 neutropenia ($p = 0.001$)	[67]
UGT1A1￼ UGT1A7￼ UGT1A9￼ UGT1A10	rs3064744￼ rs4148323	176 cancer patients	rs3064744 or rs4148323: ↓GR ($p < 0.0001$)	[153]
UGT1A1￼ ABCG2	rs4148323	45 cancer patients	rs4148323: ↑AUC$_{SN-38}$ ($p = 0.018$), ↓GR ($p = 0.006$) and 61% ↑BI ($p = 0.003$)	[154]
ABCB1	ABCB1*2	49 cancer patients	ABCB1*2: ↓CL$_{CPT-11, SN-38, APC}$ ($p = 0.0154, 0.0043, 0.0169$, respectively)	[155]

Enzymatic activities were measured by high performance liquid chromatography (HPLC).

Another study reported the effect of *DPYD* rs75017182 on DPD expression and activity and showed that heterozygous carriers presented a 35% activity reduction that was caused by alternative splicing [33].

By these means, at least four SNPs in *DPYD* have been proven deleterious: rs55886062, rs3918290, rs67376798 and rs56038477/HapB3 [30,34,156]. Studies on other variations have so far led to inconclusive or contradicting results [157].

Of late, other approaches have also been used to assess the functionality of pharmacogenetic variants. For instance, Offer et al. proposed the construction of a vector for rapid phenotypic assessment of *DPYD* variants and their relation with 5-FU sensitivity (Table 6) [29,31]. *DPYD* constructs were expressed in mammalian cells and the enzymatic activity of the expressed proteins was measured by HPLC and compared to the wild type. By these means, they could confirm that 30 of the variants caused a significant reduction in enzymatic activity. Interestingly, 19 of the variants tested displayed <25% activity. In turn, *DPYD* rs1801158, rs1801265, rs2297595, rs200687447, rs60139309 and rs114096998 had higher enzymatic activity, and therefore cells expressing these variants were more resistant to 5-FU, which may not confer susceptibility to toxicity development, but may in turn influence response rates.

In 2015, Henricks et al. proposed to assign an activity value (AV) to *DPYD* alleles, to adjust the initial dose of 5-FU. In this context, fully functional alleles had an AV = 1, reduced activity alleles had an AV = 0.5 and non-functional alleles had an AV = 0 (wild-type AV = 1; rs67376798 and rs56038477 AV = 0.5; and rs3918290 and rs55886062 AV = 0). Based on the AV of both alleles, the gene activity score (AS) is calculated, thus representing the enzymatic phenotype of the patient [30].

For genes other than *DPYD*, there is much less functional evidence (Table 6). Some research has been conducted on the relation of irinotecan PK variants. These studies were able to significantly associate polymorphisms in *ABCC1* and *ABCB1* with SN-38 exposure and the glucuronidation ratio (GR)—measured as AUC SN-38G/AUC SN-38 [73,111]. Demattia et al. investigated the possible association between *ABCG2* rs7699188 and *ABCB1* rs2032582 with irinotecan PK parameters on patients with advanced CRC by measuring plasma concentrations of irinotecan, SN38 and SN38G, but did not find any significant correlation [74]. Toffoli et al. evaluated irinotecan PK in 71 patients with metastatic CRC. They associated severe toxicity with a significantly lower GR ($p = 0.01$) and an increased biliary index (BI) ($p = 0.003$), which indicates SN-38 accumulation. Further, they reported a significant correlation between *UGT1A1*28* and lower GR ($p = 0.01$), and higher BI ($p = 0.007$) [145]. Other works showed that patients with the wild-type genotype had a significantly higher clearance of SN-38 compared to *UGT1A1*28* ($p < 0.001$), and that the homozygous genotype was significantly associated with GR ($p = 0.005$) and BI ($p = 0.014$) [151]. Iyer et al. also reported significantly lower SN-38 glucuronidation in patients with *UGT1A1*28* ($p = 0.001$) [105]. Other *UGT1A* polymorphisms, such as *UGT1A1*60* ($p = 0.005$), *UGT1A1*93* ($p < 0.0001$), *UGT1A1*6* ($p = 0.037$) and *UGT1A7*3* ($p < 0.02$), were also associated with GR and BI [73,146,150].

6. Cost-Effectiveness Analysis

Besides the need for clear evidence on the functional relevance of a pharmacogenetic biomarker, a proof of cost-effectiveness—that the pharmacogenetic strategy is more effective with an acceptable additional cost or even a cost saving—is crucial to facilitate its introduction into clinical practice and acceptance from healthcare professionals and institutions.

In 2015, Deenen et al. evaluated the safety and costs of upfront *DPYD*2A* genotyping with individualised dose adjustment treatment for fluoropyrimidines [158]. They showed that genotype-guided dosing represented a reduction in severe toxicity from 73% to 28%. Moreover, dose adjustment based on genotype produced shorter and easier to control toxicities, and a significant reduction in drug-induced death from 10% to 0%. Therefore, they demonstrated that screening for *DPYD*2A* before treatment could be lifesaving and potentially cost-efficient. Cortejoso et al. complementarily evaluated the costs of genotyping three *DPYD* variants (rs3918290, rs67376798 and rs55886062) and the management of severe neutropenia caused by fluoropyrimidines. Considering an average cost of management of EUR 3044.40 vs. EUR 6.40 per patient for *DPYD* testing, they concluded that genotyping is cost-effective if severe neutropenia is prevented in at least 2.1 cases per 1000 treated patients [159]. Given that the combined frequency of these three markers is about 1%, this provides evidence that *DPYD* testing should be considered by healthcare systems. Murphy et al. further compared the reactive vs. prospective *DPYD* genotyping of variants rs3918290, rs67376798, rs1801158 and rs55886062. Of the 134 included patients, five carried a *DPYD* variant and the costs of their hospitalisation were EUR 232,061, whereas the total cost of genotyping prior to treatment for all patients would have been only EUR 23,718. Even if patients still had to endure some ADRs, the cost would have been considerably smaller, making pharmacogenetic analysis again cost-efficient [160]. In 2019, Henricks et al. also compared the costs from prospective *DPYD* screening (rs3918290, rs67376798, rs55886062 and rs56038477) with no screening on 1103 patients receiving fluoropyrimidine-based therapy. Patients with variants rs67376798 or rs56038477 had a 25% dose reduction, while patients with rs3918290 or rs55886062 had a 50% dose reduction. They concluded that the expected costs of the screening approach were EUR 2599 vs. EUR 2650 for the non-screening approach, representing a cost saving of EUR 51 per patient. These results strongly suggested that upfront *DPYD*-guided dose individualisation does not result in extra costs, and therefore solidly supports *DPYD* screening implementation prior to fluoropyrimidine treatment as a standard of care [161]. It also constituted the basis for pharmGKB EMA guideline changes from actionable to recommended.

Gold et al. assessed the safety and costs of testing for *UGT1A1*28* before irinotecan treatment [162]. Assuming no treatment efficacy reduction, the average cost saving per patient was EUR 250. Obradovic et al. compared the standard irinotecan dose with dose reduction based on *UGT1A1* genotyping, and evaluated the cases of severe neutropenia, the number of life-years gained and the associated costs. They concluded that genotyping with dose reduction in homozygotes was cost-saving in African and Caucasian populations, but not in Asians, given the population frequency of this variant [163]. Another study by Butzke et al. compared severe neutropenia and grade 4 diarrhoea in a similar setting, to find that dosage calculations based on *UGT1A1*28* genotypes save about EUR 600 per patient [164]. More recently, Roncato et al. calculated that the costs for toxicity management per patient increased 1.4-fold for heterozygotes and 6-fold for homozygotes compared to wild-type individuals, and they were superior to the costs related to genotyping all patients before treatment [165].

7. Pharmacogenomic Testing Guidelines

Although, as we have described so far, there is a considerable amount of evidence on the effect of genetic variants on CRC chemotoxicity, translation into clinical practice is yet far from routine implementation. For now, guidelines from leading authorities, including the European Medicines Agency (EMA), the Food and Drug Administration (FDA), the private pharmacogenetic consortia, the CPIC, the Royal Dutch Association for the Advancement of Pharmacy-Pharmacogenetics Working Group (DPWG) and the Spanish Agency for Medicines and Health Products (Agencia Española de Medicamentos y Productos Sanitarios, AEMPS) have only produced a very limited list of recommendations (Table 7) [166–170].

Table 7. Current CRC pharmacogenetic guidelines for treatment administration.

Drug	Gene	Annotation by Drug Regulatory Agencies and Guidelines Recommendations				
		FDA	CPIC	AEMPS	EMA	DPWG
Fluoropyrimidines	DPYD	Actionable PGx [a] Withhold or permanently discontinue treatment in patients with evidence of acute early-onset or severe toxicity, which may indicate near complete or absence of DPD activity. No dose has been proven safe for patients with no DPD activity. There is insufficient data to recommend a specific dose in patients with partial DPD activity [170]	Actionable PGx [a] Intermediate metaboliser (individual with one normal function allele plus one no function allele, or with two decreased function alleles)—decreased DPD activity and increased risk for severe/fatal ADR. Reduce starting dose based on AS followed by titration of dose based on toxicity or therapeutic drug monitoring (if available). AS 1: Reduce dose by 50% AS 1.5: Reduce dose by 25–50%. Poor metaboliser (individual with two no function alleles, or with one no function plus one decreased function allele)—complete DPD deficiency and increased risk for severe/fatal ADR. AS 0.5: Avoid treatment, and in case alternative agents are not suitable, strongly reduce starting dose with early therapeutic drug monitoring. AS 0: Avoid treatment [167]	Testing required [b] Test for DPYD genotype (c.1905+1G>A, c.1679T>G, c.1236G>A/HapB3) and/or DPD deficiency (measure blood uracil level) before treatment. Treatment is contraindicated in patients with complete DPD deficiency. In case of partial DPD deficiency with no suitable alternative agents, reduce initial dose and monitor levels. No concrete reduction has been established [166]	Testing required [b] Test for the lack of DPD activity before treatment (measure blood uracil level, or check for DPYD variants—c.1905+1G>A, c.1679T>G, c.2846A>T y c.1236G>A/HapB3). Treatment is contraindicated in patients with complete DPD deficiency. A reduced starting dose should be considered in patients with partial DPD deficiency [169]	-
Irinotecan	UGT1A1	Actionable PGx [a] Consider reduction in starting dose for patients homozygous for the UGT1A1*28 allele. The precise dose reduction is not known and subsequent dose modifications should be considered based on individual patient tolerance to treatment [170]	-	-	-	Actionable PGx [a] Start with 70% of standard dose. If the patient tolerates it, the dose can be increased, guided by the neutrophil count [168]
Cetuximab/panitumumab	EGFR KRAS NRAS	Testing required [b] Determine EGFR expression status and confirm the absence of an RAS mutation before treatment [170]	-	-	Testing required [b] Test RAS status (KRAS and NRAS exons 2, 3 and 4) before treatment [171]	-

a: Actionable PGx—it may inform about changes in efficacy, dosage, metabolism or toxicity due to gene/protein/chromosomal variants or phenotypes, or contraindicate a drug in a subset of patients with particular variants/genotypes/phenotypes, without requiring prior testing. b: Testing required—it states that testing should be conducted before using a drug. This requirement may only be for a subset of patients.

Pharmacogenetic guidelines from CPIC for the administration of fluoropyrimidines recommend that the *DPYD* metaboliser status (based on variants rs3918290, rs67376798, rs55886062 and rs56038477) is characterised prior to treatment administration. Poor metabolisers (AS 0–0.5) either: (a) receive an alternative drug; or (b) if 5-FU/capecitabine is still considered the better suited option of treatment, it is recommended to strongly reduce the given dose and accompany with close monitoring. For intermediate metabolisers (AS 1–1.5), a 50% dose reduction is recommended [156,167]. On the other hand, the FDA only contraindicates the administration of 5-FU/capecitabine in patients with DPD deficiency, but does not directly recommend screening for DPD deficiency before treatment, neither does it distinguish heterozygous nor homozygous DPD-deficient patients (www.pharmgkb.org/gene/PA145/labelAnnotation (accessed on 07 October 2020)) [170].

As for irinotecan treatments, pharmacogenomic testing criteria are merely based on the *UGT1A1* genotype (rs3064744). DPWG recommends a 30% reduction in the standard dose if patients are *UGT1A1*28/28* [168], whereas the FDA vaguely recommends dose reduction (www.pharmgkb.org/chemical/PA450085/labelAnnotation (accessed on 07 October 2020)) [170]).

With the growing knowledge on CRC pharmacogenomics, more guidelines including other genes/variants will most likely be available in the next coming years. For instance, the *ABC* transporter genes, like *ABCC1* and *ABCB1*, have been quite studied so far and there is good evidence of their relation to the development of ADRs, both by association studies and functional assays.

8. Limitations in Pharmacogenomic Studies

In this appraisal, we have presented a comprehensive review of the field of CRC pharmacogenomics, since its early inception to the latest trends. Although remarkable findings have been produced, the road towards widespread clinical implementation is still far from over, and is inherently hindered by some of the limitations that pharmacogenetic analysis encounters. One of the main problems in pharmacogenomic studies is the extensive phenotype heterogeneity. This could be attributable to at least three different factors: (a) heterogeneity in clinical inclusion, i.e., differences in tumour staging and treatment strategies and lines (i.e., the genetic contribution to toxicity may be different in patients that have received FOLFOX as first-line treatment compared to those who have received it as second line); (b) pharmacogenomic data are not kept in a standardised manner, and it is usually hard to find in the patient's clinical record case report forms, including the appropriate scaling, timing and line of treatment, and Eastern Cooperative Oncology Group (ECOG) performance status of the patient (amongst others) should therefore be used to produce robust study designs; and (c) some ADRs, like haematological counts, can be measured quantitatively, whereas others, like diarrhoea, are subject to clinician interpretation. To overcome this, toxicity grading scales such as the Common Terminology Criteria for Adverse Events (CTCAE) should be used across studies [172].

Secondly, the influence of each therapeutical agent alone is hard, if not impossible, to assess, as the great majority of patients undergo combination therapies, and many of the ADRs are shared amongst treatments. This could be due, for instance, to the backbone presence of 5-FU in most settings but could also result from a pleiotropic effect of different drugs.

Thirdly, there has been, in general, a lack of unambiguous association findings. This could be due to the abovementioned phenotypic heterogeneity, but also other factors such as study sample sizes or population stratification issues. For instance, the overwhelming majority of studies reported in this review have been performed exclusively on Caucasian populations, and there are few published works in non-Europeans. Moreover, those that have been published in Asians show considerable differences in the allelic frequencies of the variants. Therefore, validation of findings in cohorts with appropriate statistical power is essential. On this topic, an outstanding example is the Radiogenomics Consortium, which advocates for the standardisation of toxicity data collection derived from radiation treatments. They have published guidelines for STrengthening the Reporting Of Genetic Association studies in Radiogenomics (STROGAR), which allow for multi-institutional approaches towards large-scale radiotherapy patient biorepositories and databanks. Indeed, this consortium has already successfully completed several GWAS of radiotherapy toxicity [173–177].

Fourthly, there are no implemented guidelines for the reporting of pharmacogenetic studies. There have been recent efforts to overcome this, including a publication on the STrengthening the Reporting Of Pharmacogenetic Studies (STROPS). This work produces guidelines to standardise pharmacogenetic reporting. This could be essential for the homogenisation of pharmacogenetic data leading to improved systematic reviewing and meta-analyses, hence improving the power and applicability for pharmacogenetic associations [178].

Overall, the evidence gathered so far has brilliantly supported the relevance of pharmacogenomic testing in personalised medicine approaches. Novel genomic technologies such as GWAS and NGS offer unprecedented and affordable access to genomic information that can be assessed to discover novel pharmacogenomic variants related to toxic ADRs [179,180]. Pharmacokinetic profiling has proven to be useful for the identification of patients that might benefit from modified treatment strategies and might help improve the prediction value of genetic testing. Cost-effective analyses produced so far have validated the thought that the treatment design should be designed based on pharmacogenomic data, and that these strategies are always cost-effective vs. having to palliate toxicity issues.

Nevertheless, widespread testing is still anecdotic including in regulatory guideline recommendations. Researchers must hence make additional efforts to produce sound and relevant data that can be presented to the regulatory agencies to support pre-treatment testing. Surely, we must continue working in this direction towards a more meaningful implementation of pharmacogenomics in the routine clinical practice.

Author Contributions: Conceptualisation, C.F.-R.; writing—original draft preparation, A.R.S. and C.F.-R.; writing—review and editing, A.R.S., O.M., Á.C. and C.F.-R.; supervision, C.F.-R. and Á.C.; funding acquisition, Á.C. All authors have read and agreed to the published version of the manuscript.

Funding: This research was supported by grant FIS PI 16/01057- ISCIII (to Á.C.), ISCIII PFIS grant FI17/00215 (to A.R.S.) and Fundación Olga Torres (to C.F.-R.).

Conflicts of Interest: The authors declare no conflict of interest.

References

1. Bray, F.; Ferlay, J.; Soerjomataram, I.; Siegel, R.L.; Torre, L.A.; Jemal, A. Global cancer statistics 2018: Globocan estimates of incidence and mortality worldwide for 36 cancers in 185 countries. *CA Cancer J. Clin.* **2018**, *68*, 394–424. [CrossRef] [PubMed]
2. Douillard, J.Y.; Cunningham, D.; Roth, A.D.; Navarro, M.; James, R.D.; Karasek, P.; Jandik, P.; Iveson, T.; Carmichael, J.; Alakl, M.; et al. Irinotecan combined with fluorouracil compared with fluorouracil alone. as first-line treatment for metastatic colorectal cancer: A multicentre randomised trial. *Lancet* **2000**, *355*, 1041–1047. [CrossRef]
3. de Gramont, A.; Figer, A.; Seymour, M.; Homerin, M.; Hmissi, A.; Cassidy, J.; Boni, C.; Cortes-Funes, H.; Cervantes, A.; Freyer, G.; et al. Leucovorin and fluorouracil with or without oxaliplatin as first-line treatment in advanced colorectal cancer. *J. Clin. Oncol.* **2000**, *18*, 2938–2947. [CrossRef] [PubMed]
4. Van Cutsem, E.; Cervantes, A.; Nordlinger, B.; Arnold, D. The ESMO Guidelines Working Group Metastatic colorectal cancer: ESMO clinical practice guidelines for diagnosis, treatment and follow-up. *Ann. Oncol.* **2014**, *25*, iii1–iii9. [CrossRef]
5. Iacovelli, R.; Pietrantonio, F.; Palazzo, A.; Maggi, C.; Ricchini, F.; De Braud, F.; Di Bartolomeo, M. Incidence and relative risk of grade 3 and 4 diarrhoea in patients treated with capecitabine or 5-fluorouracil: A meta-analysis of published trials. *Br. J. Clin. Pharmacol.* **2014**, *78*, 1228–1237. [CrossRef] [PubMed]
6. Schwartz, L.H.; Litière, S.; De Vries, E.; Ford, R.; Gwyther, S.; Mandrekar, S.; Shankar, L.; Bogaerts, J.; Chen, A.; Dancey, J.; et al. RECIST 1.1-Update and clarification: From the RECIST committee. *Eur. J. Cancer* **2016**, *62*, 132–137. [CrossRef]

7. Latremouille-Viau, D.; Chang, J.; Guerin, A.; Shi, S.; Wang, E.; Yu, J.; Ngai, C. The economic burden of common adverse events associated with metastatic colorectal cancer treatment in the United States. *J. Med. Econ.* **2016**, *20*, 54–62. [CrossRef]
8. Peters, E.J.; Motsinger-Reif, A.; Havener, T.M.; Everitt, L.; Hardison, N.E.; Watson, V.G.; Wagner, M.; Richards, K.L.; Province, M.A.; McLeod, H.L. Pharmacogenomic characterization of US FDA-approved cytotoxic drugs. *Pharmacogenomics* **2011**, *12*, 1407–1415. [CrossRef]
9. Watters, J.W.; Kraja, A.; Meucci, M.A.; Province, M.A.; McLeod, H.L. Genome-wide discovery of loci influencing chemotherapy cytotoxicity. *Proc. Natl. Acad. Sci. USA* **2004**, *101*, 11809–11814. [CrossRef]
10. Whirl-Carrillo, M.; McDonagh, E.M.; Hebert, J.M.; Gong, L.; Sangkuhl, K.; Thorn, C.F.; Altman, R.B.; Klein, T.E. Pharmacogenomics knowledge for personalized medicine. *Clin. Pharmacol. Ther.* **2012**, *92*, 414–417. [CrossRef]
11. Longley, D.B.; Harkin, D.P.; Johnston, P.G. 5-Fluorouracil: Mechanisms of action and clinical strategies. *Nat. Rev. Cancer* **2003**, *3*, 330–338. [CrossRef] [PubMed]
12. Food and Drug Administration. Highlights of prescribing information. *Capecitabine* **2015**. Available online: https://www.accessdata.fda.gov/drugsatfda_docs/label/2015/020896s037lbl.pdf (accessed on 13 November 2020).
13. De Matti, E.; Roncato, R.; Dalle Fratte, C.; Ecca, F.; Toffoli, G.; Cecchin, E. The use of pharmacogenetics to increase the safety of colorectal cancer patients treated with fluoropyrimidines. *Cancer Drug Resist.* **2019**, *2*, 116–130. [CrossRef]
14. Van Cutsen, E.; Twelves, C.; Cassidy, J.; Allman, D.; Bajetta, E.; Boyer, M.; Bugat, R.; Findlay, M.; Frings, S.; Jahn, M.; et al. Oral capecitabine compared with intravenous fluorouracil plus leucovorin in patients with metastatic colorectal cancer: Results of a large phase III study. *J. Clin. Oncol.* **2001**, *19*, 4097–4106. [CrossRef] [PubMed]
15. Food and Drug Administration. Highlights of prescribing information. *Oxaliplatin* **2002**. Available online: https://www.accessdata.fda.gov/drugsatfda_docs/label/2020/021492s016lbl.pdf (accessed on 13 November 2020).
16. Food and Drug Administration. Highlights of prescribing information. *Irinotecan* **2014**. Available online: https://www.accessdata.fda.gov/drugsatfda_docs/label/2014/020571s048lbl.pdf (accessed on 13 November 2020).
17. Food and Drug Administration. Highlights of prescribing information. *Cetuximab* **2009**. Available online: https://www.accessdata.fda.gov/drugsatfda_docs/label/2019/125084s273lbl.pdf (accessed on 13 November 2020).
18. Food and Drug Administration. Highlights of prescribing information. *Panitumumab* **2015**. Available online: http://www.accessdata.fda.gov/drugsatfda_docs/label/2015/125147s200lbl.pdf (accessed on 13 November 2020).
19. Food and Drug Administration. Highlights of prescribing information. *Bevacizumab* **2017**. Available online: https://www.accessdata.fda.gov/drugsatfda_docs/label/2011/125085s225lbl.pdf (accessed on 13 November 2020).
20. Thorn, C.F.; Marsh, S.; Carrillo, M.W.; McLeod, H.L.; Klein, T.E.; Altman, R.B. Pharm GKB summary: Fluoropyrimidine pathways. *Pharm. Genom.* **2011**, *21*, 237–242. [CrossRef]
21. Diasio, R.B.; Harris, B.E. *Clinical Pharmacokinetics*; Lippincott Williams and Wilkins: Philadelphia, PA, USA, 1989.
22. Raymond, E.; Chaney, S.G.; Taamma, A.; Cvitkovic, E. Oxaliplatin: A review of preclinical and clinical studies. *Ann. Oncol.* **1998**, *9*, 1053–1071. [CrossRef]
23. Marsh, S.; McLeod, H.; Dolan, E.; Shukla, S.J.; Rabik, C.A.; Gong, L.; Hernandez-Boussard, T.; Lou, X.J.; Klein, T.E.; Altman, R.B. Platinum pathway. *Pharm. Genom.* **2009**, *19*, 563–564. [CrossRef]
24. Saltz, L.B.; Cox, J.V.; Blanke, C.; Rosen, L.S.; Fehrenbacher, L.; Moore, M.J.; Maroun, J.A.; Ackland, S.P.; Locker, P.K.; Pirotta, N.; et al. Irinotecan plus Fluorouracil and Leucovorin for Metastatic Colorectal Cancer. *N. Engl. J. Med.* **2000**, *343*, 905–914. [CrossRef]
25. Wall, M.E.; Wani, M.C. Discovery to Clinic. *Ann. N. Y. Acad. Sci.* **1996**, *803*, 1–12. [CrossRef]
26. Rothenberg, M.L. Topoisomerase I inhibitors: Review and update. *Ann. Oncol.* **1997**, *8*, 837–855. [CrossRef]
27. Zhao, B.; Wang, L.; Qiu, H.; Zhang, M.; Sun, L.; Peng, P.; Yu, Q.; Yuan, X. Mechanisms of resistance to anti-EGFR therapy in colorectal cancer. *Oncotarget* **2016**, *8*, 3980–4000. [CrossRef]
28. Toffoli, G.; Giodini, L.; Buonadonna, A.; Berretta, M.; De Paoli, A.; Scalone, S.; Miolo, G.; Mini, E.; Nobili, S.; Lonardi, S.; et al. Clinical validity of a DPYD-based pharmacogenetic test to predict severe toxicity to fluoropyrimidines. *Int. J. Cancer* **2015**, *137*, 2971–2980. [CrossRef] [PubMed]
29. Offer, S.M.; Wegner, N.J.; Fossum, C.; Wang, K.; Diasio, R.B. Phenotypic profiling of DPYD variations relevant to 5-fluorouracil sensitivity using real-time cellular analysis and in vitro measurement of enzyme activity. *Cancer Res.* **2013**, *73*, 1958–1968. [CrossRef] [PubMed]

30. Henricks, L.M.; Lunenburg†, C.A.; Meulendijks, D.; Gelderblom, H.; Cats, A.; Swen, J.J.; Schellens, J.H.; Guchelaar, H. TranslatingDPYDgenotype into DPD phenotype: Using theDPYDgene activity score. *Pharmacogenomics* **2015**, *16*, 1275–1284. [CrossRef] [PubMed]
31. Offer, S.M.; Fossum, C.C.; Wegner, N.J.; Stuflesser, A.J.; Butterfield, G.L.; Diasio, R.B. Comparative Functional Analysis of DPYD Variants of Potential Clinical Relevance to Dihydropyrimidine Dehydrogenase Activity. *Cancer Res.* **2014**, *74*, 2545–2554. [CrossRef]
32. Zaanan, A.; Dumont, L.M.; Loriot, M.A.; Taieb, J.; Narjoz, C. *Clinical Pharmacology and Therapeutics*; CRC Press: Boca Raton, FL, USA, 2014.
33. Nie, Q.; Shrestha, S.; Tapper, E.E.; Trogstad-Isaacson, C.; Bouchonville, K.J.; Lee, A.M.; Wu, R.; Jerde, C.R.; Wang, Z.; Kubica, P.; et al. Quantitative Contribution of rs75017182 to Dihydropyrimidine Dehydrogenase mRNA Splicing and Enzyme Activity. *Clin. Pharmacol. Ther.* **2017**, *102*, 662–670. [CrossRef] [PubMed]
34. Meulendijks, D.; Henricks, L.M.; Sonke, G.S.; Deenen, M.J.; Froehlich, T.K.; Amstutz, U.; Largiadèr, C.R.; Jennings, B.A.; Marinaki, A.M.; Sanderson, J.D.; et al. Clinical relevance of DPYD variants c.1679T>G, c.1236G>A/HapB3, and c.1601G>A as predictors of severe fluoropyrimidine-associated toxicity: A systematic review and meta-analysis of individual patient data. *Lancet Oncol.* **2015**, *16*, 1639–1650. [CrossRef]
35. Kouwaki, M.; Hamajima, N.; Sumi, S.; Nonaka, M.; Sasaki, M.; Dobashi, K.; Kidouchi, K.; Togari, H.; Wada, Y. Identification of novel mutations in the dihydropyrimidine dehydrogenase gene in a Japanese patient with 5-fluorouracil toxicity. *Clin. Cancer Res.* **1998**, *4*, 2999–3004.
36. Falvella, F.S.; Cheli, S.; Martinetti, A.; Mazzali, C.; Iacovelli, R.; Maggi, C.; Gariboldi, M.; Pierotti, M.A.; Di Bartolomeo, M.; Sottotetti, E.; et al. DPD and UGT1A1 deficiency in colorectal cancer patients receiving triplet chemotherapy with fluoropyrimidines, oxaliplatin and irinotecan. *Br. J. Clin. Pharmacol.* **2015**, *80*, 581–588. [CrossRef]
37. Madi, A.; Fisher, D.; Maughan, T.S.; Colley, J.P.; Meade, A.M.; Maynard, J.; Humphreys, V.; Wasan, H.; Adams, R.A.; Idziaszczyk, S.; et al. Pharmacogenetic analyses of 2183 patients with advanced colorectal cancer; potential role for common dihydropyrimidine dehydrogenase variants in toxicity to chemotherapy. *Eur. J. Cancer* **2018**, *102*, 31–39. [CrossRef]
38. Vreken, P.; Van Kuilenburg, A.B.P.; Meinsma, R.; Van Gennip, A.H. Identification of novel point mutations in the dihydropyrimidine dehydrogenase gene. *J. Inherit. Metab. Dis.* **1997**, *20*, 335–338. [CrossRef]
39. O'Donnell, P.H.; Trubetskoy, V.; Nurhussein-Patterson, A.; Hall, J.P.; Nath, A.; Huo, D.; Fleming, G.F.; Ingle, J.N.; Abramson, V.G.; Morrow, P.K.; et al. Clinical evaluation of germline polymorphisms associated with capecitabine toxicity in breast cancer: TBCRC-015. *Breast Cancer Res. Treat.* **2020**, *181*, 623–633. [CrossRef] [PubMed]
40. Ruzzo, A.; Graziano, F.; Galli, F.; Galli, F.; Rulli, E.; Lonardi, S.; Ronzoni, M.; Massidda, B.; Zagonel, V.; Pella, N.; et al. Dihydropyrimidine dehydrogenase pharmacogenetics for predicting fluoropyrimidine-related toxicity in the randomised, phase III adjuvant TOSCA trial in high-risk colon cancer patients. *Br. J. Cancer* **2017**, *117*, 1269–1277. [CrossRef] [PubMed]
41. Rosmarin, D.; Palles, C.; Pagnamenta, A.; Kaur, K.; Pita, G.; Martin, M.; Domingo, E.; Jones, A.; Howarth, K.; Freeman-Mills, L.; et al. A candidate gene study of capecitabine-related toxicity in colorectal cancer identifies new toxicity variants at DPYD and a putative role for ENOSF1 rather than TYMS. *Gut* **2015**, *64*, 111–120. [CrossRef] [PubMed]
42. Pellicer, M.; García-González, X.; García, M.I.; Robles, L.; Grávalos, C.; García-Alfonso, P.; Pachón, V.; Longo, F.; Martínez, V.; Blanco, C.; et al. Identification of new SNPs associated with severe toxicity to capecitabine. *Pharmacol. Res.* **2017**, *120*, 133–137. [CrossRef] [PubMed]
43. Meulendijks, D.; Jacobs, B.A.; Aliev, A.; Pluim, D.; Van Werkhoven, E.; Deenen, M.J.; Beijnen, J.H.; Cats, A.; Schellens, J.H. Increased risk of severe fluoropyrimidine-associated toxicity in patients carrying a G to C substitution in the first 28-bp tandem repeat of the thymidylate synthase 2R allele. *Int. J. Cancer* **2015**, *138*, 245–253. [CrossRef]
44. Kristensen, M.H.; Pedersen, P.L.; Melsen, G.V.; Ellehauge, J.; Mejer, J. Variants in the dihydropyrimidine dehydrogenase, methylenetetrahydrofolate reductase and thymidylate synthase genes predict early toxicity of 5-fluorouracil in colorectal cancer patients. *J. Int. Med. Res.* **2010**, *38*, 870–883. [CrossRef]

45. Rosmarin, D.; Palles, C.; Church, D.; Domingo, E.; Jones, A.; Johnstone, E.; Wang, H.; Love, S.; Julier, P.; Scudder, C.; et al. Genetic markers of toxicity from capecitabine and other fluorouracil-based regimens: Investigation in the QUASAR2 study, systematic review, and meta-analysis. *J. Clin. Oncol.* **2014**, *32*, 1031–1039. [CrossRef]
46. Tsunoda, A.; Nakao, K.; Watanabe, M.; Matsui, N.; Ooyama, A.; Kusano, M. Associations of various gene polymorphisms with toxicity in colorectal cancer patients receiving oral uracil and tegafur plus leucovorin: A prospective study. *Ann. Oncol.* **2011**, *22*, 355–361. [CrossRef]
47. Loganayagam, A.; Arenas Hernandez, M.; Corrigan, A.; Fairbanks, L.; Lewis, C.M.; Harper, P.; Maisey, N.; Ross, P.; Sanderson, J.D.; Marinaki, A.M. Pharmacogenetic variants in the DPYD, TYMS, CDA and MTHFR genes are clinically significant predictors of fluoropyrimidine toxicity. *Br. J. Cancer* **2013**, *108*, 2505–2515. [CrossRef]
48. Lee, K.H.; Chang, H.J.; Han, S.W.; Oh, D.Y.; Im, S.A.; Bang, Y.J.; Kim, S.Y.; Lee, K.W.; Kim, J.H.; Hong, Y.S.; et al. Pharmacogenetic analysis of adjuvant FOLFOX for Korean patients with colon cancer. *Cancer Chemother. Pharm.* **2013**, *71*, 843–851. [CrossRef]
49. Jennings, B.A.; Loke, Y.K.; Skinner, J.; Keane, M.; Chu, G.S.; Turner, R.; Epurescu, D.; Barrett, A.; Willis, G. Evaluating Predictive Pharmacogenetic Signatures of Adverse Events in Colorectal Cancer Patients Treated with Fluoropyrimidines. *PLoS ONE* **2013**, *8*, 1–9. [CrossRef] [PubMed]
50. Meulendijks, D.; Henricks, L.M.; Amstutz, U.; Froehlich, T.K.; Largiadèr, C.R.; Beijnen, J.H.; de Boer, A.; Deenen, M.J.; Cats, A.; Schellens, J.H.M. Rs895819 in MIR27A improves the predictive value of DPYD variants to identify patients at risk of severe fluoropyrimidine-associated toxicity. *Int. J. Cancer* **2016**, *138*, 2752–2761. [CrossRef] [PubMed]
51. Magdy, T.; Arlanov, R.; Winter, S.; Lang, T.; Klein, K.; Toyoda, Y.; Ishikawa, T.; Schwab, M.; Zanger, U.M. ABCC11/MRP8 polymorphisms affect 5-fluorouracil-induced severe toxicity and hepatic expression. *Pharmacogenomics* **2013**, *14*, 1433–1448. [CrossRef] [PubMed]
52. Gonzalez-Haba, E.; García, M.I.; Cortejoso, L.; López-Lillo, C.; Barrueco, N.; García-Alfonso, P.; Alvarez, S.; Jiménez, J.L.; Martín, M.L.; Muñóz-Fernández, M.A.; et al. ABCB1 gene polymorphisms are associated with adverse reactions in fluoropyrimidine-treated colorectal cancer patients. *Pharmacogenomics* **2010**, *11*, 1715–1723. [CrossRef] [PubMed]
53. García-González, X.; Cortejoso, L.; García, M.I.; García-Alfonso, P.; Robles, L.; Grávalos, C.; González-Haba, E.; Marta, P.; Sanjurjo, M.; López-Fernández, L.A. Variants in CDA and ABCB1 are predictors of capecitabinerelated adverse reactions in colorectal cancer. *Oncotarget* **2015**, *6*, 6422–6430. [CrossRef]
54. Ribelles, N.; Lopez-Siles, J.; Sanchez, A.; Gonzalez, E.; Sanchez, M.; Carabantes, F.; Sanchez-Rovira, P.; Marquez, A.; Duenas, R.; Sevilla, I.; et al. A Carboxylesterase 2 Gene Polymorphism as Predictor of Capecitabine on Response and Time to Progression. *Curr. Drug Metab.* **2008**, *9*, 336–343. [CrossRef]
55. Hamzic, S.; Kummer, D.; Milesi, S.; Mueller, D.; Joerger, M.; Aebi, S.; Amstutz, U.; Largiadèr, C.R. Novel Genetic Variants in Carboxylesterase 1 Predict Severe Early-Onset Capecitabine-Related Toxicity. *Clin. Pharm. Ther.* **2017**, *102*, 796–804. [CrossRef]
56. Wheeler, H.E.; González-Neira, A.; Pita, G.; De La Torre-Montero, J.C.; Alonso, R.; Lopez-Fernandez, L.A.; Alba, E.; Martín, M.; Dolan, M.E. Identification of genetic variants associated with capecitabine-induced hand-foot syndrome through integration of patient and cell line genomic analyses. *Pharm. Genom.* **2014**, *24*, 231–237. [CrossRef]
57. Fernandez-Rozadilla, C.; Cazier, J.B.; Moreno, V.; Crous-Bou, M.; Guinó, E.; Durán, G.; Lamas, M.J.; López, R.; Candamio, S.; Gallardo, E.; et al. Pharmacogenomics in colorectal cancer: A genome-wide association study to predict toxicity after 5-fluorouracil or FOLFOX administration. *Pharm. J.* **2013**, *13*, 209–217. [CrossRef]
58. Cecchin, E.; D'Andrea, M.; Lonardi, S.; Zanusso, C.; Pella, N.; Errante, D.; De Mattia, E.; Polesel, J.; Innocenti, F.; Toffoli, G. A prospective validation pharmacogenomic study in the adjuvant setting of colorectal cancer patients treated with the 5-fluorouracil/leucovorin/oxaliplatin (FOLFOX4) regimen. *Pharm. J.* **2012**, *13*, 403–409. [CrossRef]
59. Custodio, A.; Moreno-Rubio, J.; Aparicio, J.; Gallego-Plazas, J.; Yaya, R.; Maurel, J.; Higuera, O.; Burgos, E.; Ramos, D.; Calatrava, A.; et al. Pharmacogenetic predictors of severe peripheral neuropathy in colon cancer patients treated with oxaliplatin-based adjuvant chemotherapy: A GEMCAD group study. *Ann. Oncol.* **2014**, *25*, 398–403. [CrossRef] [PubMed]

60. Stoehlmacher, J.; Park, D.J.; Zhang, W.; Yang, D.; Groshen, S.; Zahedy, S.; Lenz, H.J. A multivariate analysis of genomic polymorphisms: Prediction of clinical outcome to 5-FU/oxaliplatin combination chemotherapy in refractory colorectal cancer. *Br. J. Cancer* **2004**, *91*, 344–354. [CrossRef] [PubMed]
61. Ruzzo, A.; Graziano, F.; Galli, F.; Giacomini, E.; Floriani, I.; Galli, F.; Rulli, E.; Lonardi, S.; Ronzoni, M.; Massidda, B.; et al. Genetic markers for toxicity of adjuvant oxaliplatin and fluoropyrimidines in the phase III TOSCA trial in high-risk colon cancer patients. *Sci. Rep.* **2014**, *4*, 1–7. [CrossRef]
62. Boige, V.; Mendiboure, J.; Pignon, J.P.; Loriot, M.A.; Castaing, M.; Barrois, M.; Malka, D.; Trégouët, D.A.; Bouché, O.; Le Corre, D.; et al. Pharmacogenetic assessment of toxicity and outcome in patients with metastatic colorectal cancer treated with LV5FU2, FOLFOX, and FOLFIRI: FFCD 2000-05. *J. Clin. Oncol.* **2010**, *28*, 2556–2564. [CrossRef] [PubMed]
63. Salimzadeh, H.; Lindskog, E.B.; Gustavsson, B.; Wettergren, Y.; Ljungman, D. Association of DNA repair gene variants with colorectal cancer: Risk, toxicity, and survival. *BMC Cancer* **2020**, *20*, 1–10. [CrossRef] [PubMed]
64. Ando, Y.; Saka, H.; Ando, M.; Sawa, T.; Muro, K.; Ueoka, H.; Yokoyama, A.; Saitoh, S.; Shimokata, K.; Hasegawa, Y. Polymorphisms of UDP-glucuronosyltransferase gene and irinotecan toxicity: A pharmacogenetic analysis. *Cancer Res.* **2000**, *60*, 6921–6926. [PubMed]
65. Onoue, M.; Terada, T.; Kobayashi, M.; Katsura, T.; Matsumoto, S.; Yanagihara, K.; Nishimura, T.; Kanai, M.; Teramukai, S.; Shimizu, A.; et al. UGT1A1*6 polymorphism is most predictive of severe neutropenia induced by irinotecan in Japanese cancer patients. *Int. J. Clin. Oncol.* **2009**, *14*, 136–142. [CrossRef] [PubMed]
66. Chen, S.; Laverdiere, I.; Tourancheau, A.; Jonker, D.; Couture, F.; Cecchin, E.; Villeneuve, L.; Harvey, M.; Court, M.H.; Innocenti, F.; et al. A novel UGT1 marker associated with better tolerance against irinotecan-induced severe neutropenia in metastatic colorectal cancer patients. *Pharm. J.* **2015**, *15*, 513–520. [CrossRef]
67. Innocenti, F.; Undevia, S.D.; Iyer, L.; Chen, P.X.; Das, S.; Kocherginsky, M.; Karrison, T.; Janisch, L.; Ramírez, J.; Rudin, C.M.; et al. Genetic variants in the UDP-glucuronosyltransferase 1A1 gene predict the risk of severe neutropenia of irinotecan. *J. Clin. Oncol.* **2004**, *22*, 1382–1388. [CrossRef]
68. Côté, J.F.; Kirzin, S.; Kramar, A.; Mosnier, J.F.; Diebold, M.D.; Soubeyran, I.; Thirouard, A.S.; Selves, J.; Laurent-Puig, P.; Ychou, M. UGT1A1 polymorphism can predict hematologic toxicity in patients treated with irinotecan. *Clin. Cancer Res.* **2007**, *13*, 3269–3275. [CrossRef]
69. Lévesque, É.; Bélanger, A.S.; Harvey, M.; Couture, F.; Jonker, D.; Innocenti, F.; Cecchin, E.; Toffoli, G.; Guillemette, C. Refining the UGT1A haplotype associated with irinotecan-induced hematological toxicity in metastatic colorectal cancer patients treated with 5-fluorouracil/irinotecan-based regimens. *J. Pharm. Exp. Ther.* **2013**, *345*, 95–101. [CrossRef]
70. Han, J.-Y.; Lim, H.-S.; Park, Y.H.; Lee, S.Y.; Lee, J.S. Integrated pharmacogenetic prediction of irinotecan pharmacokinetics and toxicity in patients with advanced non-small cell lung cancer. *Lung Cancer* **2009**, *63*, 115–120. [CrossRef]
71. Chen, S.; Villeneuve, L.; Jonker, D.; Couture, F.; Laverdière, I.; Cecchin, E.; Innocenti, F.; Toffoli, G.; Lévesque, E.; Guillemette, C. ABCC5 and ABCG1 polymorphisms predict irinotecan-induced severe toxicity in metastatic colorectal cancer patients. *Pharm. Genom.* **2015**, *25*, 573–583. [CrossRef]
72. Di Martino, M.T.; Arbitrio, M.; Leone, E.; Guzzi, P.H.; Rotundo, M.S.; Ciliberto, D.; Tomaino, V.; Fabiani, F.; Talarico, D.; Sperlongano, P.; et al. Single nucleotide polymorphisms of ABCC5 and ABCG1 transporter genes correlate to irinotecan-associated gastrointestinal toxicity in colorectal cancer patients: A DMET microarray profiling study. *Cancer Biol. Ther.* **2011**, *12*, 780–787. [CrossRef]
73. Li, M.; Seiser, E.L.; Baldwin, R.M.; Ramirez, J.; Ratain, M.J.; Innocenti, F.; Kroetz, D.L. ABC transporter polymorphisms are associated with irinotecan pharmacokinetics and neutropenia. *Pharm. J.* **2018**, *18*, 35–42. [CrossRef]
74. De Mattia, E.; Toffoli, G.; Polesel, J.; D'Andrea, M.; Corona, G.; Zagonel, V.; Buonadonna, A.; Dreussi, E.; Cecchin, E. Pharmacogenetics of ABC and SLC transporters in metastatic colorectal cancer patients receiving first-line FOLFIRI treatment. *Pharm. Genom.* **2013**, *23*, 549–557. [CrossRef]
75. Hoskins, J.M.; Marcuello, E.; Altes, A.; Marsh, S.; Maxwell, T.; Van Booven, D.J.; Paré, L.; Culverhouse, R.; McLeod, H.L.; Baiget, M. Irinotecan Pharmacogenetics: Influence of Pharmacodynamic Genes. *Clin. Cancer Res.* **2008**, *14*, 1788–1796. [CrossRef]

76. Li, J.; Yu, Q.; Fu, S.; Xu, M.; Zhang, T.; Xie, C.; Feng, J.; Chen, J.; Zang, A.; Cai, Y.; et al. A novel genetic score model of UGT1A1 and TGFB pathway as predictor of severe irinotecan-related diarrhea in metastatic colorectal cancer patients. *J. Cancer Res. Clin. Oncol.* **2016**, *142*, 1621–1628. [CrossRef]
77. Takahashi, H.; Sai, K.; Saito, Y.; Kaniwa, N.; Matsumura, Y.; Hamaguchi, T.; Shimada, Y.; Ohtsu, A.; Yoshino, T.; Doi, T.; et al. Application of a Combination of a Knowledge-Based Algorithm and 2-Stage Screening to Hypothesis-Free Genomic Data on Irinotecan-Treated Patients for Identification of a Candidate Single Nucleotide Polymorphism Related to an Adverse Effect. *PLoS ONE* **2014**, *9*, e105160. [CrossRef]
78. Won, H.H.; Lee, J.; Park, J.O.; Park, Y.S.; Lim, H.Y.; Kang, W.K.; Kim, J.W.; Lee, S.Y.; Park, S.H. Polymorphic markers associated with severe oxaliplatin-induced, chronic peripheral neuropathy in colon cancer patients. *Cancer* **2012**, *118*, 2828–2836. [CrossRef]
79. Etienne-Grimaldi, M.C.; Bennouna, J.; Formento, J.L.; Douillard, J.Y.; Francoual, M.; Hennebelle, I.; Chatelut, E.; Francois, E.; Faroux, R.; El Hannani, C.; et al. Multifactorial pharmacogenetic analysis in colorectal cancer patients receiving 5-fluorouracil-based therapy together with cetuximab-irinotecan. *Br. J. Clin. Pharm.* **2012**, *73*, 776–785. [CrossRef]
80. Parmar, S.; Schumann, C.; Rüdiger, S.; Boeck, S.; Heinemann, V.; Kächele, V.; Seeringer, A.; Paul, T.; Seufferlein, T.; Stingl, J.C. Pharmacogenetic predictors for EGFR-inhibitor-associated skin toxicity. *Pharm. J.* **2013**, *13*, 181–188. [CrossRef] [PubMed]
81. Dahan, L.; Norguet, E.; Etienne-Grimaldi, M.-C.; Formento, J.-L.; Gasmi, M.; Nanni, I.; Gaudart, J.; Garcia, S.; Ouafik, L.; Seitz, J.-F.; et al. Pharmacogenetic profiling and cetuximab outcome in patients with advanced colorectal cancer. *BMC Cancer* **2011**, *11*, 496. [CrossRef]
82. Baas, J.; Krens, L.; Bohringer, S.; Mol, L.; Punt, C.; Guchelaar, H.; Gelderblom, H. Genome wide association study to identify predictors for severe skin toxicity in colorectal cancer patients treated with cetuximab. *PLoS ONE* **2018**, *13*, e0208080. [CrossRef]
83. Sibertin-Blanc, C.; Mancini, J.; Fabre, A.; Lagarde, A.; Del Grande, J.; Levy, N.; Seitz, J.F.; Olschwang, S.; Dahan, L. Vascular Endothelial Growth Factor A c.*237C>T polymorphism is associated with bevacizumab efficacy and related hypertension in metastatic colorectal cancer. *Dig. Liver Dis.* **2015**, *47*, 331–337. [CrossRef]
84. Schneider, B.P.; Wang, M.; Radovich, M.; Sledge, G.W.; Badve, S.; Thor, A.; Flockhart, D.A.; Hancock, B.; Davidson, N.; Gralow, J.; et al. Association of vascular endothelial growth factor and vascular endothelial growth factor receptor-2 genetic polymorphisms with outcome in a trial of paclitaxel compared with paclitaxel plus bevacizumab in advanced breast cancer: ECOG 2100. *J. Clin. Oncol.* **2008**, *26*, 4672–4678. [CrossRef]
85. Morita, S.; Uehara, K.; Nakayama, G.; Shibata, T.; Oguri, T.; Inada-Inoue, M.; Shimokata, T.; Sugishita, M.; Mitsuma, A.; Ando, Y. Association between bevacizumab-related hypertension and vascular endothelial growth factor (VEGF) gene polymorphisms in Japanese patients with metastatic colorectal cancer. *Cancer Chemother. Pharm.* **2013**, *71*, 405–411. [CrossRef]
86. Ma, T.; Zhu, Z.G.; Ji, Y.B.; Zhang, Y.; Yu, Y.Y.; Liu, B.Y.; Yin, H.R.; Lin, Y.Z. Correlation of thymidylate synthase, thymidine phosphorylase and dihydropyrimidine dehydrogenase with sensitivity of gastrointestinal cancer cells to 5-fluorouracil and 5-fluoro-2'-deoxyuridine. *World J. Gastroenterol.* **2004**, *10*, 172–176. [CrossRef]
87. Lecomte, T.; Ferraz, J.M.; Zinzindohoué, F.; Loriot, M.A.; Tregouet, D.A.; Landi, B.; Berger, A.; Cugnenc, P.H.; Jian, R.; Beaune, P.; et al. Thymidylate synthase gene polymorphism predicts toxicity in colorectal cancer patients receiving 5-fluorouracil-based chemotherapy. *Clin. Cancer Res.* **2004**, *10*, 5880–5888. [CrossRef]
88. Popat, S.; Matakidou, A.; Houlston, R.S. Thymidylate-synthase expression and prognosis in colorectal cancer: A systematic review and meta-analysis. *J. Clin. Oncol.* **2004**, *22*, 529–536. [CrossRef]
89. Danenberg, P.V.; Leichman, L.; Lenz, H.J.; Leichman, C.G.; Danenberg, K.D. Thymidylate Synthase Gene and Protein Expression Correlate and Are Associated with Response to 5-Fluorouracil in Human Colorectal and Gastric Tumors. *Cancer Res.* **1995**, *55*, 1407–1412.
90. De Mattia, E.; Toffoli, G. C677T and A1298C MTHFR polymorphisms, a challenge for antifolate and fluoropyrimidine-based therapy personalisation. *Eur. J. Cancer* **2009**, *45*, 1333–1351. [CrossRef] [PubMed]
91. Chua, W.; Goldstein, D.; Lee, C.K.; Dhillon, H.; Michael, M.; Mitchell, P.; Clarke, S.J.; Iacopetta, B. Molecular markers of response and toxicity to FOLFOX chemotherapy in metastatic colorectal cancer. *Br. J. Cancer* **2009**, *101*, 998–1004. [CrossRef] [PubMed]
92. Salvador-Martín, S.; García-González, X.; García, M.I.; Blanco, C.; García-Alfonso, P.; Robles, L.; Grávalos, C.; Pachón, V.; Longo, F.; Martínez, V.; et al. Clinical utility of ABCB1 genotyping for preventing toxicity in treatment with irinotecan. *Pharm. Res.* **2018**, *136*, 133–139. [CrossRef] [PubMed]

93. Glimelius, B.; Garmo, H.; Berglund, Å.; Fredriksson, L.A.; Berglund, M.; Kohnke, H.; Byström, P.; Sørbye, H.; Wadelius, M. Prediction of irinotecan and 5-fluorouracil toxicity and response in patients with advanced colorectal cancer. *Pharm. J.* **2011**, *11*, 61–71. [CrossRef] [PubMed]
94. Martin, M.; Martinez, N.; Ramos, M.; Calvo, L.; Lluch, A.; Zamora, P.; Munoz, M.; Carrasco, E.; Caballero, R.; Garcia-Saenz, J.A.; et al. Standard Versus Continuous Administration of Capecitabine in Metastatic Breast Cancer (GEICAM/2009-05): A Randomized, Noninferiority Phase II Trial With a Pharmacogenetic Analysis. *Oncologist* **2015**, *20*, 111–112. [CrossRef]
95. Rhodes, K.E.; Zhang, W.; Yang, D.; Press, O.A.; Gordon, M.; Vallböhmer, D.; Schultheis, A.M.; Lurje, G.; Ladner, R.D.; Fazzone, W.; et al. ABCB1, SLCO1B1 and UGT1A1 gene polymorphisms are associated with toxicity in metastatic colorectal cancer patients treated with first-line irinotecan. *Drug Metab. Lett.* **2007**, *1*, 23–30. [CrossRef]
96. Mathijssen, R.H.J.; Marsh, S.; Karlsson, M.O.; Xie, R.; Baker, S.D.; Verweij, J.; Sparreboom, A.; McLeod, H.L. Irinotecan pathway genotype analysis to predict pharmacokinetics. *Clin. Cancer Res.* **2003**, *9*, 3246–3253.
97. Teft, W.A.; Welch, S.; Lenehan, J.; Parfitt, J.; Choi, Y.H.; Winquist, E.; Kim, R.B. OATP1B1 and tumour OATP1B3 modulate exposure, toxicity, and survival after irinotecan-based chemotherapy. *Br. J. Cancer* **2015**, *112*, 857–865. [CrossRef]
98. Cecchin, E.; Corona, G.; Masier, S.; Biason, P.; Cattarossi, G.; Frustaci, S.; Buonadonna, A.; Colussi, A.; Toffoli, G. Carboxylesterase isoform 2 mRNA expression in peripheral blood mononuclear cells is a predictive marker of the irinotecan to SN38 activation step in colorectal cancer patients. *Clin. Cancer Res.* **2005**, *11*, 6901–6907. [CrossRef]
99. Cortejoso, L.; López-Fernández, L.A. Pharmacogenetic markers of toxicity for chemotherapy in colorectal cancer patients. *Pharmacogenomics* **2012**, *13*, 1173–1191. [CrossRef] [PubMed]
100. Qian, Y.-Y.; Liu, X.-Y.; Wu, Q.; Song, X.; Chen, X.-F.; Liu, Y.-Q.; Pei, D.; Shen, L.-Z.; Shu, Y.-Q. The ERCC1 C118T Polymorphism Predicts Clinical Outcomes of Colorectal Cancer Patients Receiving Oxaliplatin-Based Chemotherapy: A Meta-analysis Based on 22 Studies. *Asian Pac. J. Cancer Prev.* **2014**, *15*, 8383–8390. [CrossRef] [PubMed]
101. Etienne-Grimaldi, M.C.; Milano, G.; Maindrault-Gœbel, F.; Chibaudel, B.; Formento, J.L.; Francoual, M.; Lledo, G.; André, T.; Mabro, M.; Mineur, L.; et al. Methylenetetrahydrofolate reductase (MTHFR) gene polymorphisms and FOLFOX response in colorectal cancer patients. *Br. J. Clin. Pharm.* **2010**, *69*, 58–66. [CrossRef] [PubMed]
102. McLeod, H.L.; Sargent, D.J.; Marsh, S.; Green, E.M.; King, C.R.; Fuchs, C.S.; Ramanathan, R.K.; Williamson, S.K.; Findlay, B.P.; Thibodeau, S.N.; et al. Pharmacogenetic predictors of adverse events and response to chemotherapy in metastatic colorectal cancer: Results from North American Gastrointestinal Intergroup Trial N9741. *J. Clin. Oncol.* **2010**, *28*, 3227–3233. [CrossRef]
103. Gamelin, L.; Capitain, O.; Morel, A.; Dumont, A.; Traore, S.; Anne, L.B.; Gilles, S.; Boisdron-Celle, M.; Gamelin, E. Predictive factors of oxaliplatin neurotoxicity: The involvement of the oxalate outcome pathway. *Clin. Cancer Res.* **2007**, *13*, 6359–6368. [CrossRef]
104. Massacesi, C.; Terrazzino, S.; Marcucci, F.; Rocchi, M.B.; Lippe, P.; Bisonni, R.; Lombardo, M.; Pilone, A.; Mattioli, R.; Leon, A. Uridine diphosphate glucuronosyl transferase 1A1 promoter polymorphism predicts the risk of gastrointestinal toxicity and fatigue induced by irinotecan-based chemotherapy. *Cancer* **2006**, *106*, 1007–1016. [CrossRef]
105. Iyer, L.; Das, S.; Janisch, L.; Wen, M.; Ramírez, J.; Karrison, T.; Fleming, G.F.; Vokes, E.E.; Schilsky, R.L.; Ratain, M.J. UGT1A1*28 polymorphism as a determinant of irinotecan disposition and toxicity. *Pharm. J.* **2002**, *2*, 43–47. [CrossRef]
106. Liu, C.Y.; Chen, P.M.; Chiou, T.J.; Liu, J.H.; Lin, J.K.; Lin, T.C.; Chen, W.S.; Jiang, J.K.; Wang, H.S.; Wang, W.S. UGT1A1*28 polymorphism predicts irinotecan-induced severe toxicities without affecting treatment outcome and survival in patients with metastatic colorectal carcinoma. *Cancer* **2008**, *112*, 1932–1940. [CrossRef]
107. Liu, X.; Cheng, D.; Kuang, Q.; Liu, G.; Xu, W. Association of UGT1A1*28 polymorphisms with irinotecan-induced toxicities in colorectal cancer: A meta-analysis in Caucasians. *Pharm. J.* **2014**, *14*, 120–129. [CrossRef]

108. Toffoli, G.; Cecchin, E.; Gasparini, G.; D'Andrea, M.; Azzarello, G.; Basso, U.; Mini, E.; Pessa, S.; De Mattia, E.; Re, G.L.; et al. Genotype-driven phase I study of irinotecan administered in combination with fluorouracil/leucovorin in patients with metastatic colorectal cancer. *J. Clin. Oncol.* **2010**, *28*, 866–871. [CrossRef]
109. Marcuello, E.; Páez, D.; Paré, L.; Salazar, J.; Sebio, A.; Del Rio, E.; Baiget, M. A genotype-directed phase I-IV dose-finding study of irinotecan in combination with fluorouracil/leucovorin as first-line treatment in advanced colorectal cancer. *Br. J. Cancer* **2011**, *105*, 53–57. [CrossRef] [PubMed]
110. Treenert, A.; Areepium, N.; Tanasanvimon, S. Effects of ABCC2 and SLCO1B1 Polymorphisms on treatment responses in Thai metastatic colorectal cancer patients treated with Irinotecan-based chemotherapy. *Asian Pac. J. Cancer Prev.* **2018**, *19*, 2757–2764. [CrossRef] [PubMed]
111. Innocenti, F.; Kroetz, D.L.; Schuetz, E.; Dolan, M.E.; Ramírez, J.; Relling, M.; Chen, P.; Das, S.; Rosner, G.L.; Ratain, M.J. Comprehensive pharmacogenetic analysis of irinotecan neutropenia and pharmacokinetics. *J. Clin. Oncol.* **2009**, *27*, 2604–2614. [CrossRef] [PubMed]
112. Riera, P.; Salazar, J.; Virgili, A.C.; Tobeña, M.; Sebio, A.; Gallano, P.; Barnadas, A.; Páez, D. Relevance of CYP3A4*20, UGT1A1*37 and UGT1A1*28 variants in irinotecan-induced severe toxicity. *Br. J. Clin. Pharm.* **2018**, *84*, 1389–1392. [CrossRef] [PubMed]
113. Fujikura, K.; Ingelman-Sundberg, M.; Lauschke, V.M. Genetic variation in the human cytochrome P450 supergene family. *Pharm. Genom.* **2015**, *25*, 584–594. [CrossRef] [PubMed]
114. Paulík, A.; Grim, J.; Filip, S. Predictors of irinotecan toxicity and efficacy in treatment of metastatic colorectal cancer. *Acta Medica* **2012**, *55*, 153–159. [CrossRef]
115. Sunakawa, Y.; Yang, D.; Moran, M.; Astrow, S.H.; Tsuji, A.; Stephens, C.; Zhang, W.; Cao, S.; Takahashi, T.; Denda, T.; et al. Combined assessment of EGFR-related molecules to predict outcome of 1st-line cetuximab-containing chemotherapy for metastatic colorectal cancer. *Cancer Biol. Ther.* **2016**, *17*, 751–759. [CrossRef]
116. Pander, J.; Gelderblom, H.; Antonini, N.F.; Tol, J.; van Krieken, J.H.J.M.; van der Straaten, T.; Punt, C.J.A.; Guchelaar, H.J. Correlation of FCGR3A and EGFR germline polymorphisms with the efficacy of cetuximab in KRAS wild-type metastatic colorectal cancer. *Eur. J. Cancer* **2010**, *46*, 1829–1834. [CrossRef]
117. Lambrechts, D.; Moisse, M.; Delmar, P.; Miles, D.W.; Leighl, N.; Escudier, B.; Van Cutsem, E.; Bansal, A.T.; Carmeliet, P.; Scherer, S.J.; et al. Genetic markers of bevacizumab-induced hypertension. *Angiogenesis* **2014**, *17*, 685–694. [CrossRef]
118. Etienne-Grimaldi, M.C.; Formento, P.; Degeorges, A.; Pierga, J.Y.; Delva, R.; Pivot, X.; Dalenc, F.; Espié, M.; Veyret, C.; Formento, J.L.; et al. Prospective analysis of the impact of VEGF-A gene polymorphisms on the pharmacodynamics of bevacizumab-based therapy in metastatic breast cancer patients. *Br. J. Clin. Pharm.* **2011**, *71*, 921–928. [CrossRef]
119. Le, D.T.; Durham, J.N.; Smith, K.N.; Wang, H.; Bartlett, B.R.; Aulakh, L.K.; Lu, S.; Kemberling, H.; Wilt, C.; Luber, B.S.; et al. Mismatch repair deficiency predicts response of solid tumors to PD-1 blockade. *Science* **2017**, *357*, 409–413. [CrossRef] [PubMed]
120. Food and Drug Administration. FDA Grants Accelerated Approval to Ipilimumab for MSI-H or dMMR Metastatic Colorectal Cancer. Available online: https://www.fda.gov/drugs/resources-information-approved-drugs/fda-grants-accelerated-approval-ipilimumab-msi-h-or-dmmr-metastatic-colorectal-cancer (accessed on 30 October 2020).
121. Food and Drug Administration. FDA Approves Pembrolizumab for First-Line Treatment of MSI-H/dMMR Colorectal Cancer. Available online: https://www.fda.gov/drugs/drug-approvals-and-databases/fda-approves-pembrolizumab-first-line-treatment-msi-hdmmr-colorectal-cancer (accessed on 30 October 2020).
122. Bins, S.; Basak, E.A.; El Bouazzaoui, S.; Koolen, S.L.W.; De Hoop, E.O.; Van Der Leest, C.H.; Van Der Veldt, A.A.M.; Sleijfer, S.; Debets, R.; Van Schaik, R.H.N.; et al. Association between single-nucleotide polymorphisms and adverse events in nivolumab-treated non-small cell lung cancer patients. *Br. J. Cancer* **2018**, *118*, 1296–1301. [CrossRef] [PubMed]
123. Al-Samkari, H.; Snyder, G.D.; Nikiforow, S.; Tolaney, S.M.; A Freedman, R.; Losman, J.-A. Haemophagocytic lymphohistiocytosis complicating pembrolizumab treatment for metastatic breast cancer in a patient with the PRF1A91V gene polymorphism. *J. Med. Genet.* **2018**, *56*, 39–42. [CrossRef] [PubMed]

124. Queirolo, P.; Dozin, B.; Morabito, A.; Banelli, B.; Carosio, R.; Fontana, V.; Ferrucci, P.F.; Martinoli, C.; Cocorocchio, E.; Ascierto, P.A.; et al. CTLA-4 gene variant-1661A>G may predict the onset of endocrine adverse events in metastatic melanoma patients treated with ipilimumab. *Eur. J. Cancer* **2018**, *97*, 59–61. [CrossRef]
125. Oguri, T.; Mitsuma, A.; Inada-Inoue, M.; Morita, S.; Shibata, T.; Shimokata, T.; Sugishita, M.; Nakayama, G.; Uehara, K.; Hasegawa, Y.; et al. Genetic polymorphisms associated with oxaliplatin-induced peripheral neurotoxicity in Japanese patients with colorectal cancer. *Int. J. Clin. Pharm. Ther.* **2013**, *51*, 475–481. [CrossRef]
126. Terrazzino, S.; Argyriou, A.A.; Cargnin, S.; Antonacopoulou, A.G.; Briani, C.; Bruna, J.; Velasco, R.; Alberti, P.; Campagnolo, M.; Lonardi, S.; et al. Genetic determinants of chronic oxaliplatin-induced peripheral neurotoxicity: A genome-wide study replication and meta-analysis. *J. Peripher. Nerv. Syst.* **2015**, *20*, 15–23. [CrossRef]
127. Motsinger-Reif, A.A.; Jorgenson, E.; Relling, M.V.; Kroetz, D.L.; Weinshilboum, R.; Cox, N.J.; Roden, D.M. Genome-wide association studies in pharmacogenomics:successes and lessons. *Pharm. Genom.* **2013**, *23*, 1744–6872. [CrossRef]
128. Singleton, A.B.; Hardy, J.; Traynor, B.J.; Houlden, H. Towards a complete resolution of the genetic architecture of disease. *Trends Genet.* **2010**, *26*, 438–442. [CrossRef]
129. Manolio, T.A.; Collins, F.S.; Cox, N.J.; Goldstein, D.B.; Hindorff, L.A.; Hunter, D.J.; McCarthy, M.I.; Ramos, E.M.; Cardon, L.R.; Chakravarti, A.; et al. Finding the missing heritability of complex diseases. *Nature* **2009**, *461*, 747–753. [CrossRef]
130. Scientific, T.F. Axiom Spain Biobank Array. Available online: http://www.usc.es/cegen/wp-content/uploads/2019/08/COL32017-1217-Axiom-Spain-EN_FLR_FINAL.pdf. (accessed on 7 October 2020).
131. Mizzi, C.; Peters, B.; Mitropoulou, C.; Mitropoulos, K.; Katsila, T.; Agarwal, M.R.; Van Schaik, R.H.N.; Drmanac, R.; Borg, J.; Patrinos, G.P. Personalized pharmacogenomics profiling using whole-genome sequencing. *Pharmacogenomics* **2014**, *15*, 1223–1234. [CrossRef]
132. Apellániz-Ruiz, M.; Lee, M.Y.; Sánchez-Barroso, L.; Gutiérrez-Gutiérrez, G.; Calvo, I.; García-Estévez, L.; Sereno, M.; García-Donás, J.; Castelo, B.; Guerra, E.; et al. Whole-exome sequencing reveals defective CYP3A4 variants predictive of paclitaxel dose-limiting neuropathy. *Proc. Clin. Cancer Res.* **2015**, *21*, 322–328. [CrossRef] [PubMed]
133. Kozyra, M.; Ingelman-Sundberg, M.; Lauschke, V.M. Rare genetic variants in cellular transporters, metabolic enzymes, and nuclear receptors can be important determinants of interindividual differences in drug response. *Genet. Med.* **2017**, *19*, 20–29. [CrossRef] [PubMed]
134. Santos, M.; Niemi, M.; Hiratsuka, M.; Kumondai, M.; Ingelman-Sundberg, M.; Lauschke, V.M.; Rodríguez-Antona, C. Novel copy-number variations in pharmacogenes contribute to interindividual differences in drug pharmacokinetics. *Genet. Med.* **2018**, *20*, 622–629. [CrossRef] [PubMed]
135. Ingelman-Sundberg, M.; Mkrtchian, S.; Zhou, Y.; Lauschke, V.M. Integrating rare genetic variants into pharmacogenetic drug response predictions. *Hum. Genom.* **2018**, *12*, 1–12. [CrossRef] [PubMed]
136. Schaller, L.; Lauschke, V.M. The genetic landscape of the human solute carrier (SLC) transporter superfamily. *Hum. Genet.* **2019**, *138*, 1359–1377. [CrossRef] [PubMed]
137. Van Staveren, M.C.; Jan Guchelaar, H.; Van Kuilenburg, A.B.P.; Gelderblom, H.; Maring, J.G. Evaluation of predictive tests for screening for dihydropyrimidine dehydrogenase deficiency. *Pharm. J.* **2013**, *13*, 389–395. [CrossRef] [PubMed]
138. Van Kuilenburg, A.B.P.; Häusler, P.; Schalhorn, A.; Tanck, M.W.T.; Proost, J.H.; Terborg, C.; Behnke, D.; Schwabe, W.; Jabschinsky, K.; Maring, J.G. Evaluation of 5-fluorouracil pharmacokinetics in cancer patients with a c.1905+1G>A Mutation in DPYD by means of a bayesian limited sampling strategy. *Clin. Pharm.* **2012**, *51*, 163–174. [CrossRef]
139. Maring, J.G.; Van Kuilenburg, A.B.P.; Haasjes, J.; Piersma, H.; Groen, H.J.M.; Uges, D.R.A.; Van Gennip, A.H.; De Vries, E.G.E. Reduced 5-FU clearance in a patient with low DPD activity due to heterozygosity for a mutant allele of the DPYD gene. *Br. J. Cancer* **2002**, *86*, 1028–1033. [CrossRef]
140. Offer, S.M.; Lee, A.M.; Mattison, L.K.; Fossum, C.; Wegner, N.J.; Diasio, R.B. A DPYD Variant (Y186C) in Individuals of African Ancestry Is Associated With Reduced DPD Enzyme Activity. *Clin. Pharm. Ther.* **2013**, *94*, 158–166. [CrossRef]

141. Morel, A.; Boisdron-Celle, M.; Fey, L.; Soulie, P.; Craipeau, M.C.; Traore, S.; Gamelin, E. Clinical relevance of different dihydropyrimidine dehydrogenase gene single nucleotide polymorphisms on 5-fluorouracil tolerance. *Mol. Cancer Ther.* **2006**, *5*, 2895–2904. [CrossRef]
142. Van Kuilenburg, A.; Hausler, P.; Schalhorn, A.; Tanck, M.; Proost, J.H.; Terborg, C.; Behnke, D.; Schwabe, W.; Jabschinsky, K.; Maring, J.G. Evaluation of 5-FU pharmacokinetics in cancer patients with DPD deficiency using a Bayesian limited sampling strategy. *Ther. Drug Monit.* **2011**, *33*, 478.
143. Zhang, H.; Li, Y.-M.; Zhang, H.; Jin, X. DPYD*5 gene mutation contributes to the reduced DPYD enzyme activity and chemotherapeutic toxicity of 5-FU. *Med. Oncol.* **2007**, *24*, 251–258. [CrossRef] [PubMed]
144. Sáez-Belló, M.; Mangas-Sanjuán, V.; Martínez-Gómez, M.A.; López-Montenegro Soria, M.Á.; Climente-Martí, M.; Merino-Sanjuán, M. Evaluation of ABC gene polymorphisms on the pharmacokinetics and pharmacodynamics of capecitabine in colorectal patients: Implications for dosing recommendations. *Br. J. Clin. Pharm.* **2020**, online. [CrossRef] [PubMed]
145. Toffoli, G.; Cecchin, E.; Corona, G.; Russo, A.; Buonadonna, A.; D'Andrea, M.; Pasetto, L.M.; Pessa, S.; Errante, D.; De Pangher, V.; et al. The role of UGT1A1*28 polymorphism in the pharmacodynamics and pharmacokinetics of irinotecan in patients with metastatic colorectal cancer. *J. Clin. Oncol.* **2006**, *24*, 3061–3068. [CrossRef] [PubMed]
146. Cecchin, E.; Innocenti, F.; D'Andrea, M.; Corona, G.; De Mattia, E.; Biason, P.; Buonadonna, A.; Toffoli, G. Predictive role of the UGT1A1, UGT1A7, and UGT1A9 genetic variants and their haplotypes on the outcome of metastatic colorectal cancer patients treated with fluorouracil, leucovorin, and irinotecan. *J. Clin. Oncol.* **2009**, *27*, 2457–2465. [CrossRef]
147. Labriet, A.; De Mattia, E.; Cecchin, E.; Lévesque, É.; Jonker, D.; Couture, F.; Buonadonna, A.; D'Andrea, M.; Villeneuve, L.; Toffoli, G.; et al. Improved progression-free survival in irinotecan-treated metastatic colorectal cancer patients carrying the HNF1A coding variant p.I27L. *Front. Pharm.* **2017**, *8*, 712. [CrossRef]
148. Fujita, K.I.; Nagashima, F.; Yamamoto, W.; Endo, H.; Sunakawa, Y.; Yamashita, K.; Ishida, H.; Mizuno, K.; Matsunaga, M.; Araki, K.; et al. Association of ATP-binding cassette, sub-family C, number 2 (ABCC2) genotype with pharmacokinetics of irinotecan in Japanese patients with metastatic colorectal cancer treated with irinotecan plus infusional 5-fluorouracil/leucovorin (FOLFIRI). *Biol. Pharm. Bull.* **2008**, *31*, 2137–2142. [CrossRef]
149. Paoluzzi, L.; Singh, A.S.; Price, D.K.; Danesi, R.; Mathijssen, R.H.J.; Verweij, J.; Figg, W.D.; Sparreboom, A. Influence of genetic variants in UGT1A1 and UGT1A9 on the in vivo glucuronidation of SN-38. *J. Clin. Pharm.* **2004**, *44*, 854–860. [CrossRef]
150. Sai, K.; Saeki, M.; Saito, Y.; Ozawa, S.; Katori, N.; Jinno, H.; Hasegawa, R.; Kaniwa, N.; Sawada, J.; Komamura, K.; et al. UGT1A1 haplotypes associated with reduced glucuronidation and increased serum bilirubin in irinotecan-administered Japanese patients with cancer*1. *Clin. Pharm. Ther.* **2004**, *75*, 501–515. [CrossRef]
151. De Jong, F.A.; Scott-Horton, T.J.; Kroetz, D.L.; McLeod, H.L.; Friberg, L.E.; Mathijssen, R.H.; Verweij, J.; Marsh, S.; Sparreboom, A. Irinotecan-induced diarrhea: Functional significance of the polymorphic ABCC2 transporter protein. *Clin. Pharm. Ther.* **2007**, *81*, 42–49. [CrossRef]
152. de Jong, F.A.; Kehrer, D.F.S.; Mathijssen, R.H.J.; Creemers, G.; de Bruijn, P.; van Schaik, R.H.N.; Planting, A.S.T.; van der Gaast, A.; Eskens, F.A.L.M.; Janssen, J.T.P.; et al. Prophylaxis of Irinotecan-Induced Diarrhea with Neomycin and Potential Role for UGT1A1*28 Genotype Screening: A Double-Blind, Randomized, Placebo-Controlled Study. *Oncologist* **2006**, *11*, 944–954. [CrossRef] [PubMed]
153. Minami, H.; Sai, K.; Saeki, M.; Saito, Y.; Ozawa, S.; Suzuki, K.; Kaniwa, N.; Sawada, J.I.; Hamaguchi, T.; Yamamoto, N.; et al. Irinotecan pharmacokinetics/pharmacodynamics and UGT1A genetic polymorphisms in Japanese: Roles of UGT1A1*6 and *28. *Pharm. Genom.* **2007**, *17*, 497–504. [CrossRef] [PubMed]
154. Jada, S.R.; Lim, R.; Wong, C.I.; Shu, X.; Lee, S.C.; Zhou, Q.; Goh, B.C.; Chowbay, B. Role of UGT1A1*6, UGT1A1*28 and ABCG2 c.421C>A polymorphisms in irinotecan-induced neutropenia in Asian cancer patients. *Cancer Sci.* **2007**, *98*, 1461–1467. [CrossRef] [PubMed]
155. Sai, K.; Kaniwa, N.; Itoda, M.; Saito, Y.; Hasegawa, R.; Komamura, K.; Ueno, K.; Kamakura, S.; Kitakaze, M.; Shirao, K.; et al. Haplotype analysis of ABCB1/MDR1 blocks in a Japanese population reveals genotype-dependent renal clearance of irinotecan. *Pharmacogenetics* **2003**, *13*, 741–757. [CrossRef]

156. Henricks, L.M.; Lunenburg, C.A.T.C.; de Man, F.M.; Meulendijks, D.; Frederix, G.W.J.; Kienhuis, E.; Creemers, G.-J.; Baars, A.; Dezentjé, V.O.; Imholz, A.L.T.; et al. DPYD genotype-guided dose individualisation of fluoropyrimidine therapy in patients with cancer: A prospective safety analysis. *Lancet Oncol.* **2018**, *19*, 1459–1467. [CrossRef]
157. Kleibl, Z.; Fidlerova, J.; Kleiblova, P.; Kormunda, S.; Bilek, M.; Bouskova, K.; Sevcik, J.; Novotny, J. Influence of dihydropyrimidine dehydrogenase gene (DPYD) coding sequence variants on the development of fluoropyrimidine-related toxicity in patients with high-grade toxicity and patients with excellent tolerance of fluoropyrimidine-based chemotherapy. *Neoplasma* **2009**, *56*, 303–316. [CrossRef]
158. Deenen, M.J.; Meulendijks, D.; Cats, A.; Sechterberger, M.K.; Severens, J.L.; Boot, H.; Smits, P.H.; Rosing, H.; Mandigers, C.M.; Soesan, M.; et al. Upfront Genotyping of DPYD*2A to Individualize Fluoropyrimidine Therapy: A Safety and Cost Analysis. *J. Clin. Oncol.* **2016**, *34*, 227–234. [CrossRef]
159. Cortejoso, L.; García-González, X.; García, M.I.; García-Alfonso, P.; Sanjurjo, M.; López-Fernández, L.A. Cost-effectiveness of screening for DPYD polymorphisms to prevent neutropenia in cancer patients treated with fluoropyrimidines. *Pharmacogenomics* **2016**, *17*, 979–984. [CrossRef]
160. Murphy, C.; Byrne, S.; Ahmed, G.; Kenny, A.; Gallagher, J.; Harvey, H.; O'Farrell, E.; Bird, B. Cost Implications of Reactive Versus Prospective Testing for Dihydropyrimidine Dehydrogenase Deficiency in Patients with Colorectal Cancer: A Single-Institution Experience. *Dose-Response* **2018**, *16*, 16. [CrossRef]
161. Henricks, L.M.; Lunenburg, C.A.; De Man, F.M.; Meulendijks, D.; Frederix, G.W.; Kienhuis, E.; Creemers, G.-J.; Baars, A.; Dezentjé, V.O.; Imholz, A.L.; et al. A cost analysis of upfront DPYD genotype–guided dose individualisation in fluoropyrimidine-based anticancer therapy. *Eur. J. Cancer* **2019**, *107*, 60–67. [CrossRef]
162. Gold, H.T.; Hall, M.J.; Blinder, V.; Schackman, B.R. Cost effectiveness of pharmacogenetic testing for uridine diphosphate glucuronosyltransferase 1A1 before irinotecan administration for metastatic colorectal cancer. *Cancer* **2009**, *115*, 3858–3867. [CrossRef] [PubMed]
163. Obradovic, M.; Mrhar, A.; Kos, M. Cost-effectiveness of UGT1A1 genotyping in second-line, high-dose, once every 3 weeks irinotecan monotherapy treatment of colorectal cancer. *Pharmacogenomics* **2008**, *9*, 539–549. [CrossRef] [PubMed]
164. Butzke, B.; Oduncu, F.S.; Severin, F.; Pfeufer, A.; Heinemann, V.; Giesen-Jung, C.; Stollenwerk, B.; Rogowski, W.H. The cost-effectiveness of UGT1A1 genotyping before colorectal cancer treatment with irinotecan from the perspective of the German statutory health insurance. *Acta Oncol.* **2016**, *55*, 318–328. [CrossRef] [PubMed]
165. Roncato, R.; Cecchin, E.; Montico, M.; De Mattia, E.; Giodini, L.; Buonadonna, A.; Solfrini, V.; Innocenti, F.; Toffoli, G. Cost Evaluation of Irinotecan-Related Toxicities Associated With the UGT1A1*28 Patient Genotype. *Clin. Pharm. Ther.* **2017**, *102*, 123–130. [CrossRef]
166. Agencia Española de Medicamentosy Produtos Sanitarios Fluorouracilo, Capecitabina, Tegafury Flucitosina en Pacientes con Déficit de Dihidropirimidina Deshidrogenasa. Available online: https://www.aemps.gob.es/informa/notasinformativas/medicamentosusohumano-3/seguridad-1/2020-seguridad-1/fluorouracilo-capecitabina-tegafur-y-flucitosina-en-pacientes-con-deficit-de-dihidropirimidina-deshidrogenasa/ (accessed on 24 September 2020).
167. Amstutz, U.; Henricks, L.M.; Offer, S.M.; Barbarino, J.; Schellens, J.H.; Swen, J.J.; Klein, T.E.; McLeod, H.L.; Caudle, K.E.; Diasio, R.B.; et al. Clinical Pharmacogenetics Implementation Consortium (CPIC) Guideline for Dihydropyrimidine Dehydrogenase Genotype and Fluoropyrimidine Dosing: 2017 Update. *Clin. Pharm. Ther.* **2018**, *103*, 210–216. [CrossRef]
168. The Pharmacogenetics Working Group. UGT1A1: Irinotecan. Available online: https://www.g-standaard.nl/risicoanalyse/B0001694.PDF (accessed on 24 September 2020).
169. European Medicines Agency. Recommendations on DPD Testing Prior to Treatment with Fluorouracil, Capecitabine, Tegafur and Flucytosine. Available online: https://www.ema.europa.eu/en/news/ema-recommendations-dpd-testing-prior-treatment-fluorouracil-capecitabine-tegafur-flucytosine (accessed on 24 September 2020).
170. Food and Drug Administration. Table of Pharmacogenomic Biomarkers in Drug Labeling. Available online: https://www.fda.gov/media/124784/download (accessed on 24 September 2020).
171. European Medicines Agency. Erbitux (cetuximab). *Am. J. Neuroradiol.* **2010**, *31*, 626–627.

172. Cancer Therapy Evaluation Program. Common Terminology Criteria for Adverse Events (CTCAE).v.5.0. Available online: https://ctep.cancer.gov/protocoldevelopment/electronic_applications/docs/ctcae_v5_quick_reference_5x7.pdf (accessed on 23 July 2020).
173. Kerns, S.L.; Fachal, L.; Dorling, L.; Barnett, G.C.; Baran, A.; Peterson, D.R.; Hollenberg, M.; Hao, K.; Narzo, A.D.; Ahsen, M.E.; et al. Radiogenomics Consortium Genome-Wide Association Study Meta-Analysis of Late Toxicity After Prostate Cancer Radiotherapy. *J. Natl. Cancer Inst.* **2020**, *112*, 179–190. [CrossRef]
174. Barnett, G.C.; Thompson, D.; Fachal, L.; Kerns, S.; Talbot, C.; Elliott, R.M.; Dorling, L.; Coles, C.E.; Dearnaley, D.P.; Rosenstein, B.S.; et al. A genome wide association study (GWAS) providing evidence of an association between common genetic variants and late radiotherapy toxicity. *Radiother. Oncol.* **2014**, *111*, 178–185. [CrossRef]
175. Fachal, L.; Gómez-Caamaño, A.; Barnett, G.C.; Peleteiro, P.; Carballo, A.M.; Calvo-Crespo, P.; Kerns, S.L.; Sánchez-García, M.; Lobato-Busto, R.; Dorling, L.; et al. A three-stage genome-wide association study identifies a susceptibility locus for late radiotherapy toxicity at 2q24.1. *Nat. Genet.* **2014**, *46*, 891–894. [CrossRef]
176. Kerns, S.L.; Stock, R.G.; Stone, N.N.; Blacksburg, S.R.; Rath, L.; Vega, A.; Fachal, L.; Gómez-Caamaño, A.; De Ruysscher, D.; Lammering, G.; et al. Genome-wide association study identifies a region on chromosome 11q14.3 associated with late rectal bleeding following radiation therapy for prostate cancer. *Radiother. Oncol.* **2013**, *107*, 372–376. [CrossRef]
177. Kerns, S.L.; Dorling, L.; Fachal, L.; Bentzen, S.; Pharoah, P.D.; Barnes, D.R.; Gómez-Caamaño, A.; Carballo, A.M.; Dearnaley, D.P.; Peleteiro, P.; et al. Meta-analysis of Genome Wide Association Studies Identifies Genetic Markers of Late Toxicity Following Radiotherapy for Prostate Cancer. *EBioMedicine* **2016**, *10*, 150–163. [CrossRef] [PubMed]
178. Richardson, M.; Kirkham, J.; Dwan, K.; Sloan, D.J.; Davies, G.R.; Jorgensen, A.L. STrengthening the Reporting of Pharmacogenetic Studies: Development of the STROPS guideline. *PLoS Med.* **2020**, *17*, e1003344. [CrossRef]
179. Hegde, M.; Santani, A.; Mao, R.; Ferreira-Gonzalez, A.; Weck, K.E.; Voelkerding, K.V. Development and validation of clinical whole-exome and whole-genome sequencing for detection of germline variants in inherited disease. *Arch. Pathol. Lab. Med.* **2017**, *141*, 798–805. [CrossRef] [PubMed]
180. Zhou, Y.; Fujikura, K.; Mkrtchian, S.; Lauschke, V.M. Computational methods for the pharmacogenetic interpretation of next generation sequencing data. *Front. Pharm.* **2018**, *9*, 1–17. [CrossRef]

Publisher's Note: MDPI stays neutral with regard to jurisdictional claims in published maps and institutional affiliations.

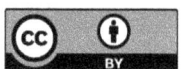

© 2020 by the authors. Licensee MDPI, Basel, Switzerland. This article is an open access article distributed under the terms and conditions of the Creative Commons Attribution (CC BY) license (http://creativecommons.org/licenses/by/4.0/).

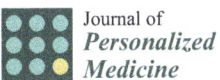

Review

Genetic Determinants in *HLA* and Cytochrome P450 Genes in the Risk of Aromatic Antiepileptic-Induced Severe Cutaneous Adverse Reactions

Ali Fadhel Ahmed [1], Chonlaphat Sukasem [2,3,4,5], Majeed Arsheed Sabbah [6], Nur Fadhlina Musa [7], Dzul Azri Mohamed Noor [1] and Nur Aizati Athirah Daud [1,7,*]

1. Discipline of Clinical Pharmacy, School of Pharmaceutical Sciences, Universiti Sains Malaysia, Pulau Pinang 11800, Malaysia; alifadhel1131990@student.usm.my or alifadhel1131990@gmail.com (A.F.A.); dzulazri@usm.my (D.A.M.N.)
2. Department of Pathology, Faculty of Medicine Ramathibodi Hospital, Mahidol University, Bangkok 10400, Thailand; chonlaphat.suk@mahidol.ac.th
3. Laboratory for Pharmacogenomics, Somdech Phra Debaratana Medical Center (SDMC), Ramathibodi Hospital, Bangkok 10400, Thailand
4. The Thai Severe Cutaneous Adverse Drug Reaction (THAI-SCAR) Research Group, Chulalongkorn University, Bangkok 10330, Thailand
5. Advanced Research and Development Laboratory, Bumrungrad International Hospital, Bangkok 10110, Thailand
6. Forensic DNA for Research and Training Centre, Alnahrain University, Baghdad 64074, Iraq; majeedbio@gmail.com
7. Human Genome Center, School of Medical Sciences, Universiti Sains Malaysia, Kubang Kerian, Kota Bharu 16150, Malaysia; fadhlina@usm.my
* Correspondence: aizati@usm.my or aizati.daud@gmail.com

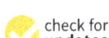

Citation: Ahmed, A.F.; Sukasem, C.; Sabbah, M.A.; Musa, N.F.; Mohamed Noor, D.A.; Daud, N.A.A. Genetic Determinants in *HLA* and Cytochrome P450 Genes in the Risk of Aromatic Antiepileptic-Induced Severe Cutaneous Adverse Reactions. *J. Pers. Med.* **2021**, *11*, 383. https://doi.org/10.3390/jpm11050383

Academic Editor: Luis A. López-Fernández

Received: 5 March 2021
Accepted: 28 April 2021
Published: 7 May 2021

Publisher's Note: MDPI stays neutral with regard to jurisdictional claims in published maps and institutional affiliations.

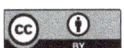

Copyright: © 2021 by the authors. Licensee MDPI, Basel, Switzerland. This article is an open access article distributed under the terms and conditions of the Creative Commons Attribution (CC BY) license (https://creativecommons.org/licenses/by/4.0/).

Abstract: Adverse drug reaction (ADR) is a pressing health problem, and one of the main reasons for treatment failure with antiepileptic drugs. This has become apparent in the event of severe cutaneous adverse reactions (SCARs), which can be life-threatening. In this review, four hypotheses were identified to describe how the immune system is triggered in the development of SCARs, which predominantly involve the human leukocyte antigen (HLA) proteins. Several genetic variations in HLA genes have been shown to be strongly associated with the susceptibility to developing SCARs when prescribed carbamazepine or phenytoin. These genetic variations were also shown to be prevalent in certain populations. Apart from the HLA genes, other genes proposed to affect the risk of SCARs are genes encoding for CYP450 drug-metabolising enzymes, which are involved in the pharmacokinetics of offending drugs. Genetic variants in CYP2C9 and CYPC19 enzymes were also suggested to modulate the risk of SCARs in some populations. This review summarizes the literature on the manifestation and aetiology of antiepileptic-induced SCARs, updates on pharmacogenetic markers associated with this reaction and the implementation of pre-emptive testing as a preventive strategy for SCARs.

Keywords: HLA; cutaneous adverse drug reaction; SCAR; genetic polymorphism; antiepileptics; CYP450 enzymes

1. Introduction

An adverse drug reaction (ADR) is defined as a noxious or unintended response of the body to regular exposure to chemical materials such as drugs, for the purpose of prophylaxis, diagnosis or therapy of a disease, or modification of physiological functions of organs [1]. ADRs are common at the community level and account for about 6.5% of all hospitalized cases, and incur increased attention, health care and community costs in 15% of patients. Statistics in the United States of America indicate that ADRs are responsible for more than 100,000 deaths annually, making ADR the sixth leading cause of death in the States, with similar statistics seen in the United Kingdom [2,3].

Several antiepileptic drugs (AEDs) are commonly associated with adverse skin reactions [4]. Severe and life-threatening skin reactions are referred to as severe cutaneous adverse reactions (SCARs) [5]. SCARs which occur following the use of certain drugs are a type of delayed hypersensitivity reaction that is idiosyncratic, unpredictable and dose-independent. SCARs account for 15–20% of all adverse drug reactions, which include Stevens-Johnson syndrome (SJS), toxic epidermal necrolysis (TEN) and drug reaction with eosinophilia and systemic symptoms (DRESS). Statistics indicate that the annual incidence of SJS is 1.2–6.0 per million, while the incidence of TEN is 0.4–1.2 per million annually [6,7]. Both reactions are characterized by high mortality and morbidity rates despite the low incidence, as the mortality rate for SJS is 1–5% while for TEN it is 25–30% [8,9]. SCARs are most commonly observed among patients taking carbamazepine (CBZ), phenytoin (PHT) and lamotrigine, and typically occur within the first three months of initiation [8].

Knowledge of patients' genetic information might help in preventing antiepileptic-induced SCARs. Several genetic variations, especially in the genes encoding for human leukocyte antigen HLA-A, HLA-B and cytochrome P450 enzymes have been significantly associated with a higher risk of developing a SCAR [9–11]. Identifying the type of SCAR is also essential for determining the HLA alleles and the P450 isoforms associated with this hypersensitivity syndrome. The findings of this association will shed light on the predisposing genetic risk factors in SCARs and provide a means for preventive measures, such as a pre-emptive screening of HLA and CYP450 markers before the initiation of drug treatment [12]. This is in line with the emerging approach of precision medicine where prescribed medication takes individual genetic variability into consideration. This review further focuses on the genetic variations of several genes involved in the mechanism of antiepileptic-induced SCARs, and the potential contribution of pre-emptive testing as part of the genotype-guided therapeutics for the prevention of SCARs.

2. Severe Cutaneous Adverse Drug Reactions (SCARs) and AEDs Use

SCARs linked with the use of medications are a type of delayed hypersensitivity reaction that is idiosyncratic, non-predictable and independent of dose. SCARs pose a challenge in the clinical management of patients, as they are related to increased mortality and morbidity, long-term subsequent medical events and high healthcare costs [13].

Skin rash is a common manifestation of ADR in affected individuals. SCARs constitute a large variety of clinical phenotypes, from maculopapular exanthema (MPE) to hypersensitivity syndrome (HSS), SJS, TEN, DRESS and acute generalized acute exanthematous pustulosis (AGEP) [14]. A milder form of cutaneous adverse reaction is MPE, a rash that is mild, self-limited and usually resolved after the offending drugs are withdrawn. Unlike MPE, SCARs have serious morbidity, involve systemic manifestation and pose high mortality [15].

About 3% of patients on antiepileptic drugs may develop cutaneous eruptions [16]. A mild form of MPE may occur in about 2.8% of AED users, with phenytoin, lamotrigine and carbamazepine displaying the highest rates (5.9%, 4.8% and 3.7%, respectively), and these reactions may resolve naturally within 3–20 days [17]. Meanwhile, more severe types of cutaneous ADRs including HSS, SJS, TEN and DRESS are less common [18,19]. The histopathology of MPE, DRESS and SJS/TEN is predominated with exocytosis and lymphocyte and macrophage infiltration. In severe cases of SJS/TEN, extensive keratinocyte necrosis is observed. The severity of inflammatory infiltrate and epidermal manifestation increases from MPE to DRESS and SJS/TEN [18].

3. Clinical Manifestations of SCARs

SJS and TEN are characterized by sloughing of the skin, mucosal membranes and the surface of the eye via immune mechanisms that lead to cell death or necrosis [19]. The early stages of SJS/TEN clinical manifestation include fever, malaise, flu-like symptoms, and also symptoms involving eyes, ear, nose and throat for a few days or up to 2 weeks prior to cutaneous manifestations. Cutaneous manifestations of SJS begin with skin pain or a burning sensation (Figure 1A,B). It first appears on the face, pre-sternal area of the upper trunk and extremities, and involves erythroderma, purpura, pustules and swelling of the affected area [20]. Symptoms are typically manifested in the proximal parts of the extremities, while the distal parts are relatively spared [21]. In a short period of time, erythematous macules or diffuse erythema will develop over the trunk and extremities. As the red areas develop, the central dusty necrotic areas expand with the subsequent growth of bullae. As the disease progresses, the layers of the full-thickness epidermis will separate, exposing dark red, moist dermis resembling extreme second-degree burns [22,23].

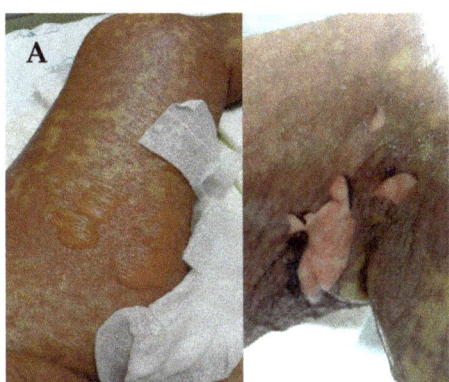 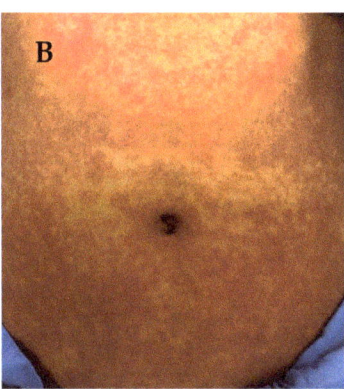

Figure 1. (**A**) Manifestations of Stevens-Johnson syndrome (SJS) and toxic epidermal necrolysis (TEN), in which the skin begins to blister and peel. Erythroderma, extensive skin lesions, aggressive detachment of the epidermis and erosion of mucous membranes can be observed; (**B**) dermatologic manifestations of drug reaction with eosinophilia and systemic symptoms (DRESS) typically consist of diffuse pruritic macular and urticarial rash. Facial oedema and periorbital areas with scale and crust around the nose and lip can be found. All patients have provided informed consent before being enrolled and provided the pictures.

A positive Nikolsky sign is significant diagnostic evidence and precedes the occurrence of life-threatening events [24,25]. There is less than 10% and over 30% epidermal detachment in SJS and TEN, respectively. Any disorder with between 10% and 29% epidermal detachment is typically diagnosed as overlapping with SJS/TEN [26]. The clinical presentation of these reactions may also differ among individuals. In one confirmed case of SJS, only mucosal membrane lesions without skin lesions were present in a 14 year-old child [27]. Mucosal membrane involvement may occur in 85% to 95% of SJS and TEN patients; while involvement of conjunctivae, mucous membranes of the nares, mouth, oropharynx, anorectal junction, vulvovaginal area and urethral meatus may occur in 85% to 95% of SJS and TEN patients [28].

Early diagnosis of SCARs that helps in the identification of the culprit drugs is important in the acute stages of the reaction. A prompt recognition helps to improve the management of the disease and limits long-term sequelae. Classification of SCARs is also important in identifying causal drugs. Studies have shown that the interval between drug intake and SCARs onset differ according to the type of SCARs. SJS/TEN has a shorter latency period compared to DRESS [29]. Assessment scores and tools developed to assist in investigation of SCARs to determine clinical patterns and identify causal drugs are discussed in the following section.

4. Phenotyping and Causality of SCARs

The clinical phenotype of SCARs is defined by the disease characteristics (i.e., phenotypic traits) that explain discrepancies between persons with the reactions in terms of clinically significant outcomes (such as symptoms, extent and severity of rash, involvement of other organs, as well as laboratory and clinical parameters) [29,30]. Clinical phenotyping of SCARs was proposed by RegiSCAR (European Registry of Severe Cutaneous Adverse Reactions), a multinational collaborative research consortium previously known as EuroSCAR [31]. The RegiSCAR group operates as a registry of clinical data and biological samples, and provides continuous surveillance on new drugs and guidelines for SCARs. The aim of this group is to promote the safe use of drugs while reducing the medical and economic burden of SCARs on public health. To prevent misdiagnosis, RegiSCAR defined consensus diagnosis criteria for each SCAR phenotype. SCAR cases were investigated using standardized questionnaires to obtain detailed information on clinical phenotypes, including collecting clinical photographs and skin biopsies and associated medical conditions. Other phenotypes like type of skin rash, hospitalization and organ involvement are also included in the assessment criteria in the diagnosis of HSS/DRESS [29].

In the determination drug causality, the assessment criteria include non-genetic factors such as drug exposure, rechallenge, disease aetiology and previous report of similar cases [31]. The RegiSCAR group reported that the causality of SCARs could be attributed to other high-risk medications and that misdiagnoses were frequent. Overlapping SCAR phenotypes were rare, as SJS and TEN are known to be variants of the same disease, while SJS/TEN and DRESS are two distinct diseases [29,32].

Several algorithms were used to perform the causality assessment of SCARs objectively, as a standardized approach is important to establish an accurate and reproducible diagnosis. The algorithms used for drug causality assessment in cutaneous ADRs include the Naranjo algorithm, the French pharmacovigilance causality score test and the RUCAM algorithm [31,33]. From the RegiSCAR findings, a specific algorithm for drug causality was constructed, known as the drug causality algorithm for epidermal necrolysis (ALDEN), which has gained prominence as it is frequently applied in recent SJS and TEN cases [31].

Assessing drug causality is also a challenge due to incomplete reporting of drug exposure. Generally, for SCARs assessment, it relies mainly on cutaneous manifestation and clinical presentation, duration of the eruptions, associated symptoms and latency time between starting the drug and eruption onset. The distribution and physical examination of the skin lesions coupled with skin biopsy for histological testing are important for the accurate and quick diagnosis of SJS/TEN, as a diagnosis of SJS/TEN within 7 days of onset is associated with improved survival [18]. Using the study data, several parameters were considered in the estimation of drug risk, prognosis indexes, disease outcome and effects on treatments for SCARs. Other ongoing investigations include phenotype determination, lymphocytes' antigenic specificity and susceptibility genes and associated single-nucleotide polymorphisms (SNPs) [34].

Not all individuals exposed to the offending drugs are affected, which might indicate a genetic predisposition towards this effect. Progress in the field of genetics has broadened our knowledge and ability to prevent ADR events by identifying the genetic markers responsible for such reactions among the affected patients [35]. Genetic markers found to be linked to an increased risk of SCARs are genes encoding for human leukocyte antigen (HLA), drug transporter proteins (e.g., ABCB1, SLCO1B1), drug-metabolizing enzymes (cytochrome P450), glucose-6-phosphate dehydrogenase (G6PD) and nucleoside diphosphate linked moiety X-type motif 15 (NUDT15) [36]. The following sections focus on genetic markers in HLA genes and genes encoding for cytochrome P450 enzymes.

5. Human Leukocyte Antigen (HLA) and Its Role in ADRs

The major histocompatibility complex (MHC) is a group of proteins on the cell surface that mediate immunological reaction to foreign molecules or antigens entering the body [37]. The MHC binds to foreign molecules and displays them on the surface of cells for recognition by corresponding T cells, followed by the release of immunological mediators as a response. Human MHC, also known as human leukocyte antigen (HLA) complex, is encoded by over 200 genes located on the short arm of chromosome 6 (6p21.3) [38]. HLA complex is divided into three major classes: class I, type II and class III. Class I consists of three genes: HLA-A, HLA-B and HLA-C. The HLA class I molecules are expressed on the membranes of most karyocytes and can provide CD8+ T cell endogenous peptides, the cytotoxic T cells. Meanwhile, class II MHC consists of six primary genes: HLA-DPA1, HLA-DPB1, H1LA-DQA1, HLADQB1, HLA-DRA and HLA-DRB1. The HLA class II is only expressed on immune cell surfaces such as exogenous peptides to CD4+ T-helper cells and dendritic cells. Occasionally, cross-presentation may occur, such as in viral infections [39].

All cells responsible for presenting peptides to immune cells express HLA class I in their surfaces. In general, old proteins are broken down from cells by a continuous process of collecting peptides to make new ones. Some of the broken peptide fragments bind with MHC molecules and are recognized by the body's immune cells as "self-molecules". If the broken cell has a pathogen, the pathogen peptides that bind to the molecules of the MHC are known as foreign (nonself) peptides and activate an immune response against the disease-causing antigens [40].

HLA genes are highly polymorphic, and the proteins bind to multiple types of peptides to be recognized as either "self-antigens" or "foreign antigens." Genetic differences in HLA genes play a crucial role in determining the susceptibility of an individual to autoimmune diseases and other infections. It also plays a vital role in the success of organ transplants, as genetic compatibility of the HLA genes between the donor and the recipient is very important [34]. Several recent studies have also shown a significant correlation between HLA proteins and the risk of idiosyncratic ADRs [41,42]. The following sections discuss the proposed immune response related to SCARs and the genetic polymorphisms of several genes linked to the risk of SCAR caused by AEDs.

6. The Hypothesis of Immune Response in SCARs

ADRs are divided into type A, which is predictable, and type B, which is idiosyncratic [43–45]. Type A ADRs are directly caused by the pharmacology of drugs and commonly occur in a dose-dependent relationship; type B ADRs are not related to the pharmacology or dosage of drugs [44–46]. Idiosyncratic ADRs can be immune-mediated or non-immune-mediated [41]. Immune-mediated ADRs are rarely noticed during clinical trials and are difficult to predict. There are some rare cases where the drug induces an immune response by interacting with MHC molecules, but not much is known about the exact mechanisms associated with such ADRs [41,47].

Researchers developed four hypotheses to understand how the immune system is activated in an HLA-molecule-dependent manner in the development of SCARs: (i) the "hapten/prohapten" theory, (ii) the "p-i" concept, (iii) the "altered peptide repertoire" model and (iv) the "altered T cell receptor (TCR) repertoire" model [48,49]. Figure 2 illustrates the proposed mechanism of immune response in SCARs.

The first hypothesis, "hapten/prohapten", suggests that a drug or its reactive compound can bind covalently to an endogenous peptide to form an antigenic hapten–carrier complex. The concept of this model is to establish covalent bonds between the medication or its reactive metabolites, self-peptides and HLA molecules. This is accompanied by the activation of drug-specific immune responses [50]. The second concept of pharmacological interaction with immune receptors, the "p-i" concept, assumes that the drug or its reactive metabolites may be directly, inversely or disproportionately linked to HLA and/or TCR without binding to the antigen peptide. This suggests that there is a pharmacological interaction with immune receptors, which implies stimulation of the immune system by noncovalent binding of a drug to T-cell receptors for antigens (p-i TCR) or human leukocyte antigens (p-i HLA). The consequences of these interactions are heterogeneous; clinically, it can lead to T-cell-mediated reactions such as Stevens-Johnson syndrome/toxic epidermal necrolysis, drug rash with eosinophilia and systemic symptoms, acute generalized exanthematous pustulosis and maculopapular eruptions. If the drug binds to the TCR, it can become stimulatory, and additional interaction with HLA/peptide complexes is necessary for full stimulation. In the "p-i" model, it is assumed that the classic antigen-processing pathway in antigen-presenting cells may be bypassed. The third model, the "altered peptide repertoire" model, proposes that the drug is bound closely to "self-peptides" and is presented in the form of a peptide repertoire given to HLA and TCR [50]. The drug is not related directly to HLA in the "altered peptide repertoire" model. For example, the "altered TCR repertoire" explains that a drug (e.g., sulfamethoxazole) binds to a certain TCR, changes the TCR conformation and has the ability to produce an HLA–self-peptide complex that triggers an immune response [50]. In the model of "altered TCR repertoire", TCR acts as the initial molecular drug interaction. With the link of an offending drug presented to the HLA molecule or TCR, the HLA–drug–TCR combination can stimulate the activation of cell signalling pathways and result in an expansion of cytotoxic T lymphocytes.

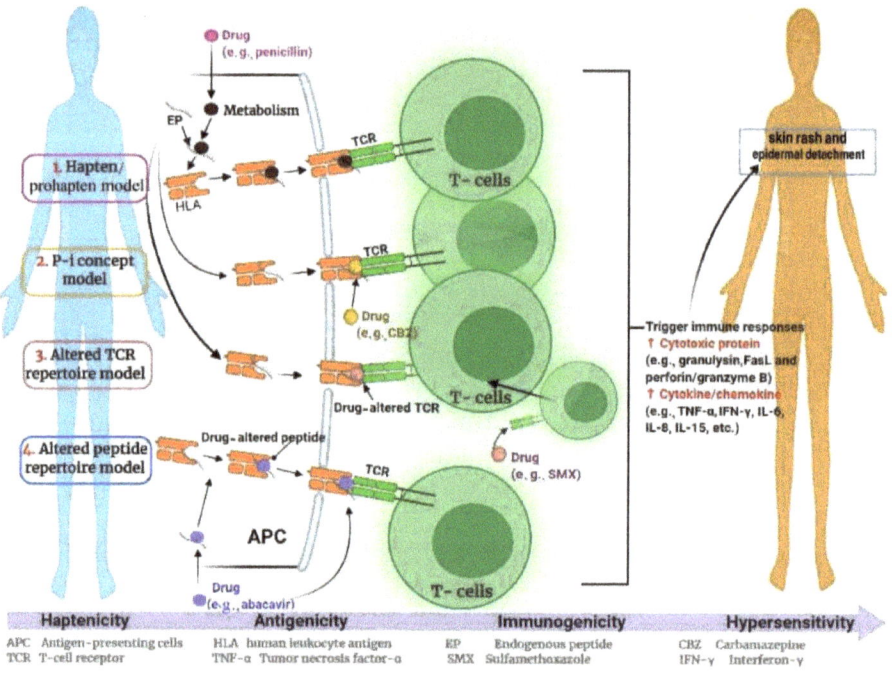

Figure 2. The hypothesis pertaining to the immune response mechanism during severe cutaneous adverse reaction.

7. Genetic Polymorphisms of HLA Genes

The MHC region has been associated with more diseases than any other region in the human genome. The MHC region is densely clustered with genes that have a strong linkage disequilibrium, making it challenging to pinpoint the exact causative variant and the related function. Disease resistance has been proposed to drive the evolution in MHC variation. By taking amino acid residue 57 of HLADQB in type I diabetes as an example, although autoimmune diseases are demonstrated to be associated with changes in the groove residues, it is still not fully understood how the changes mediate autoimmune diseases [51]. In humans, the HLA complex region might be the most polymorphic region. The polymorphisms in this region are not widely spread out, but are concentrated in the region encoding the peptide-binding groove. In the case of HLA class I, $\alpha 1$ and $\alpha 2$ domains involve variable amino acid residues and are the determinants of antigenic specificities of molecules. Of all the HLA genes, HLA-B is known to be the most polymorphic, with more than 4000 alleles [48,49].

Aside from its association to diseases, the HLA allele polymorphisms have been studied extensively to draw inferences about human migration and genetic diversity among different populations. For example, HLA-B*15, the most polymorphic allele in HLA-B locus, has a non-symmetrical distribution in the Asian population, whereby the alleles in northeast Asia are more prevalent in the global population. In contrast, the alleles found in the Southeast Asian (SEA) population are more specific to the SEA region. For example, the most common allele in B*15 lineage, HLA- B*15:01, is more prevalent in northeast Asia, whereas HLA-B*15:02 is more prevalent in the south of Asia spreading southwards into SEA. The distribution of HLA-B*15:02 supports the human migratory route into SEA [52,53]. HLA-B*15:13 is more specific, and is observed within the Indonesian archipelago of SEA, while HLA-A*31:01 is present in more than 15% of people with Japanese, Native American, South Indian (e.g., Tamil Nadu) and Arabic ancestry, in up to 10% of people with Han Chinese, Korean, European, Latin American and other Indian ancestry, and in up to 5% of African-Americans [9,50,54].

8. HLA Alleles and SCARs Induced by AEDs

SCARs are unpredictable and not dose-dependent. Substantial progress for underlying SCAR mechanisms has been made with the discovery of the association between HLA alleles and SCARs. In this section, we summarize recent updates in the identification of genetic markers involved in SCARs or hypersensitivity reactions induced by aromatic AEDs). The reported findings are summarized and listed in Table 1, while the frequency of each allele is presented in Table 2.

Table 1. Ethnicity and phenotype specific association between HLA allele and AED-induced SCARs.

AEDs	HLA Alleles	Population/Ethnicity	Phenotype	Reference
Carbamazepine	HLA-A*02:01	Iranian	SJS	[55]
	HLA-A*31:01	Caucasian Japanese	DRESS MPE SJS/TEN	[56–60]
		Korean	DRESS, SJS/TEN	[60]
		Han Chinese	DRESS, MPE,	
	HLA-A*51:01	Iranian	SJS	[55]
	HLA-B*15:02	Han Chinese Thai Malay Indian Vietnamese Indonesian	SJS/TEN	[9,51,61–64]
	HLA-B*15:08	Indian	SJS/TEN	[65]
	HLA-B*15:11	Japanese Korean	SJS/TEN	[66] [58]
	HLA-B*15:18	Japanese	SJS/TEN	[67]
	HLA-B*15:21	Filipino	SJS/TEN	[68]
Phenytoin	HLA-B*15:02	Han Chinese Thai Malay	SJS/TEN	[69] [70] [71]
	HLA-B*15:13	Malay	SJS/TEN	[71]
Lamotrigine	HLA-B*15:01	Han Chinese	SJS/TEN	[69] [72]
Phenobarbital	HLA-B*13:01	Thai Han Chinese	SJS/TEN	[73]
	HLA–B*51:01	Japanese	SJS/TEN	[11]

Abbreviations. SJS: Stevens-Johnson syndrome; TEN: toxic epidermal necrolysis; DRESS: drug reaction with eosinophilia and systemic symptoms; MPE: maculopapular exanthema.

Table 2. HLA-A and HLA-B allele frequency for various ethnicities.

HLA Alleles	Population/Ethnicity	Allele Frequency	Reference
HLA-A			
HLA-A*02:01	Iranian	0.202	[74]
	Caucasian	0.0214	[75]
HLA-A*31:01	Japanese	0.084	[76]
	Korean	0.0562	[77]
	Han Chinese	0.0307	[78]
HLA-B			
HLA-B*13:01	Thai	0.210–0.0410	[79,80]
	Han Chinese	0.0405	[81]
HLA-B*15:01	Han Chinese	0.038	[82]
HLA-B*15:02	Han Chinese	0.0190–0.1240	[82,83]
	Thai	0.084	[84]
	Malay	0.1225	[85]
	Indian	0.013	[86]
	Vietnamese	0.135	[87]
	Indonesian	0.122	[88]
HLA-B*15:11	Japanese	0.0088	[76]
	Korean	0.0166	[77]
HLA-B*15:13	Malay	0.0599	[85]
HLA-B*15:18	Japanese	0.0152	[89]
HLA-B*15:21	Filipino	0.01	[90]
HLA-B*51:01	Japanese	0.07–0.9	[91]

8.1. Carbamazepine-Induced SCARs

Carbamazepine (CBZ) is a drug widely used to treat epilepsy, bipolar disorder and trigeminal neuralgia [64,92,93]. While usually well-tolerated, up to 10% of patients may have a cutaneous ADR [93]. The only effective intervention in this situation is withdrawal or prevention of the use of this medication [7]. The clinical symptoms of CBZ-induced SCARs are similar to anticonvulsant hypersensitivity syndrome with an immune-based and genetic predisposition [11].

Previous reports demonstrated that carriers of the HLA-B*15:02 allele were associated with approximately a 100-fold risk of developing SJS/TEN with the use of CBZ15 [15,63,94–96]. The first documentation of the strong association (OR > 1000) between HLA-B*15:02 and SJS induced by CBZ was among Han Chinese patients [51,59]. Other reports among Malaysians, Han Chinese and Thai patients indicated that patients with CBZ-induced SJS carried HLA-B*15:02 alleles, while some patients also carried the HLA-B*15:21 allele [62,97,98]. One study among Han Chinese identified that 100% (44/44) of patients using CBZ therapy and presented with SJS/TEN syndrome were carrying the HLA-B*15:02 allele, while only 3% (1/301) of the CBZ -tolerant patients were HLA-B*15:02-positive [71]. Meanwhile, several studies reported a relationship between HLA-B*15:02 and SJS/TEN resulting from the use of CBZ therapy in many populations, including Africans, Koreans, Malaysians, Japanese, Caucasians and Indians [39].

The association between HLA-B*15:02 and CBZ-induced SJS/TEN is both ethnicity- and phenotype-specific. This association was successfully recorded in Han Chinese patients, and in Asian populations including Malays, Thais and Indians [62,99,100]. However, it was not commonly observed amongst Japanese and Caucasian patients [63,96,97]. Inconsistency and variation in the allele frequency between population groups is frequently observed. For example, the allele frequency of HLA-B*15: 02 was high amongst several Asian populations (0.12–0.157 in Malays, 0.057–0.145 in Han Chinese and 0.085–0.275 in Thais) but lower in other populations such as Koreans (0.004), Europeans (0.01–0.02) and Japanese (0.002) [101]. For other types of cutaneous ADRs like eosinophilia and systemic symptoms (DRESS), there were no reports on their risk associated with HLA-B alleles with the use of CBZ [71,102,103].

The established association between HLA-B*15:02 and the risk of CBZ-induced SCARs warrants preventative measures to ensure the safe use of this medication. Based on previous reports on the risk of this allele in patients receiving CBZ, the FDA and European Medicines Agency included warnings on drug labels advising the need for genotyping among patients from certain areas of Asia before starting CBZ therapy [104]. A pre-emptive screening for HLA-B*15:02 was introduced in some countries, and its clinical utility was demonstrated recently by a prospective cohort study in Taiwan [105]. In this study, around 4800 patients were genotyped, and 7.7% were positive for HLA-B*15:02. The patients were prescribed an alternative therapy to CBZ, and no patients developed SJS in the study, contrary to the expected ten cases based on past incidences [106]. A study in Thailand also found that the genotyping for HLA-B*15:02 was cost-effective in preventing the occurrence of SCARs [107].

Several HLA alleles constitute the HLA-B75 serotype commonly found in Southeast Asian populations, for example, HLA-B*15:21, HLA-B*13:01 and HLA-B*15:21 [78]. HLA-A*31:01 alleles were significantly associated with CBZ-DRESS in Europeans ($p < 0.001$; OR 57.6, 95% CI 11.0–340) [59]. The pathogenesis of these CBZ hypersensitivity reactions requires further research, as it remains unclear whether HLA-B*15:02 represents the true causal allele or if it is in linkage disequilibrium with another causal variant.

8.2. Phenytoin-Induced SCAR

Phenytoin is a commonly prescribed AED that can cause cutaneous ADRs, ranging from MPE to life-threatening SCARs such as DRESS and SJS/TEN [103]. A previous study showed a confirmed association between HLA-B*15:02 and phenytoin-induced SJS/TEN in Malay patients (61.5% (8/13 cases) vs. 21.9% (7/32 controls), OR 5.71; $p = 0.016$) and showed a significant association between HLA-B*15:13 and both phenytoin-induced SJS/TEN (53.8% (7/13 cases), OR 11.28; $p = 0.003$) and phenytoin-induced DRESS (100% (3/3 cases), OR 59.00; $p = 0.003$) [71].

Several studies reported the association between HLA-B*15:02 and phenytoin-induced SJS/TEN in the Han Chinese population [69,100]. Furthermore, a study by Hung et. al. found a genetic risk with several other alleles, including HLA-B*15:02, HLA-B*13:01, Cw*08:01 and DRB1*16:02 in a similar population [59]. Cw*08:01 is within the haplotype of B*15:02, and therefore its association can be explained by linkage disequilibrium. On the other hand, despite a statistically significant association for HLA-B*13:01 and DRB1*16:02 alleles [59], the sample size was reported to be small. The association between B*15:02 allele and phenytoin-induced SCARs could not be replicated in some other studies [103,108], while only one study reported the association between HLA-B*56:02 and phenytoin-related SCARs, including DRESS and SJS/TEN [108]. In the European population, there was no association found between HLA-A*31:01 and phenytoin-induced cutaneous ADRs [9,109].

8.3. Lamotrigine-Induced SJS/TEN SCARs

Lamotrigine is a new-generation AED, and several alleles have been associated with lamotrigine-induced SCARs. In Thai patients, HLA-A*02:07 and HLA-B*15:02 were associated with an increased risk of lamotrigine-induced cutaneous ADRs, while associations were also found between HLA-A*33:03, HLA-B*15:02, HLA-B*44:03 and lamotrigine-induced MPE [9]. Meanwhile, there are contradictory findings on the association between HLA-B*15:02 and lamotrigine-induced SJS/TEN [59,69,72,100]. In the Han Chinese population, one study found an association between HLA-A*33:03 and HLA-B*15:02 and lamotrigine-induced MPE [110]. A recent study among Koreans reported that individuals expressing the HLA-B*44:03 allele may be highly susceptible to lamotrigine-induced SJS/TEN [111]. These alleles were suggested for use as screening markers to prevent cutaneous ADRs before the initiation of lamotrigine [110].

In the European population, a weak association was found between HLA-B*38 and lamotrigine-induced SJS/TEN (OR 80; $p < 10^{-6}$) [112]. In other studies, several other alleles (i.e., HLA-B*5801, A*6801, Cw*0718, DQB1*0609 and DRB1*1301) were found to be weakly associated with lamotrigine-induced SCARs, but these results would need to be confirmed in a larger independent sample [113,114]. Another study failed to identify any single major HLA-related genetic risk factor for lamotrigine-induced SCARs in patients of European origin [113].

8.4. Phenobarbital-Induced SJS/TEN SCARs

Phenobarbital is one of the major causes of hypersensitivity to aromatic anticonvulsants in children. Patients with phenobarbital hypersensitivity may present with maculopapular rashes or SCARs, including SJS, TEN or DRESS. The incidence of aromatic anticonvulsant hypersensitivity is estimated to vary from 1/1000 to 1/10,000 [115], with a high mortality rate, especially in patients with SCARs [116]. Phenobarbital, the first-line anticonvulsant that is commonly used in seizure disorders in Thai children, is also one of the most common causes of SCARs in Thailand. Recently, there has been increasing evidence of the role of pharmacogenetics in predicting anticonvulsant-induced SCARs. However, there have only been a limited number of studies investigating the association between HLA genotypes and phenobarbital hypersensitivity. A small study from Japan demonstrated the association of HLA-B*51:01 and phenobarbital-induced SJS/TEN [117]. Eight patients who developed SJS/TEN reactions with the use of phenobarbital were recruited from the Japan Severe Adverse Reactions (JSAR) research group and RIKEN. One of them also had also received phenytoin. The onset of reaction after the initiation of the drug was 15.1 ± 7.1 days, which was slightly longer than those with reactions induced by phenytoin. Compared to healthy Japanese volunteers (n = 2878), six out of these eight patients carried HLA-B*51:01 and a significant association was observed between this allele and phenobarbital-induced SJS/TEN (OR 16.71, 95% CI 3.66–83.1) [117].

There is a potential cross-reactivity between use of aromatic AEDs in developing SCARs, possibly explained by the 'hapten hypothesis' mentioned earlier. Several studies have reported cases of patients with similar reactions following the use of two aromatic AEDs, while also presenting with the HLA-B*15:02 allele. A study by Locharernkul et al. [70] reported cases of MPE in three patients with the use of both CBZ and PHT. Meanwhile, Wang et al. found cross-reactivity towards aromatic AEDs in two Han Chinese patients who were both positive for HLA-B*15:02 [118]. Despite these reports, there is no definitive assumption on the magnitude and risk of AED-related cross-reactivity, partly because the use of another aromatic AED would have been avoided if the patients had a previous history of AED-induced SCARs.

9. Cytochrome P450 Enzymes and the Risk of SCAR

Cytochrome P450 is a superfamily of enzymes, including three main CYP families, CYP1, CYP2 and CYP3, which is responsible for the metabolism of a wide range of drugs [119,120]. Human beings have 57 CYP genes and 33 pseudogenes arranged into 18 families and 42 subfamilies. The P450 isoforms vary in abundance in the liver; however, CYP2C9, CYP2D6 and CYP3A4 account for 60–70% of all phase I biotransformations of drugs [121,122].

CYP2C9 and CYP2C19 are two of the most studied enzymes with clinically significant genetic variations (Table 3). The CYP2C9 gene is highly polymorphic, with at least 60 variants found in different populations [122]. CYP2C9*2 and *3 alleles have been associated with reduced enzymatic activity compared to the wild-type allele (CYP2C9*1) by 12% and 5% for *2 and *3, respectively [123]. Both alleles differ from the wild type by a single point mutation; CYP2C9*2 is characterized by a C416T SNP in exon three, resulting in an Arg144Cys amino acid substitution, whereas CYP2C9*3 expresses A1061C in exon 7, causing an Ile359Leu substitution [123].

Both of these alleles have proven to be determinants of significantly impaired metabolism of many CYP2C9 substrates, including phenytoin [124,125]. Phenotyping experiments showed that on a single dose of phenytoin, carriers build up approximately 30% higher serum levels compared to a person homozygous for the wild-type allele [126]. Since phenytoin has a narrow therapeutic index, this may have implications for the effect of the drug. A genome-wide-association study (GWAS) followed by direct sequencing of the CYP2C9 gene in patients from Taiwan, Malaysia and Japan showed that the missense variant CYP2C9*3 was associated with a 93–95% reduction in phenytoin clearance and that patients had phenytoin-induced SCARs. In addition to the CYP2C9 genotype, factors such as renal insufficiency, hepatic dysfunction and the concurrent use of substances that compete with or inhibit the enzymes contribute to variations in phenytoin clearance and/or to the risk of developing adverse effects, as delayed clearance of phenytoin was observed in the absence of CYP2C9C*3 [71].

In a study of 60 epileptic Dutch patients, the results demonstrated a strong association between the CYP2C9 allelic variables and the phenytoin dose requirements. The allele frequencies reported in this population were 76.7% for CYP2C9*1, 14.2% for CYP2C9*2 and 9.2% for CYP2C9*3, which were comparable to the frequencies reported in other studies of Caucasian populations [127]. Genotyping was suggested to be carried out at for any patients who might be prescribed phenytoin. Dosage adjustment based on the CYP2C9 genotype, especially prior to therapy, would be beneficial to lower the risk of concentration-dependent drug intoxication in carriers [127]. The defective CYP2C9 and/or CYP2C19 alleles could affect not only the pharmacokinetics but also the pharmacodynamics of phenytoin and CBZ therapy [128]. The FDA-approved drug label for phenytoin states that consideration should be given to avoiding phenytoin as an alternative for carbamazepine in individuals positive for HLA-B*15:02 because variant CYP2C9 alleles may contribute to unusually high levels of phenytoin [129]. For CYP2C19, three polymorphic alleles, CYP2C19*1 (wild type), CYP2C19*2 and CYP2C19*3, were identified to be relevant in the changes in drug metabolism. There were interethnic differences in CYP2C19 alleles observed in the Asian populations, particularly among the Chinese [9] and Japanese [130]. In a study conducted by Manuyakorn among Thai patients treated with CBZ and PHT, although the result was not statistically significant (OR 2.5, 95% CI 0.96–67.3; $p = 0.06$) [11], he showed that the patients with CYP2C19*2 variant had a higher likelihood of developing SCARs compared to patients with wild-type CYP2C19. It was also found that the CYP-catalysed metabolism of antiepileptics was increased in children [9,11].

Table 3. Cytochrome P450 allele frequency for various ethnicities.

AEDs	Population/ Ethnicity	Genetic Variation	Allele Frequency	References
Carbamazepine	Thai	CYP2C19*2	0.29	[11]
	Korean	CYP3A5*3	0.237	[131,132]
	Japanese	CYP3A5	7	[128,133]
Phenytoin	Japanese	CYP2C9	0	[134]
	Caucasian	CYP2C9*2	0.15	[127]
	Caucasian	CYP2C9*3	0.07	[127]
	Indian	CYP2C19*2	4.5	[135,136]
		CYP2C19*3	10.1	
	Thai	CYP2C 19*2	0.27	[102,137]
	Thai	CYP2C19*3	0.02	[102,137]
	Malay	CYP2C9*1	0.9407	[134,138]
Phenobarbital	Japanese	CYP2C19	0.26	[139]
	Japanese	CYP2C9	0.966	[140]

10. Clinical Application of Pharmacogenetic Testing in the Prevention of SCARs

Genetic testing is able to predict a patient's risk of developing ADRs, especially SCARs, and this knowledge could facilitate further strategies to avoid this complication. Pharmacogenetic testing is a type of genetic test consisting of a panel of genes important for the pharmacokinetics and pharmacodynamics of a drug, and is an attractive option for pre-emptive screening upon the initiation of a drug. This test can be used to identify individuals who are at risk of severe idiosyncratic adverse events, those who may not benefit from the therapy (e.g., non-responders) and the metabolism profile (e.g., fast versus slower metabolizers), which would ultimately allow for the individualization of drug dosage. This information would be useful in determining the choice of therapy and alternative strategies for treatment. Although there has been great interest in pharmacogenetics, there is a large gap in the knowledge on actionable variants (results which can change treatment), and the use of genetic testing in the clinical setting is limited to a few variants and drugs.

At present, several pharmacogenetic markers associated with drug hypersensitivity have been successfully identified and utilised in clinical practice. Growing evidence suggests that for patients with documented high genetic risks, pharmacogenomic testing is an efficient preventive tool. Currently, national health insurance organizations in Taiwan, Hong Kong, Singapore, Thailand and mainland China have approved pre-emptive genetic testing for the HLA-B*15:02 allele among new CBZ users [141,142]. Moreover, the U.S. FDA also suggests that HLA-B*15:02 testing be performed before patients are treated with oxcarbazepine. In addition to HLA-B*15:02, testing of the HLA-A*31:01 allele before the initiation of CBZ was also proposed among patients of Asian descent.

Screening for pharmacogenetic markers before the initiation of CBZ and PHT was shown to be cost-effective in addressing the risks of ADR. As examples, countries like Thailand, Singapore and Taiwan had performed pharmacogenetic screening for HLA alleles, and have shown significant reduction in the number of SJS/TEN cases reported with the use of risky drugs, not only limited to AEDs. As an example, HLA screening prior to the use of CBZ was implemented by the Singaporean Health Sciences Authority (HSA) in 2013 [141,142]. As a result of this national screening, a significant reduction of SJS/TEN cases was observed among patients on CBZ, from a baseline of ~18 cases per year (within 4 years) to only one case per year, just four years after the implementation of the HLA testing service [143,144]. In a Taiwanese study conducted on 4877 epilepsy patients prior to the initiation of CBZ, 7.7% of them were found to be positive for HLA-B*15:02. After 2 months of monitoring for symptoms of cutaneous reactions, a mild, transient rash was found to develop in 4.3% of the subjects, but SJS/TEN did not develop in any of the HLA-B*15:02-negative subjects receiving the same drug. This was a significant reduction from the historical incidence of 0.23% in one year [143].

Meanwhile, in Thailand, pre-emptive genetic testing is also offered at Ramathibodi Hospital in Bangkok prior to the prescription of antiepileptics and other relevant drugs (Figure 3). The population frequency of HLA allele risk, predictive value, cost of genotyping and cost of alternative drugs were postulated to be the key factors influencing cost-effectiveness. Moreover, the availability and accessibility of these alternative drugs are crucial in maintaining the relevance of this pre-emptive testing and to safeguard patients.

Clinical Pharmacogenetics Implementation Consortium (CPIC) publishes genotype-based drug guidelines to help clinicians better understand how genetic test results could be used to optimize drug therapy. CPIC is focused on well-known examples of pharmacogenomic associations that have been implemented in selected clinical settings. Each CPIC guideline adheres to a standardized format and includes a standard system for grading evidence linking genotypes to phenotypes, and assigning a level of strength to each prescription recommendation. CPIC guidelines contain the necessary information to help clinicians translate patient-specific diplotypes for each gene into clinical phenotypes or drug dosage groups [144].

Several countries have implemented the pre-emptive pharmacogenetic screening of HLA allele for SCAR prevention, including Thailand, Singapore and Taiwan, as mentioned above. These countries have shown significant reductions in the number of SJS/TEN cases reported with the use of risky drugs, not only limited to AEDs. These implementation initiatives were shown to be supported by the authorities, and were incorporated as part of pharmacovigilance programs. Indeed, proactive steps should be taken to bridge pharmacogenetic knowledge and clinical application, particularly in the scope of preventable adverse drug reactions.

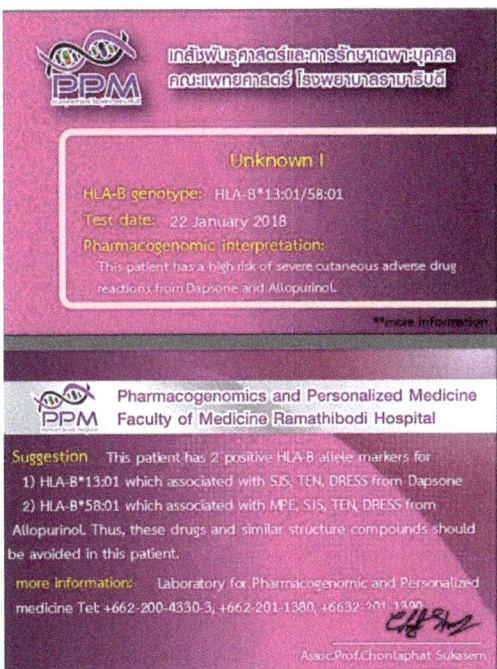

Figure 3. The pharmacogenetic card as part of pharmacogenetic implementation practice in Thailand. Patients' pharmacogenetic information is entered into the pharmacogenetic card, a purple rectangle and wallet-sized card that they carry around and show to their future healthcare providers, such as physicians and pharmacists.

11. Conclusions

Cutaneous adverse drug reaction is a significant health burden, especially SCARs, which can be life threatening. Several immunological response mechanisms have been proposed to be involved in these reactions. Based on the current evidence, genetic screening is the best way forward as a preventive strategy against SCAR risks. An improved understanding of the mechanistic pathways of drug-induced SCARs and the pharmacokinetics of the offending drugs may provide insight into other potential markers in determining the risk of SCARs. While other possibly relevant genetic markers may be associated with AED-induced SCARs (e.g., variations in CYP2C19 genes), only a few HLA gene markers are currently included in pre-emptive genetic tests prior to the initiation of these drugs. In line with efforts towards precision medicine, continuous research in discovering genetic markers and performing cost–benefit analyses of pre-emptive screening may further facilitate preventive strategies in clinical practice.

Author Contributions: A.F.A., N.A.A.D. and D.A.M.N. conceived and designed the concept of the manuscript; A.F.A. drafted the manuscript; N.A.A.D., D.A.M.N., C.S., M.A.S. and N.F.M. revised the manuscript critically for important intellectual content. All authors have read and agreed to the published version of the manuscript.

Funding: This review was supported by Short Term Grant Universiti Sains Malaysia (304.PFAR-MASI.6315398) and The International Research Network-The Thailand Research Fund (IRN60W003).

Institutional Review Board Statement: Not applicable.

Informed Consent Statement: Not applicable.

Data Availability Statement: Not applicable. This review did not report any new data.

Acknowledgments: We would like to acknowledge Faculty of Medicine Ramathibodi Hospital, Mahidol University, and the contribution of Mohammed Ahmed Imran Ak Kaif in the preparation of the manuscript.

Conflicts of Interest: The authors declare no conflict of interest.

References

1. WHO. *International Drug Monitoring: The Role of National Centres, Report of a WHO Meeting [Held in Geneva from 20 to 25 September 1971]*; World Health Organization Technical Report Series No. 498; World Health Organization: Geneva, Switzerland, 1972.
2. Lazarou, J.; Pomeranz, B.H.; Corey, P.N. Incidence of adverse drug reactions in hospitalized patients: A meta-analysis of prospective studies. *JAMA* **1998**, *279*, 1200–1205. [CrossRef]
3. Pirmohamed, M.; James, S.; Meakin, S.; Greene, C.; Scott, A.K.; Walley, T.J.; Farrar, K.; Parks, B.K.; Breckenridge, A.M. Adverse drug reactions as cause of admission to hospital: Prospective analysis of 18 820 patients. *BMJ* **2004**, *329*, 15–19. [CrossRef]
4. Mori, F.; Blanca-Lopez, N.; Caubet, J.; Demoly, P.; Du Toit, G.; Gomes, E.R.; Kuyucu, S.; Romano, A.; Soyer, O.; Tsabouri, S.; et al. Delayed hypersensitivity to antiepileptic drugs in children. *Pediatr. Allergy Immunol.* **2021**, *32*, 425–436. [CrossRef]
5. Alfares, I.; Javaid, M.S.; Chen, Z.; Anderson, A.; Antonic-Baker, A.; Kwan, P. Sex Differences in the Risk of Cutaneous Adverse Drug Reactions Induced by Antiseizure Medications: A Systematic Review and Me-ta-analysis. *CNS Drugs* **2021**, *35*, 161–176. [CrossRef] [PubMed]
6. Chia, F.L.; Leong, K.P. Severe cutaneous adverse reactions to drugs. *Curr. Opin. Allergy Clin. Immunol.* **2007**, *7*, 304–309. [CrossRef] [PubMed]
7. Roujeau, J.-C.; Kelly, J.P.; Naldi, L.; Rzany, B.; Stern, R.S.; Anderson, T.; Auquier, A.; Bastuji-Garin, S.; Correia, O.; Locati, F.; et al. Medication Use and the Risk of Stevens–Johnson Syndrome or Toxic Epidermal Necrolysis. *N. Engl. J. Med.* **1995**, *333*, 1600–1608. [CrossRef]
8. Iriki, H.; Adachi, T.; Mori, M.; Tanese, K.; Funakoshi, T.; Karigane, D.; Shimizu, T.; Okamoto, S.; Keisuke, N. Toxic epidermal necrolysis in the absence of circulating T cells: A possi-ble role for resident memory T cells. *J. Am. Acad. Dermatol.* **2014**, *71*, e214–e216. [CrossRef] [PubMed]
9. Sukasem, C.; Pratoomwun, J.; Satapornpong, P.; Klaewsongkram, J.; Rerkpattanapipat, T.; Reknimitr, P.; Lertpichiktul, P.; Puangpetch, A.; Nakkam, N.; Konyoung, P.; et al. Genetic association of co–trimoxazole–induced se-vere cutaneous adverse reactions is phenotype–specific: HLA class I genotypes and haplotypes. *Clin. Pharmacol. Ther.* **2020**, *108*, 1078–1089. [CrossRef]
10. Tong, H.; Phan, N.V.T.; Nguyen, T.T.; Nguyen, D.V.; Vo, N.S.; Le, L. Review on Databases and Bioinformatic Approaches on Pharmacogenomics of Adverse Drug Reactions. *Pharmacogenomics Pers. Med.* **2021**, *14*, 61–75. [CrossRef]
11. Manuyakorn, W.; Siripool, K.; Kamchaisatian, W.; Pakakasama, S.; Visudtibhan, A.; Vilaiyuk, S.; Rujirawat, T.; Benjaponpitak, S. Phenobarbital–induced severe cutaneous ad-verse drug reactions are associated with CYP2C19* 2 in Thai children. *Pediatr. Allergy Immunol.* **2013**, *24*, 299–303. [CrossRef] [PubMed]
12. Chan, F.L.; Dodiuk-Gad, R.P. Implementation of Genetic Screening to Prevent Severe Cutaneous Ad-verse Drug Reactions Is Crucial—Rebuttal from the Devil's Antagonist. *JAMA Dermatol.* **2020**, *156*, 220–221. [CrossRef]
13. Thong, B.Y.-H.; Tan, T.-C. Epidemiology and risk factors for drug allergy. *Br. J. Clin. Pharmacol.* **2011**, *71*, 684–700. [CrossRef] [PubMed]
14. Krivoy, N.; Taer, M.; Neuman, M.G. Antiepileptic drug-induced hypersensitivity syndrome reactions. *Curr. Drug Saf.* **2006**, *1*, 289–299. [CrossRef]
15. Mehta, M.; Shah, J.; Khakhkhar, T.; Shah, R.; Hemavathi, K.G. Anticonvulsant hypersensitivity syn-drome associated with carbamazepine administration: Case series. *J. Pharmacol. Pharmacother.* **2014**, *5*, 59.
16. Anwar, T.M.; Faris, P.M. A Systematic Review on Lamotrigine Induced Skin Rashes. *J. Drug Deliv. Ther.* **2021**, *11*, 146–151. [CrossRef]
17. Roujeau, J.-C. The Spectrum of Stevens-Johnson Syndrome and Toxic Epidermal Necrolysis: A Clinical Classification. *J. Investig. Dermatol.* **1994**, *102*, 28S–30S. [CrossRef] [PubMed]
18. Duong, T.A.; Valeyrie-Allanore, L.; Wolkenstein, P.; Chosidow, O. Severe cutaneous adverse reactions to drugs. *Lancet* **2017**, *390*, 1996–2011. [CrossRef]
19. Pavlos, R.; Mallal, S.; Phillips, E. HLA and pharmacogenetics of drug hypersensitivity. *Pharmacogenomics* **2012**, *13*, 1285–1306. [CrossRef]
20. Choudhary, S.; McLeod, M.; Torchia, D.; Romanelli, P. Drug Reaction with Eosinophilia and Systemic Symptoms (DRESS) Syndrome. *J. Clin. Aesthetic Dermatol.* **2013**, *6*, 31–37.
21. Auquier-Dunant, A.; Mockenhaupt, M.; Naldi, L.; Correia, O.; Schröder, W.; Roujeau, J.-C. Correlations Between Clinical Patterns and Causes of Erythema Multiforme Majus, Stevens-Johnson Syndrome, and Toxic Epidermal Necrolysis. *Arch. Dermatol.* **2002**, *138*, 1019–1024. [CrossRef] [PubMed]
22. Irwin, M.F.; Arthur, Z.E.; Klauss, W.K.; Frank, A.; Lowell, A.G.S.K. *Fitzpatrick's Dermatology in General Medicine*, 5th ed.; McGraw Hill: New York, NY, USA, 1999.
23. Hall, J.B.; Schmidt, G.A.; Wood, L.D.H. *Principles of Critical Care*, 4th ed.; McGraw-Hill: New York, NY, USA, 1999.
24. Fritsch, P.O.; Sidoroff, A. Drug-Induced Stevens-Johnson Syndrome/Toxic Epidermal Necrolysis. *Am. J. Clin. Dermatol.* **2000**, *1*, 349–360. [CrossRef] [PubMed]

25. Creamer, D.; Walsh, S.; Dziewulski, P.; Exton, L.; Lee, H.; Dart, J.; Setterfield, J.; Bunker, C.; Ardern-Jones, M.; Watson, K.; et al. UK guidelines for the management of Stevens–Johnson syndrome/toxic epidermal necrolysis in adults 2016. *J. Plast. Reconstr. Aesthetic Surg.* **2016**, *69*, e119–e153. [CrossRef] [PubMed]
26. French, L.E.; Trent, J.T.; Kerdel, F.A. Use of intravenous immunoglobulin in toxic epidermal necrolysis and Stevens–Johnson syndrome: Our current understanding. *Int. Immunopharmacol.* **2006**, *6*, 543–549. [CrossRef]
27. Vanfleteren, I.; Van Gysel, D.; De Brandt, C. Stevens-Johnson Syndrome: A Diagnostic Challenge in the Absence of Skin Lesions. *Pediatr. Dermatol.* **2003**, *20*, 52–56. [CrossRef] [PubMed]
28. Tomy, M.; Hui, L.I. Severe cutaneous adverse drug reactions: A review on epidemiology, etiology, clinical manifestation and pathogenesis. *Chin. Med. J.* **2008**, *121*, 756–761. [CrossRef]
29. Kardaun, S.; Sidoroff, A.; Valeyrie-Allanore, L.; Halevy, S.; Davidovici, B.; Mockenhaupt, M.; Roujeau, J. Variability in the clinical pattern of cutaneous side-effects of drugs with systemic symptoms: Does a DRESS syndrome really exist? *Br. J. Dermatol.* **2007**, *156*, 609–611. [CrossRef]
30. Han, M.K.; Agusti, A.; Calverley, P.M.; Celli, B.R.; Criner, G.; Curtis, J.L.; Fabbri, L.M.; Goldin, J.G.; Jones, P.W.; Macnee, W.; et al. Chronic obstructive pulmonary disease phenotypes: The future of COPD. *Am. J. Respir. Crit. Care Med.* **2010**, *182*, 598–604. [CrossRef]
31. Sassolas, B.; Haddad, C.; Mockenhaupt, M.; Dunant, A.; Liss, Y.; Bork, K.; Haustein, U.F.; Vieluf, D.; Roujeau, J.C.; Louet, H.L. ALDEN, an algorithm for assessment of drug causal-ity in Stevens–Johnson syndrome and toxic epidermal necrolysis: Comparison with case–control analysis. *Clin. Pharmacol. Ther.* **2010**, *88*, 60–68. [CrossRef] [PubMed]
32. Bastuji-Garin, S.; Rzany, B.; Stern, R.S.; Shear, N.H.; Naldi, L.; Roujeau, J.-C. Clinical Classification of Cases of Toxic Epidermal Necrolysis, Stevens-Johnson Syndrome, and Erythema Multiforme. *Arch. Dermatol.* **1993**, *129*, 92–96. [CrossRef]
33. Bégaud, B.; Evreux, J.C.; Jouglard, J.; Lagier, G. Imputation of the unexpected or toxic effects of drugs. Actualization of the method used in France. *Therapy* **1985**, *40*, 111–118.
34. Palmieri, T.L.; Greenhalgh, D.G.; Saffle, J.R.; Spence, R.J.; Peck, M.D.; Jeng, J.C.; Mozingo, D.W.; Yowler, C.J.; Sheridan, R.L.; Ahrenholz, D.H.; et al. A Multicenter Review of Toxic Epidermal Necrolysis Treated in U.S. Burn Centers at the End of the Twentieth Century. *J. Burn. Care Rehabil.* **2002**, *23*, 87–96. [CrossRef]
35. Alfirevic, A.P.M. Genomics of adverse drug reactions. *Trends Pharmacol. Sci.* **2017**, *38*, 100–109. [CrossRef] [PubMed]
36. Hung, C.W.W.C.S. *Genetics of Adverse Drug Reactions*; John Wiley Sons: Hoboken, NJ, USA, 2017.
37. Lin, M.; Xu, H.; Shi, Y.; Da, L.-T. Antigenic Peptide Loading into Major Histocompatibility Complex Class I Is Driven by the Substrate N-Terminus. *CCS Chem.* **2021**, *2021*, 979–994. [CrossRef]
38. Naranjo, A.C.; Busto, U.; Sellers, E.M.; Sandor, P.; Ruiz, I.; Roberts, A.E.; Janecek, E.; Domecq, C.; Greenblatt, D.J. A method for estimating the probability of adverse drug reactions. *Clin. Pharmacol. Ther.* **1981**, *30*, 239–245. [CrossRef] [PubMed]
39. Lim, K.S.; Kwan, P.; Tan, C.T. Association of HLA-B* 1502 allele and carbamazepine-induced severe adverse cutaneous drug reaction among Asians, a review. *Neurol. Asia* **2008**, *13*, 15–21.
40. Cresswell, P.; Ackerman, A.L.; Giodini, A.; Peaper, D.R.; Wearsch, P.A. Mechanisms of MHC class I-restricted antigen processing and cross-presentation. *Immunol. Rev.* **2005**, *207*, 145–157. [CrossRef] [PubMed]
41. Pirmohamed, M.; Naisbitt, D.J.; Gordon, F.; Park, B.K. The danger hypothesis—potential role in idiosyncratic drug reactions. *Toxicology* **2002**, *181*, 55–63. [CrossRef]
42. Daly, K.A. Human leukocyte antigen (HLA) pharmacogenomic tests: Potential and pitfalls. *Curr. Drug Metab.* **2014**, *15*, 196–201. [CrossRef] [PubMed]
43. Zazzara, M.B.; Palmer, K.; Vetrano, D.L.; Carfì, A.; Graziano, O. Adverse drug reactions in older adults: A narrative review of the literature. *Eur. Geriatr. Med.* **2021**. online ahead of print. [CrossRef]
44. Bharadwaj, M.; Illing, P.; Theodossis, A.; Purcell, A.W.; Rossjohn, J.; McCluskey, J. Drug Hypersensitivity and Human Leukocyte Antigens of the Major Histocompatibility Complex. *Annu. Rev. Pharmacol. Toxicol.* **2012**, *52*, 401–431. [CrossRef]
45. Edwards, I.R.; Aronson, J.K. Adverse drug reactions: Definitions, diagnosis, and management. *Lancet* **2000**, *356*, 1255–1259. [CrossRef]
46. Becquemont, L. HLA: A pharmacogenomics success story. *Pharmacogenomics* **2010**, *11*, 277–281. [CrossRef] [PubMed]
47. Karnes, J.H.; Miller, M.A.; White, K.D.; Konvinse, K.C.; Pavlos, R.K.; Redwood, A.J.; Peter, J.G.; Lehloenya, R.; Mallal, S.A.; Phillips, E.J.; et al. Applications of Immunopharmacogenomics: Predicting, Preventing, and Understanding Immune-Mediated Adverse Drug Reactions. *Annu. Rev. Pharmacol. Toxicol.* **2019**, *59*, 463–486. [CrossRef] [PubMed]
48. Robinson, J.; Barker, D.J.; Georgiou, X.; Cooper, A.M.; Flicek, P.; Marsh, E.S.G. IPD-IMGT/HLA Database. *Nucleic Acids Res.* **2019**, *48*, D948–D955. [CrossRef] [PubMed]
49. Robinson, J.; Halliwell, J.A.; Hayhurst, J.D.; Flicek, P.; Parham, P.; Marsh, S.G.E. The IPD and IMGT/HLA database: Allele variant databases. *Nucleic Acids Res.* **2015**, *43*, D423–D431. [CrossRef] [PubMed]
50. Dean, L. *Carbamazepine Therapy and HLA Genotype*; NCBI: Bethesda, MD, USA, 2018.
51. Pappas, D.J.; Lizee, A.; Paunic, V.; Beutner, K.R.; Motyer, A.; Vukcevic, D.; Leslie, S.; Biesiada, J.; Meller, J.; Taylor, K.D.; et al. Significant variation between SNP-based HLA imputations in diverse populations: The last mile is the hardest. *Pharm. J.* **2018**, *18*, 367–376. [CrossRef]
52. Di, D.; Sanchez-Mazas, A. Challenging views on the peopling history of East Asia: The story according to HLA markers. *Am. J. Phys. Anthr.* **2011**, *145*, 81–96. [CrossRef]

53. Solberg, O.D.; Mack, S.J.; Lancaster, A.K.; Single, R.M.; Tsai, Y.; Sanchez-Mazas, A.; Thomson, G. Balancing selection and heterogeneity across the classical human leukocyte antigen loci: A meta-analytic review of 497 population studies. *Hum. Immunol.* **2008**, *69*, 443–464. [CrossRef]
54. Chang, C.-C.; Too, C.-L.; Murad, S.; Hussein, S.H. Association of HLA-B*1502 allele with carbamazepine-induced toxic epidermal necrolysis and Stevens-Johnson syndrome in the multi-ethnic Malaysian population. *Int. J. Dermatol.* **2011**, *50*, 221–224. [CrossRef] [PubMed]
55. Esmaeilzadeh, H.; Farjadian, S.; Alyasin, S.; Nemati, H.; Nabavizadeh, H.; Esmaeilzadeh, E. Epidemiology of Severe Cutaneous Adverse Drug Reaction and Its HLA Association among Pediatrics. *Iran. J. Pharm. Res. IJPR* **2019**, *18*, 506–522.
56. McCormack, M.; Alfirevic, A.; Bourgeois, S.; Farrell, J.J.; Kasperavičiūtė, D.; Carrington, M.; Sills, G.J.; Marson, T.; Jia, X.; De Bakker, P.I.; et al. HLA-A*3101 and Carbamazepine-Induced Hypersensitivity Reactions in Europeans. *N. Engl. J. Med.* **2011**, *364*, 1134–1143. [CrossRef] [PubMed]
57. Ozeki, T.; Mushiroda, T.; Yowang, A.; Takahashi, A.; Kubo, M.; Shirakata, Y.; Ikezawa, Z.; Iijima, M.; Shiohara, T.; Hashimoto, K.; et al. Genome-wide association study identifies HLA-A*3101 allele as a genetic risk factor for carbamazepine-induced cutaneous adverse drug reactions in Japanese population. *Hum. Mol. Genet.* **2010**, *20*, 1034–1041. [CrossRef] [PubMed]
58. Kim, S.-H.; Lee, K.W.; Song, W.-J.; Kim, S.-H.; Jee, Y.-K.; Lee, S.-M.; Kang, H.-R.; Park, H.-W.; Cho, S.-H.; Park, S.-H.; et al. Carbamazepine-induced severe cutaneous adverse reactions and HLA genotypes in Koreans. *Epilepsy Res.* **2011**, *97*, 190–197. [CrossRef] [PubMed]
59. Genin, E.; Chen, D.-P.; Hung, S.-I.; Sekula, P.; Schumacher, A.M.; Chang, P.-Y.; Tsai, S.-H.; Wu, T.-L.; Bellón, T.; Tamouza, R.; et al. HLA-A*31:01 and different types of carbamazepine-induced severe cutaneous adverse reactions: An international study and meta-analysis. *Pharmacogenomics J.* **2014**, *14*, 281–288. [CrossRef]
60. Hung, S.-I.; Chung, W.-H.; Jee, S.-H.; Chen, W.-C.; Chang, Y.-T.; Lee, W.-R.; Hu, S.-L.; Wu, M.-T.; Chen, G.-S.; Wong, T.-W.; et al. Genetic susceptibility to carbamazepine-induced cutaneous adverse drug reactions. *Pharmacogenetics Genom.* **2006**, *16*, 297–306. [CrossRef]
61. Chung, W.-H.; Hung, S.-I.; Hong, H.-S.; Hsih, M.-S.; Yang, L.-C.; Ho, H.C.; Wu, J.Y.; Chen, Y.-T. A marker for Stevens–Johnson syndrome. *Nature* **2004**, *428*, 486. [CrossRef]
62. Tassaneeyakul, W.; Tiamkao, S.; Jantararoungtong, T.; Chen, P.; Lin, S.-Y.; Chen, W.-H.; Konyoung, P.; Khunarkornsiri, U.; Auvichayapat, N.; Pavakul, K.; et al. Association between HLA-B*1502 and carbamazepine-induced severe cutaneous adverse drug reactions in a Thai population. *Epilepsia* **2010**, *51*, 926–930. [CrossRef]
63. Nguyen, D.V.; Chu, H.C.; Nguyen, D.V.; Phan, M.H.; Craig, T.; Baumgart, K.; van Nunen, S. HLA-B* 1502 and carbamazepine-induced severe cutaneous adverse drug reactions in Vietnamese. *Asia Pac. Allergy* **2015**, *5*, 68–77. [CrossRef]
64. Yuliwulandari, R.; Shin, J.G.; Kristin, E.; Suyatna, F.D.; Prahasto, I.D.; Prayuni, K.; Mahasirimongkol, S.; Cavallari, L.H.; Mitropoulou, C.; Patrinos, G.P.; et al. Cost-effectiveness analysis of genotyping for HLA-B*15:02 in Indonesian patients with epilepsy using a generic model. *Pharm. J.* **2021**. online ahead of print. [CrossRef]
65. Hung, C.-C.; Chang, W.-L.; Ho, J.-L.; Tai, J.J.; Hsieh, T.-J.; Huang, H.-C.; Hsieh, Y.-W.; Liou, H.-H. Association of polymorphisms in EPHX1, UGT2B7, ABCB1, ABCC2, SCN1A and SCN2A genes with carbamazepine therapy optimization. *Pharmacogenomics* **2012**, *13*, 159–169. [CrossRef]
66. Kaniwa, N.; Saito, Y.; Aihara, M.; Matsunaga, K.; Tohkin, M.; Kurose, K.; Furuya, H.; Takahashi, Y.; Muramatsu, M.; Kinoshita, S.; et al. HLA-B*1511 is a risk factor for carbamazepine-induced Stevens-Johnson syndrome and toxic epidermal necrolysis in Japanese patients. *Epilepsia* **2010**, *51*, 2461–2465. [CrossRef]
67. Kaniwa, N.; Saito, Y.; Aihara, M.; Matsunaga, K.; Tohkin, M.; Kurose, K.; Sawada, J.-I.; Furuya, H.; Takahashi, Y.; Muramatsu, M.; et al. HLA-B locus in Japanese patients with anti-epileptics and allopurinol-related Stevens–Johnson syndrome and toxic epidermal necrolysis. *Pharmacogenomics* **2008**, *9*, 1617–1622. [CrossRef] [PubMed]
68. Sun, Y.; Ye, X.; Fan, Y.; Wang, L.; Luo, X.; Liu, H.; Gao, X.; Gong, Z.; Wang, Y.; Qiu, W.; et al. High Detection Rate of Copy Number Variations Using Capture Sequencing Data: A Retrospective Study. *Clin. Chem.* **2020**, *66*, 455–462. [CrossRef] [PubMed]
69. Cheung, Y.; Cheng, S.; Chan, E.J.M.; Lo, S.V.; Ng, M.H.L.; Kwan, P. HLA–B alleles associated with severe cutaneous reactions to antiepileptic drugs in Han Chinese. *Epilepsia* **2013**, *54*, 1307–1314. [CrossRef] [PubMed]
70. Locharernkul, C.; Loplumlert, J.; Limotai, C.; Korkij, W.; Desudchit, T.; Tongkobpetch, S.; Kangwanshiratada, O.; Hirankarn, N.; Suphapeetiporn, K.; Shotelersuk, V. Carbamazepine and phenytoin induced Stevens-Johnson syndrome is associated with HLA-B*1502 allele in Thai population. *Epilepsia* **2008**, *49*, 2087–2091. [CrossRef] [PubMed]
71. Chang, C.-C.; Ng, C.-C.; Too, C.-L.; Choon, S.-E.; Lee, C.-K.; Chung, W.-H.; Hussein, S.H.; Lim, K.-S.; Murad, S. Association of HLA-B*15:13 and HLA-B*15:02 with phenytoin-induced severe cutaneous adverse reactions in a Malay population. *Pharm. J.* **2016**, *17*, 170–173. [CrossRef]
72. Zeng, T.; Long, Y.-S.; Min, F.-L.; Liao, W.-P.; Shi, Y.-W. Association of HLA-B*1502 allele with lamotrigine-induced Stevens-Johnson syndrome and toxic epidermal necrolysis in Han Chinese subjects: A meta-analysis. *Int. J. Dermatol.* **2014**, *54*, 488–493. [CrossRef]
73. Tempark, T.; Satapornpong, P.; Rerknimitr, P.; Nakkam, N.; Saksit, N.; Wattankrai, P.; Jantararoungtong, T.; Koomdee, N.; Mahakkanukrauh, A.; Tassaneeyakul, W.; et al. Dapsone-induced severe cutaneous adverse drug reactions are strongly linked with HLA-B* 13: 01 allele in the Thai population. *Pharmacogenet. Genom.* **2017**, *27*, 429–437. [CrossRef]
74. Allele Frequency Net Database. Available online: http://www.allelefrequencies.net/pop6001c.asp?pop_id=1801 (accessed on 30 April 2021).

75. Hagenlocher, Y.; Willburger, B.; Behrens, G.A.; Schmidt, A.H.; Ioffe, Y.; Sauter, J. 6-Locus HLA allele and haplotype frequencies in a population of 1075 Russians from Karelia. *Hum. Immunol.* **2019**, *80*, 95–96. [CrossRef]
76. Ikeda, N.; Kojima, H.; Nishikawa, M.; Hayashi, K.; Futagami, T.; Tsujino, T.; Kusunoki, Y.; Fujii, N.; Suegami, S.; Miyazaki, Y.; et al. Determination of HLA-A, -C, -B, -DRB1 allele and haplotype frequency in Japanese population based on family study. *Tissue Antigens* **2015**, *85*, 252–259. [CrossRef]
77. Huh, J.Y.; Yi, D.Y.; Eo, S.; Cho, H.; Park, M.H.; Kang, M.S. HLA–A,–B and–DRB 1 polymorphism in K oreans defined by sequence–based typing of 4128 cord blood units. *Int. J. Immunogenet.* **2013**, *40*, 515–523. [CrossRef]
78. Qin, Q.P.; Su, F.; Yan, X.W.; Xing, Z.; Meng, P.; Chengya, W.; Jie, S. Distribution of human leucocyte antigen–A,–B and–DR alleles and haplotypes at high resolution in the population from Jiangsu province of China. *Int. J. Immunogenet.* **2011**, *38*, 475–481. [CrossRef] [PubMed]
79. Chandanayingyong, D.; Stephens, H.A.; Klaythong, R.; Sirikong, M.; Udee, S.; Longta, P.; Chantangpol, R.; Bejrachandra, S.; Rungruang, E. HLA-A, -B, -DRB1, -DQA1, and -DQB1 polymorphism in thais. *Hum. Immunol.* **1997**, *53*, 174–182. [CrossRef]
80. Pimtanothai, N.; Charoenwongse, P.; Mutirangura, A.; Hurley, C. Distribution of HLA-B alleles in nasopharyngeal carcinoma patients and normal controls in Thailand. *Tissue Antigens* **2002**, *59*, 223–225. [CrossRef]
81. Pan, Q.-Q.; Fan, S.; Wang, X.-Y.; Pan, M.; Zhao, X.; Zhou, X.-Y.; Wang, C.-Y.; Shen, J. The distribution of human leukocyte antigen-A, -B, and -DRB1 alleles and haplotypes based on high-resolution genotyping of 167 families from Jiangsu Province, China. *Hum. Immunol.* **2011**, *72*, 872–876. [CrossRef] [PubMed]
82. Hong, W.; Fu, Y.; Chen, S.; Wang, F.; Ren, X.; Xu, A. Distributions of HLA class I alleles and haplotypes in Northern Han Chinese. *Tissue Antigens* **2005**, *66*, 297–304. [CrossRef]
83. Yao, Y.; Shi, L.; Matsushita, M.; Yu, L.; Lin, K.; Tao, Y.; Huang, X.; Yi, W.; Oka, T.; Tokunaga, K.; et al. Distribution of HLA-A, -B, -Cw, and -DRB1 alleles and haplotypes in an isolated Han population in Southwest China. *Tissue Antigens* **2009**, *73*, 561–568. [CrossRef]
84. Romphruk, A.V.; Romphruk, A.; Kongmaroeng, C.; Klumkrathok, K.; Paupairoj, C.; Leelayuwat, C. HLA class I and II alleles and haplotypes in ethnic Northeast Thais. *Tissue Antigens* **2010**, *75*, 701–711. [CrossRef] [PubMed]
85. Tan, L.-K.; Mohd-Farid, B.; Salsabil, S.; Heselynn, H.; Wahinuddin, S.; Lau, I.-S.; Gun, S.-C.; Nor-Suhaila, S.; Eashwary, M.; Mohd-Shahrir, M.S.; et al. HLA-A, -B, -C, -DRB1 and -DQB1 alleles and haplotypes in 951 Southeast Asia Malays from Peninsular Malaysia. *Hum. Immunol.* **2016**, *77*, 818–819. [CrossRef]
86. Seshasubramanian, V.; Manisekar, N.K.; Sathishkannan, A.D.; Naganathan, C.; Nandakumar, Y.; Narayan, S. Malayalam speaking population from South India: Common five-locus haplotypes in Malayalam speaking population. *HLA* **2018**, *92*, 432–434. [CrossRef]
87. Hoa, B.K.; Hang, N.T.L.; Kashiwase, K.; Ohashi, J.; Lien, L.T.; Horie, T.; Shojima, J.; Hijikata, M.; Sakurada, S.; Satake, M.; et al. HLA-A, -B, -C, -DRB1 and -DQB1 alleles and haplotypes in the Kinh population in Vietnam. *Tissue Antigens* **2007**, *71*, 127–134. [CrossRef] [PubMed]
88. Yuliwulandari, R.; Sachrowardi, Q.; Nakajima, H.; Kashiwase, K.; Hirayasu, K.; Mabuchi, A.; Sofro, A.S.M.; Tokunaga, K. Association of HLA-A, -B, and -DRB1 with pulmonary tuberculosis in western Javanese Indonesia. *Hum. Immunol.* **2010**, *71*, 697–701. [CrossRef]
89. Itoh, Y.; Mizuki, N.; Shimada, T.; Azuma, F.; Itakura, M.; Kashiwase, K.; Kikkawa, E.; Kulski, J.K.; Satake, M.; Inoko, H. High-throughput DNA typing of HLA-A, -B, -C, and -DRB1 loci by a PCR–SSOP–Luminex method in the Japanese population. *Immunogenetics* **2005**, *57*, 717–729. [CrossRef]
90. Available online: http://allelefrequencies.net/pop6001c.asp?pop_id=1231 (accessed on 30 April 2021).
91. Bannai, M.; Tokunaga, K.; Imanishi, T.; Harihara, S.; Fujisawa, K.; Juji, T.; Omoto, K. HLA class II alleles in Ainu living in Hidaka district, Hokkaido, northern Japan. *Am. J. Phys. Anthr.* **1996**, *101*, 1–9. [CrossRef]
92. Cruccu, G.; Gronseth, G.; Alksne, J.; Argoff, C.; Brainin, M.; Burchiel, K.; Nurmikko, T.; Zakrewska, J.M.; American Academy of Neurology Society; European Federation of Neurological Society. AAN-EFNS guidelines on trigeminal neuralgia management. *Eur. J. Neurol.* **2008**, *15*, 1013–1028. [CrossRef]
93. Marson, A.G.; Al-Kharusi, A.M.; Alwaidh, M.; Appleton, R.; Baker, A.G.; Chadwick, D.W.; Cramp, C.; Cockerell, O.C.; Cooper, P.N.; Doughty, J.; et al. The SANAD study of effectiveness of carbamazepine, gabapentin, lamotrigine, oxcarbazepine, or topiramate for treatment of partial epilepsy: An unblinded randomised controlled trial. *Lancet* **2007**, *369*, 1000–1015. [CrossRef]
94. Fan, W.-L.; Shiao, M.-S.; Hui, R.C.-Y.; Su, S.-C.; Wang, C.-W.; Chang, Y.-C.; Chung-Yee, H.R. HLA Association with Drug-Induced Adverse Reactions. *J. Immunol. Res.* **2017**, *2017*, 3186328. [CrossRef] [PubMed]
95. Khosama, H.; Budikayanti, A.; Khor, A.H.P.; Lim, K.S.; Ng, C.-C.; Mansyur, I.G.; Harahap, A.; Ranakusuma, T.A.R.; Tan, C.T. HLA-B* 1502 and carbamazepine induced Stevens-Johnson syndrome/toxic epidermal necrolysis in Indonesia. *Neurol. Asia* **2017**, *22*, 113–116.
96. Yip, V.L.; Marson, A.G.; Jorgensen, A.L.; Pirmohamed, M.; Alfirevic, A. HLA Genotype and Carbamazepine-Induced Cutaneous Adverse Drug Reactions: A Systematic Review. *Clin. Pharmacol. Ther.* **2012**, *92*, 757–765. [CrossRef] [PubMed]
97. Van Nguyen, D.; Vidal, C.; Chu, H.C.; van Nunen, S. Developing pharmacogenetic screening methods for an emergent country: Vietnam. *World Allergy Organ. J.* **2019**, *12*, 100037. [CrossRef]
98. Jaruthamsophon, K.; Tipmanee, V.; Sangiemchoey, A.; Sukasem, C.; Limprasert, P. HLA-B*15:21 and carbamazepine-induced Stevens-Johnson syndrome: Pooled-data and in silico analysis. *Sci. Rep.* **2017**, *7*, 45553. [CrossRef] [PubMed]

99. Mehta, T.Y.; Prajapati, L.M.; Mittal, B.; Joshi, C.G.; Sheth, J.J.; Patel, D.B.; Dave, D.M.; Goyal, R.K. Association of HLA-B* 1502 allele and carbamazepine-induced Stevens-Johnson syndrome among Indians. *Indian J. Dermatol. Venereol. Leprol.* **2009**, *75*, 579. [CrossRef] [PubMed]
100. Man, C.B.; Kwan, P.; Baum, L.; Yu, E.; Lau, K.; Cheng, A.S.; Ng, M.H. Association between HLA-B*1502 Allele and Antiepileptic Drug-Induced Cutaneous Reactions in Han Chinese. *Epilepsia* **2007**, *48*, 1015–1018. [CrossRef] [PubMed]
101. Kano, Y.; Hirahara, K.; Asano, Y.; Shiohara, T. HLA-B allele associations with certain drugs are not confirmed in Japanese patients with severe cutaneous drug reactions. *Acta Derm. Venereol.* **2008**, *88*, 616–618. [PubMed]
102. Sukasem, C.; Chaichan, C.; Nakkrut, T.; Satapornpong, P.; Jaruthasopom, K.; Janatraroungtong, T.; Koomdee, N.; Sriritttha, S.; Medhasi, S.; Oo-Puthinan, S.; et al. Association between HLA-B alleles and carbamazepine-induced macu-lopapular exanthema and severe cutaneous reactions in Thai patients. *J. Immunol. Res.* **2018**, *2018*, 2780272. [CrossRef]
103. Tangamornsuksan, W.; Chaiyakunapruk, N.; Somkrua, R.; Lohitnavy, M.; Tassaneeyakul, W. Relationship between the HLA-B* 1502 allele and carbamazepine-induced Stevens-Johnson syndrome and toxic epidermal necrolysis: A systematic re-view and meta-analysis. *JAMA Dermatol.* **2013**, *149*, 1025–1032. [CrossRef]
104. Ferrell, P.B.; McLeod, H.L. Carbamazepine, HLA-B* 1502 and risk of Stevens–Johnson syndrome and toxic epidermal necrolysis: US FDA recommendations. *Pharmacogenomics* **2008**, *9*, 1543–1546. [CrossRef] [PubMed]
105. Wang, Q.; Zhou, J.-Q.; Zhou, L.-M.; Chen, Z.-Y.; Fang, Z.-Y.; Chen, S.-D.; Yang, L.-B.; Cai, X.-D.; Dai, Q.-L.; Hong, H.; et al. Association between HLA-B*1502 allele and carbamazepine-induced severe cutaneous adverse reactions in Han people of southern China mainland. *Seizure* **2011**, *20*, 446–448. [CrossRef]
106. Yip, V.L.M.; Alfirevic, A.; Pirmohamed, M. Genetics of Immune-Mediated Adverse Drug Reactions: A Comprehensive and Clinical Review. *Clin. Rev. Allergy Immunol.* **2015**, *48*, 165–175. [CrossRef]
107. Locharernkul, C.; Shotelersuk, V.; Hirankarn, N. HLA-B* 1502 screening: Time to clinical practice. *Epilepsia* **2010**, *51*, 936–938. [CrossRef]
108. Tassaneeyakul, W.; Prabmeechai, N.; Sukasem, C.; Kongpan, T.; Konyoung, P.; Chumworathayi, P.; Tiamkao, S.; Khunarkornsiri, U.; Kulkantrakorn, K.; Saksit, N.; et al. Associations between HLA class I and cytochrome P450 2C9 genetic polymorphisms and phenytoin-related severe cutaneous adverse reactions in a Thai population. *Pharm. Genom.* **2016**, *26*, 225–234. [CrossRef] [PubMed]
109. McCormack, M.; Urban, T.J.; Shianna, K.V.; Walley, N.; Pandolfo, M.; Depondt, C.; Chaila, E.; O'Conner, G.; Kasperaviciute, D.; Radtke, R.A.; et al. Genome-wide mapping for clinically relevant predictors of lamotrigine-and phenytoin-induced hypersensitivity reactions. *Pharmacogenomics* **2012**, *13*, 399–405. [CrossRef] [PubMed]
110. Koomdee, N.; Pratoomwun, J.; Jantararoungtong, T.; Teeramoke, V.; Tassaneeyakul, W.; Klaewsongkram, J.; Rerkpattanpipat, T.; Santon, S.; Puangpetch, A.; Intusome, U.; et al. Association of HLA-A and HLA-B alleles with lamotrigi-ne-induced cutaneous adverse drug reactions in the Thai population. *Front. Pharmacol.* **2017**, *8*, 879. [CrossRef]
111. Gerogianni, K.; Tsezou, A.; Dimas, K. Drug-induced skin adverse reactions: The role of pharmacogenomics in their pre-vention. *Mol. Diagn. Ther.* **2018**, *22*, 297–314. [CrossRef]
112. Lonjou, C.; Borot, N.; Sekula, P.; Ledger, N.; Thomas, L.; Halevy, S.; Naldi, L.; Bouwes-Bavinck, J.-N.; Sidoroff, A.; de Toma, C.; et al. A European study of HLA-B in Stevens–Johnson syndrome and toxic epidermal necrolysis related to five high-risk drugs. *Pharmacogenetics Genom.* **2008**, *18*, 99–107. [CrossRef] [PubMed]
113. Kazeem, G.R.; Cox, C.; Aponte, J.; Messenheimer, J.; Brazell, C.; Nelsen, A.C.; Nelson, M.R.; Foot, E. High-resolution HLA genotyping and severe cutaneous adverse reactions in lamotrigine-treated patients. *Pharm. Genom.* **2009**, *19*, 661–665. [CrossRef]
114. Park, H.J.; Kim, S.R.; Leem, D.W.; Moon, I.J.; Koh, S.B.; Park, K.H.; Park, J.-W.; Lee, J.-H. Clinical features of and genetic predisposition to drug-induced Stevens–Johnson syndrome and toxic epidermal necrolysis in a single Korean tertiary institution patients—investigating the relation between the HLA-B* 4403 allele and lamotrigine. *Eur. J. Clin. Pharmacol.* **2015**, *71*, 35–41. [CrossRef] [PubMed]
115. Knowles, S.R.; Dewhurst, N.; Shear, N.H. Anticonvulsant hypersensitivity syndrome: An update. *Expert Opin. Drug Saf.* **2012**, *11*, 767–778. [CrossRef]
116. Yang, C.-Y.; Dao, R.-L.; Lee, T.-J.; Lu, C.-W.; Hung, S.-I.; Chung, W.-H. Severe cutaneous adverse reactions to antiepileptic drugs in Asians. *Neurology* **2011**, *77*, 2025–2033. [CrossRef]
117. Kaniwa, N.; Sugiyama, E.; Saito, Y.; Kurose, K.; Maekawa, K.; Hasegawa, R.; Furuya, H.; Ikeda, H.; Takahashi, Y.; Muramatsu, M.; et al. Specific HLA types are associated with antiepileptic drug-induced Stevens-Johnson syndrome and toxic epidermal necrolysis in Japanese subjects. *Pharmacogenomics* **2013**, *14*, 1821–1831. [CrossRef]
118. Wang, J.; Zhang, J.; Wu, X.; Yu, P.; Hong, Z. HLA-B*1502 allele is associated with a cross-reactivity pattern of cutaneous adverse reactions to antiepileptic drugs. *J. Int. Med. Res.* **2012**, *40*, 377–382. [CrossRef] [PubMed]
119. Akkaif, M.A.; Sha'aban, A.; Daud, N.A.A.; Ng, M.L.; Ibrahim, B. Investigate the Strategy of Using Pharmacogenetics and Pharmacometabonomics to the Personalization of Ticagrelor Antiplatelet Therapy. *Syst. Rev. Pharm.* **2020**, *11*, 1100–1107.
120. Nebert, D.W.; Russell, D.W. Clinical importance of the cytochromes P450. *Lancet* **2002**, *360*, 1155–1162. [CrossRef]
121. Akkaif, M.A.; Daud, N.A.A.; Sha'aban, A.; Ng, M.L.; Kader, M.A.S.A.; Noor, D.A.M.; Ibrahim, B. The Role of Genetic Polymorphism and Other Factors on Clopidogrel Re-sistance (CR) in an Asian Population with Coronary Heart Disease (CHD). *Molecules* **2021**, *26*, 1987. [CrossRef]

122. Gaedigk, A.; Ingelman–Sundberg, M.; Miller, N.A.; Leeder, J.S.; Whirl-Carillo, M.; Klein, T.E.; PharmVar Steering Committee. The Pharmacogene Variation (PharmVar) Consortium: Incorporation of the human cytochrome P450 (CYP) allele nomenclature database. *Clin. Pharmacol. Ther.* **2018**, *103*, 399–401. [CrossRef]
123. Aithal, G.P.; Day, C.P.; Kesteven, P.J.; Daly, A.K. Association of polymorphisms in the cytochrome P450 CYP2C9 with warfarin dose requirement and risk of bleeding complications. *Lancet* **1999**, *353*, 717–719. [CrossRef]
124. Miners, J.O.; Birkett, D.J. Cytochrome P4502C9: An enzyme of major importance in human drug metabolism. *Br. J. Clin. Pharmacol.* **1998**, *45*, 525–538. [CrossRef]
125. Odani, A.; Hashimoto, Y.; Otsuki, Y.; Uwai, Y.; Hattori, H.; Furusho, K.; Inui, K. Genetic polymorphism of the CYP2C subfamily and its effect on the pharma-cokinetics of phenytoin in Japanese patients with epilepsy. *Clin. Pharmacol. Ther.* **1997**, *62*, 287–292. [CrossRef]
126. Aynacioglu, A.S.; Brockmöller, J.; Bauer, S.; Sachse, C.; Güzelbey, P.; Öngen, Z.; Nacak, M.; Roots, I. Frequency of cytochrome P450 CYP2C9 variants in a Turkish population and functional relevance for phenytoin. *Br. J. Clin. Pharmacol.* **1999**, *48*, 409–415. [CrossRef]
127. van der Weide, J.; Steijns, L.S.W.; van Weelden, M.J.M.; de Haan, K. The effect of genetic polymorphism of cytochrome P450 CYP2C9 on phenytoin dose requirement. *Pharmacogenet. Genom.* **2001**, *11*, 287–291. [CrossRef]
128. Saruwatari, J.; Ishitsu, T.; Nakagawa, K. Update on the genetic polymorphisms of drug-metabolizing enzymes in an-tiepileptic drug therapy. *Pharmaceuticals* **2010**, *3*, 2709–2732. [CrossRef] [PubMed]
129. Morton Grove IMGPI. PHENYTOIN Suspension. Available online: https://dailymed.nlm.nih.gov/dailymed/drugInfo.cfm?setid=efd93f07-818b-41ae-abd6-49ec5175311a (accessed on 30 April 2021).
130. Yang, Z.; Cui, H.; Hasi, T.; Jia, S.; Gong, M.; Su, X. Genetic polymorphisms of cytochrome P450 enzymes 2C9 and 2C19 in a healthy Mongolian population in China. *Genet. Mol. Res.* **2010**, *9*, 1844–1851. [CrossRef]
131. Park, P.-W.; Seo, Y.H.; Ahn, J.Y.; Kim, K.-A.; Park, J.-Y. Effect ofCYP3A5*3genotype on serum carbamazepine concentrations at steady-state in Korean epileptic patients. *J. Clin. Pharm. Ther.* **2009**, *34*, 569–574. [CrossRef] [PubMed]
132. Lee, J.S.; Cheong, H.S.; Kim, L.H.; Kim, J.O.; Seo, D.W.; Kim, Y.H.; Chung, M.W.; Han, S.Y.; Shin, H.D. Screening of Genetic Polymorphisms of CYP3A4 and CYP3A5 Genes. *Korean J. Physiol. Pharmacol.* **2013**, *17*, 479–484. [CrossRef]
133. Seo, T.; Nakada, N.; Ueda, N.; Hagiwara, T.; Hashimoto, N.; Nakagawa, K.; Ishitsu, T. Effect of CYP3A5*3 on carbamazepine pharmacokinetics in Japanese patients with epilepsy. *Clin. Pharmacol. Ther.* **2006**, *79*, 509–510. [CrossRef] [PubMed]
134. Chung, W.-H.; Chang, W.-C.; Lee, Y.-S.; Wu, Y.-Y.; Yang, C.-H.; Ho, H.-C.; Chen, M.-J.; Lin, J.-Y.; Hui, R.C.-Y.; Ho, J.-C.; et al. Genetic Variants Associated With Phenytoin-Related Severe Cutaneous Adverse Reactions. *JAMA* **2014**, *312*, 525–534. [CrossRef]
135. Samidorai, A.; Charles, N.S.C.; Babu, S.P.K.K.; Ramesh, V. Cytochrome P450 CYP2C9 gene polymorphism in phenytoin induced gingival enlargement: A case report. *J. Pharm. Bioallied Sci.* **2013**, *5*, 237–239. [CrossRef]
136. Silvado, C.E.; Terra, V.C.; Twardowschy, C.A. CYP2C9 polymorphisms in epilepsy: Influence on phenytoin treatment. *Pharmacogenomics Pers. Med.* **2018**, *11*, 51–58. [CrossRef] [PubMed]
137. Phabphal, K.; Geater, A.; Limapichart, K.; Sathirapanya, P.; Setthawatcharawanich, S. Role of CYP2C9 polymorphism in phenytoin-related metabolic abnormalities and subclinical atherosclerosis in young adult epileptic patients. *Seizure* **2013**, *22*, 103–108. [CrossRef]
138. Seng, K.C.; Gin, G.G.; Sangkar, J.V.; Phipps, M.E. Frequency of cytochrome P450 2C9 (CYP2C9) alleles in three ethnic groups in Malaysia. *Asia Pac. J. Mol. Biol. Biotechnol.* **2003**, *11*, 83–91.
139. Saruwatari, J.; Ishitsu, T.; Seo, T.; Shimomasuda, M.; Okada, Y.; Goto, S.; Nagata, R.; Takashima, A.; Yoshida, S.; Yoshida, S.; et al. The clinical impact of cytochrome P450 polymorphisms on anti-epileptic drug therapy. *Epilepsy Seizure* **2010**, *3*, 34–50. [CrossRef]
140. Goto, S.; Seo, T.; Murata, T.; Nakada, N.; Ueda, N.; Ishitsu, T.; Nakagawa, K. Population Estimation of the Effects of Cytochrome P450 2C9 and 2C19 Polymorphisms on Phenobarbital Clearance in Japanese. *Ther. Drug Monit.* **2007**, *29*, 118–121. [CrossRef] [PubMed]
141. Toh, D.S.L.; Tan, L.L.; Aw, D.C.W.; Pang, S.M.; Lim, S.H.; Thirumoorthy, T.; Lee, H.Y.; Tay, Y.K.; Tan, S.K.; Vasudevan, A.; et al. Building pharmacogenetics into a pharmacovigilance program in Singapore: Using serious skin rash as a pilot study. *Pharm. J.* **2014**, *14*, 316–321. [CrossRef]
142. White, K.D.; Abe, R.; Ardern-Jones, M.; Beachkofsky, T.; Bouchard, C.; Carleton, B.; Chodosh, J.; Cibotti, R.; Davis, R.; Denny, J.C.; et al. SJS/TEN 2017: Building Multidisciplinary Networks to Drive Science and Translation. *J. Allergy Clin. Immunol. Pr.* **2018**, *6*, 38–69. [CrossRef] [PubMed]
143. Chen, P.; Lin, J.-J.; Lu, C.-S.; Ong, C.-T.; Hsieh, P.F.; Yang, C.-C.; Tai, C.-T.; Wu, S.-L.; Lu, C.-H.; Hsu, Y.-C.; et al. Carbamazepine-Induced Toxic Effects and HLA-B*1502 Screening in Taiwan. *New Engl. J. Med.* **2011**, *364*, 1126–1133. [CrossRef] [PubMed]
144. Fan, M.; Bousman, C.A. Commercial Pharmacogenetic Tests in Psychiatry: Do they Facilitate the Implementation of Pharmacogenetic Dosing Guidelines? *Pharmacopsychiatry* **2020**, *53*, 174–178. [CrossRef]

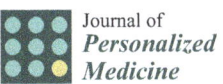

Journal of Personalized Medicine

Article

Association of *HLA-B*51:01*, *HLA-B*55:01*, *CYP2C9*3*, and Phenytoin-Induced Cutaneous Adverse Drug Reactions in the South Indian Tamil Population

Shobana John [1], Karuppiah Balakrishnan [2], Chonlaphat Sukasem [3,4], Tharmarajan Chinnathambi Vijay Anand [5], Bhutorn Canyuk [6] and Sutthiporn Pattharachayakul [1,*]

1. Department of Clinical Pharmacy, Faculty of Pharmaceutical Sciences, Prince of Songkla University, Songkhla, Hat Yai 90110, Thailand; john.shobana@gmail.com
2. Department of Immunology, School of Biological Sciences, Madurai Kamaraj University, Madurai 625021, Tamil Nadu, India; immunobala@mkuniversity.org
3. Division of Pharmacogenomics and Personalized Medicine, Department of Pathology, Faculty of Medicine, Ramathibodi Hospital, Mahidol University, Bangkok 10400, Thailand; chonlaphat.suk@mahidol.ac.th
4. Laboratory for Pharmacogenomics, SomdechPhraDebaratana Medical Center (SDMC), Ramathibodi Hospital, Bangkok 10400, Thailand
5. Department of Neurology, Meenakshi Mission Hospital and Research Center, Madurai 625107, Tamil Nadu, India; tcvijayanand@gmail.com
6. Department of Pharmaceutical Chemistry, Faculty of Pharmaceutical Sciences, Prince of Songkla University, Songkhla, Hat Yai 90110, Thailand; cbhutorn@pharmacy.psu.ac.th
* Correspondence: sutthiporn@pharmacy.psu.ac.th; Tel.: +66-(0)74288816-7 or +66-(0)74288821; Fax: +66-(0)-7421-8503

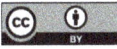

Citation: John, S.; Balakrishnan, K.; Sukasem, C.; Anand, T.C.V.; Canyuk, B.; Pattharachayakul, S. Association of *HLA-B*51:01*, *HLA-B*55:01*, *CYP2C9*3*, and Phenytoin-Induced Cutaneous Adverse Drug Reactions in the South Indian Tamil Population. *J. Pers. Med.* **2021**, *11*, 737. https://doi.org/10.3390/jpm11080737

Academic Editor: Luis A. López-Fernández

Received: 1 July 2021
Accepted: 26 July 2021
Published: 28 July 2021

Publisher's Note: MDPI stays neutral with regard to jurisdictional claims in published maps and institutional affiliations.

Copyright: © 2021 by the authors. Licensee MDPI, Basel, Switzerland. This article is an open access article distributed under the terms and conditions of the Creative Commons Attribution (CC BY) license (https://creativecommons.org/licenses/by/4.0/).

Abstract: Phenytoin (PHT) is one of the most commonly reported aromatic anti-epileptic drugs (AEDs) to cause cutaneous adverse reactions (CADRs), particularly severe cutaneous adverse reactions (SCARs). Although human leukocyte antigen *(HLA)-B*15:02* is associated with PHT-induced Steven Johnson syndrome/toxic epidermal necrosis (SJS/TEN) in East Asians, the association is much weaker than it is reported for carbamazepine (CBZ). In this study, we investigated the association of pharmacogenetic variants of the HLA B gene and *CYP2C9*3* with PHT-CADRs in South Indian epileptic patients. This prospective case-controlled study included 25 PHT-induced CADRs, 30 phenytoin-tolerant patients, and 463 (HLA-B) and 82 (*CYP2C9*3*) normal-controls from previous studies included for the case and normal-control comparison. Six SCARs cases and 19 mild-moderate reactions were observed among the 25 cases. Pooled data analysis was performed for the *HLA B*51:01* and PHT-CADRs associations. The Fisher exact test and multivariate binary logistic regression analysis were used to identify the susceptible alleles associated with PHT-CADRs. Multivariate analysis showed that *CYP2C9*3* was significantly associated with overall PHT-CADRs (OR = 12.00, 95% CI 2.759–84.87, p = 003). In subgroup analysis, *CYP2C9*3* and *HLA B*55:01* were found to be associated with PHT-SCARs (OR = 12.45, 95% CI 1.138–136.2, p = 0.003) and PHT-maculopapular exanthema (MPE) (OR = 4.041, 95% CI 1.125–15.67, p = 0.035), respectively. Pooled data analysis has confirmed the association between *HLA B*51:01*/PHT-SCARs (OR = 6.273, 95% CI 2.24–16.69, p = <0.001) and *HLA B*51:01*/PHT-overall CADRs (OR = 2.323, 95% CI 1.22–5.899, p = 0.037). In this study, neither the case nor the control groups had any patients with *HLA B*15:02*. The risk variables for PHT-SCARs, PHT-overall CADRs, and PHT-MPE were found to be *HLA B*51:01*, *CYP2C9*3*, and *HLA B*55:01*, respectively. These alleles were identified as the risk factors for the first time in the South Indian Tamil population for PHT-CADRs. Further investigation is warranted to establish the clinical relevance of these alleles in this population with larger sample size.

Keywords: HLA B; *CYP2C9*3*; cutaneous adverse drug reactions (CADRs); anti-epileptic drugs (AEDS); phenytoin (PHT); genetic risk factors; South India; India

1. Introduction

Phenytoin (PHT) is still the most effective treatment for generalized tonic-clonic seizures (GTCS) despite newer anti-epileptic drugs' (AED) availability [1,2]. However, cutaneous adverse drug reactions (CADRs) may limit its use; the estimated relative risk of PHT-severe cutaneous adverse reactions (SCARs) was reported to be 13% [3]. The prevalence of CADRs ranges from 2–5% in India [4]. Further, PHT and carbamazepine (CBZ) are the worst offenders of CADRs, with incidence rates of 13 and 18%, respectively [5]. The contributing factors to CADRs can be both genetic and non-genetic. In 2004, the association between *HLA B*15:02* and CBZ-Steven Johnson syndrome/toxic epidermal necrosis (SJS/TEN) was reported among the Han Chinese populations [6]. Later this association has been confirmed with PHT-SJS/TEN in the Thai and Chinese Asian population [7,8]. As a result, the FDA issued a warning for *HLA B*15:02*/PHT-SJS/TEN cross-reactivity. However, the strength of this association is weaker than CBZ-SJS/TEN and not demonstrated well enough in many populations [9,10].

Polymorphisms in genes that encode drug-metabolizing enzymes, in addition to HLA-B alleles, play a key role in the initiation of CADRs by slowing drug metabolism. PHT is metabolized primarily by CYP 450 in phase I reactions and mostly by UDP-glucuronosyl transferase (UGT) in phase II reactions. The enzymes *CYP2C9* and *CYP2C19* are responsible for 90% and 10% of the metabolism of PHT, respectively [11]. In CYP2C9, 2* and 3* variants are responsible for reduced PHT clearance [12,13].

Due to distinct waves of immigration, dissimilar genetic patterns in the Indian population have been extensively documented: North Indians are genetically closer to Caucasians, whilst Central Indians are closer to Asians than the European group [14,15]. The South Indians, or Dravidians, who are distributed on the southern side of India (peninsular India), are the original inhabitants of the Indian sub-continent; thus, the distribution of polymorphic alleles is not homogenous [16,17]. For example, the frequency of *HLA B*15:02* is lower (0%) among West Coast Parsi and higher (6%) among Pawra in the Khandesh region [18,19]. Similarly, the frequency of *CYP2C9*3* varies by location in India: a higher frequency (7–9%) is seen in the Dravidian population, whereas the prevalence is relatively low (0–2%) in the North Indian population [20].

A few studies in India have reported the association of HLA alleles and AEDs induced CADRs [21–24], and one study from South India reported a high serum PHT concentration in healthy volunteers carrying *CYP2C9*3* [19]. There has been little research into the genetic risk factors for PHT-CADRs in the South Indian Tamils, who inhabit primarily in Tamil Nadu, India, and also scantily in Malaysia, Sri Lanka, Singapore, and Mauritius. We aimed to look at the relationship between HLA-B alleles, *CYP2C9*3*, and PHT-CADRs in the South Indian Tamil population for the first time in this study.

2. Methodology

2.1. Study Design and Settings

This study was conducted as a prospective case-controlled study over a period of 13-months in the Neurology-Outpatient Department (OPD), Neurology ward, and Neurology-Intensive Care Unit (ICU) of Meenakshi Mission Hospital and Research Center (MMHRC) in Madurai, Tamil Nadu, India. This study was approved by the Institutional Ethics Committee Board of MMHRC (MMHRC/IEC/07/2018). DNA analysis of both cases and tolerant controls was performed at the Immunology Department, School of Biological Sciences, Madurai Kamaraj University, Madurai, Tamil Nadu, India (Figure 1).

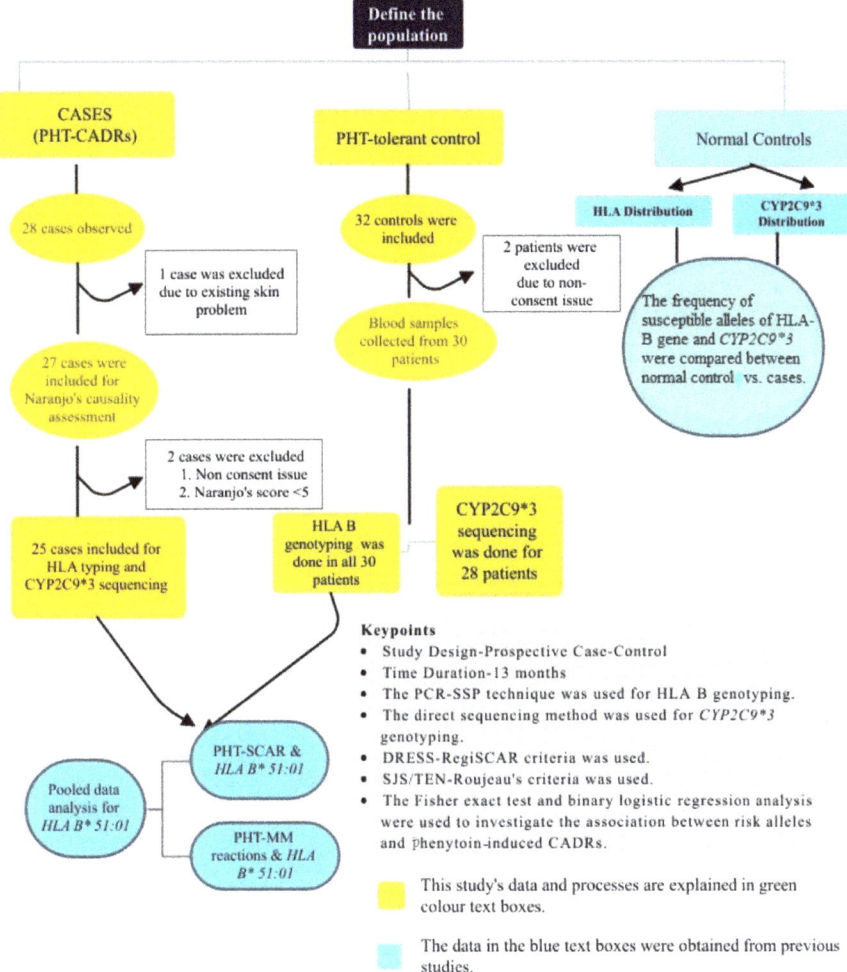

Figure 1. Flowchart of study design.

2.2. Participants

Patients who had reported CADRs within 12 weeks of using PHT were included in the study. Patients on PHT for more than 3 months and had no signs or symptoms of CADRs were considered tolerant controls. The patients who signed the consent form and agreed to give 3 mL of whole blood were included. Patients experiencing other PHT-ADRs and with established skin problems, such as psoriasis and contact dermatitis, were eliminated. Normal-control data was retrieved only from South Indian populations, but no such restrictions were kept for pooled data analysis.

The dermatologist at MMHRC diagnosed all of the PHT-CADRs as well as additional diagnostic criteria, such as the temporal relationship with phenytoin, clinical morphology of the skin, and mucosal and systemic involvement. SJS/TEN, acute generalized exanthematous pustulosis (AGEP), exfoliative dermatitis (ED), drug rash with eosinophilia and systemic symptoms (DRESS) reactions were considered as SCARs. The remaining reactions with no/less mucosal involvement were considered to be mild-moderate reactions in this study [25]. Maculopapular exanthema was defined as a rash characterized by fine pink macules/papules/lesions on the skin with no mucosal or systemic involvement (MPE) [26]. Acneiform drug eruption was defined as a monomorphic eruption without comedones (AFDE) [27].

Fixed drug eruption (FDE) was defined as a single round and oral, sharply demarcated, red-lined lesion with a diameter of 1–10 cm [28]. PHT-lichenoid drug eruption was defined as skin lesions characterized by scaling and hypertrophic pigmentation, generally in combination with oral eruption (LDE) [29]. Patients with rapidly developing dark purpuric macules, atypical target lesions, blisters accompanied by mucosal and skin detachment were diagnosed with SJS, according to Roujeau's criteria [30]. The RegiSCAR criteria were used to diagnose DRESS and DHS, which included an acute skin rash with at least one internal organ lymphadenopathy; hematologic abnormalities, such as eosinophilia and atypical lymphocytosis; and fever [25]. Patients with erythematic inflammatory skin disease, scaling on the cutaneous surface of the skin, thickened skin, itching, swollen lymph nodes, fever, and fluid loss were considered as PHT-ED [31].

Once the patient was identified as a case or control, the consent form was handed to them along with a patient information document created in the local language of Tamil. The normal-control data for the HLA-B association study was obtained from Leenam Dedhia et al. (2015), who investigated HLA diversity and its significance in South Indians [32]. The normal control data for *CYP2C9*3* and PHT-CADRs association testing is from the published literature (Nahar R et al. 2013) [33].

2.3. Causality Assessment

The causality of PHT-CADRs was assessed using Naranjo's scale, with patients scoring 9 (definite) and 5–8 (probable) included in this study [34]. Patients reported with DRESS were included if the RegiSCAR score was definite >5 and probable (4–5) [35]. The ALDEN score was used to assess the drug's causality with SJS: patients scoring very probable >6 or probable 4–5 were included [36].

2.4. Genotyping

2.4.1. DNA Extraction/HLA-B Genotyping

DNA was extracted from 3mL of peripheral blood using the salting-out method [37,38]. A UV spectrophotometer was used to measure the concentration and purity of DNA by measuring its optical density (OD) at 260 nm. The polymerase chain reactions-sequence-specific primer technique was used to genotype HLA-B. (PCR-SSP) (Applied Biosystems Verti-Thermal cycler, Thermo Fisher Scientific, Waltham, MA, USA) [39].

2.4.2. CYP2C9*3 Sequencing

The reference DNA sequence of the target variant *CYP2C9*3* was retrieved (rs1057910), and the genomic DNA was amplified using the selected forward primer from chromosome passion at 94981018 to 94981037 bp (GTGCATCTGTAACCATCCTC) and the reverse complementary primer from chromosome passion at 94981455 to 94981476 bp (GAGTTATGCACTTCTCTCACCC). The PCR DNA was purified according to the manufacturer's protocol by MinElute PCR Purification Kit (Cat. No. 28006, Qiagen, Valencia, CA, USA) and sequenced using a 3500 automatic DNA segmentation analyser (3730 DNA analyzer, Applied Biosystems, Thermo Fisher Scientific, Waltham, MA, USA). Sequence scanner software was used to obtain sequential sequencing.

2.5. Statistical Analysis

To compare the demographics and clinical features of the case and control groups, a Student's t-test was performed. The Fisher exact or Pearson chi-square tests were used if the demographics are categorical variables. The OR was calculated to see if there was an association between specific pharmacogenetic risk factors and PHT-CADRs. The Fisher exact test was used to get the p-value. Woolf's logit method was used for any cells in a contingency table that had zero. The bivariate analysis was carried out on alleles with a prevalence of more than 5% in the case group. To examine the association of various risk alleles with PHT-induced CADRs, PGx variants that exhibit significant association in bivariate analysis were included in a multivariate binary logistic regression analysis.

We used pooled data analysis for the *HLA B*51:01* to boost the study's power. The *HLA B*51:01* case and tolerant control data were obtained from one of the North Indian studies that reported the relationship between HLA alleles and AED-induced CADRs [20].

All the statistical analysis was performed using GraphPad Prism 8. After Bonferroni correction, a *p*-value 0.008 (<0.05/6—two-tailed) was considered significant.

3. Results

3.1. Patient Demographics

This study included 30 PHT-tolerant and 25 PHT-induced CADRs epileptic cases in this study. Six (23.07%) of the 25 cases were SCARs, including two cases of SJS, three cases of DRESS, and one case of ED. The remaining 19 cases (76.92%) were mild-moderate reactions, comprised of 15 MPE, 2 AFDE, 1 LDE, and 1 FDE. The case group included 14 males and 11 females with a mean age of 40.60 ± 18.15 years, while the PHT-tolerant group included 18 males and 12 females with a mean age of 36.21 ± 14.71 years. Epilepsy, seizure, cerebrovascular accidents, and CNS infections were the common indications for PHT in both the case and tolerant groups (Table 1) (Supplementary Table S1).

Table 1. Patient demographics and clinical manifestations of PHT-CADRs and PHT-tolerant group.

Parameters		PHT-Induced CADRsN (%)		Total (25)	Tolerant (30)	*p* Value
		Severe (6)	MPE and other Mild-Moderate Reactions [c] (19)			
Age	<20	02 (33.33)	1 (5.26)	3 (12)	5 (16.66)	0.71
	21–40	01 (16.66)	8 (42.10)	9 (36)	11 (36.66)	0.80
	41–60	2 (33.33)	6 (31.57)	8 (32)	12 (40)	0.26
	>60	2 (33.33)	3 (15.78)	5 (20)	02 (6.66)	0.12
Mean age ± SD		44.5 ± 21.77	39.75 ± 1.414	42.15 ± 3.35	36.21 ± 14.71	0.36 [a]
No of comorbidities (Mean)		2 ± 0.00	1 ± 1.05	1.54 ± 0.82	037 ± 0.75	0.01
Gender	Male	04 (66.66)	10 (52.63)	14 (56)	18 (60)	0.59 [b]
	Female	02 (33.33)	09	11 (44)	12 (40)	
Onset latency (days)		9–26	7–42	7–42	-	-
Indications	Seizure	3 (50)	9 (47.36)	12 (48)	11 (36.66)	-
	Epilepsy	2 (33.33)	8 (42.10)	10 (40)	16 (53.33)	-
	CVA	1 (16.66)	1 (5.26)	02 (8)	03 (10)	-
	Others	0	1 (5.26)	01 (4)	-	-
Social History	Alcohol (Yes)	1 (16.66)	6 (31.57)	7 (28)	8 (26.66)	>0.99
	Smoking (Yes)	0	3 (15.78)	3 (12)	1 (3.33)	0.31
Causality scores	Naranjo's	7	5–7	5–7	-	-
	RegiSCARS	>5	-	>5	-	-
	ALDEN	7–8		7–8	-	-

Table 1. Cont.

Parameters			PHT-Induced CADRsN (%)		Total (25)	Tolerant (30)	p Value
			Severe (6)	MPE and other Mild-Moderate Reactions c (19)			
CM/Skin		Itching	1 (16.66)	13 (68.42)	14 (56)	-	-
		Pap. Rash/Redness	6 (100)	19 (100)	25 (25)	-	-
		Papules/Pustules	4 (66.66)	04 (21.05)	08 (32)	-	-
		Blistering/Peeling	2 (33.33)	0	02 (8)	-	-
		Erythema P/P	3 (50)	0	03 (12)	-	-
CM/Mucosa		Eye	6 (100)	2 (10.52)	08 (32)	-	-
		Oral Mucosa	6 (100)	0	06 (24)	-	-
		Genital	4 (66.66)	0	04 (16)	-	-
		Anogenital	2 (33.33)	0	02 (8)	-	-
		F.Edema	4 (66.66)	2 (10.52)	06 (24)	-	-
CM/Systemic abnormalities		Fever	6 (100)	3 (10.52)	09 (36)	-	-
Liver							
AST IU/L (Mean ± SD)	SJS/DRESS/ED		96.50 ± 9.192/183.7 ± 96.66/185	-	-	-	-
ALT IU/L (Mean ± SD)	SJS/DRESS/ED		72.00 ± 12.73/241.3 ± 139.9/131	-	-	-	-
Alk.Phosphatase	SJS/DRESS/ED		117.5 ± 17.68/331.0 ± 128.7/401	-	-	-	-
Haematological abn.							
WBC (Mean ± SD)	SJS/DRESS/ED		5200 ± 424.3/11200 ± 2458/8000/µL	-	-	-	-
Lymphocytes (M %)	SJS/DRESS/ED		17%/56%/-	-	-	-	-
Eosinophil (M %)	SJS/DRESS/ED		09/12/-	-	-	-	-
Lymphadnopathy	SJS/DRESS/ED		Absent/3/Absent	-	-	-	-
AEDs Combination		PHT+VPA	2 (33.33)	2 (10.00)	4 (15.38)	6 (18.75)	>0.999
		PHT+LEV	2 (33.33)	5 (25.00)	7 (26.92)	4 (12.50)	0.1935
		PHT+VPA+LEV	-	1 (5.00)	1 (03.84)	-	0.4576
		Others	2 (33.33)	2 (10.00)	4 (15.38)	0	-

SJS, Steven Johnson syndrome; DRESS, drug reactions eosinophilia systemic syndrome; ED, exfoliative dermatitis; MPR, maculo-papular rash; c FDE, fixed drug eruption; LDE, lichenoid drug eruption; AFDE, acneiform drug eruption were in others category, a p value was calculated by independent Student's t test, b p-value calculated by Fisher's exact test.

The CYP2C9 normal-control data from the previous study included 82 healthy people (40 males and 42 females) from Dravidian or South Indian populations, such as Tamils (25), Andhra Pradesh (32), and Kerala [35]. This study included the data of 463 HLA-B normal-controls (Tamils) that was retrieved from past literature [34]. A total of 52 PHT-CADRs patients (31 MPE, 7 SJS/TEN, 8 DRESS, and 5 FDE) and 100 PHT-tolerant control patients with ages ranging from 6 to 72 were included in the pooled analysis. There were 22/30 and 41/59 females and males in their case and tolerant groups, respectively [20].

3.2. Clinical Features of PHT-CADRs

The itching was more common among mild-moderate reactions (13/20) than SCARs (1/6). Maculopapular rash/exanthematous rash or lesions/skinredness/burning sensation or warmth while touching were the most common cutaneous clinical manifestations in mild-moderate reactions (6/6 in SCARs and 13/20). Papules, pustules, blisters, and erythema were other serious features of skin reactions that were more common with SCARs (4/6) than mild to moderate reactions (5/20). The most commonly impacted mucosal sites were the mouth, eyes, genitals, and anogenital mucosa. SCARs were the only ones that showed systemic involvement. The most commonly affected systems were the liver and hematological systems. All three DRESS patients showed lymphadenopathy, abnormal lymphocytes, and eosinophilia. In one ED patient, neutrophilic leukocytosis was observed (Table 1).

The onset latency period ranged from 7 to 42 days, with a mean of 21.7 days. In Naranjo's causation assessment, all cases received a likely score of ≥5. According to the RegiSCAR and ALDEN criteria, all DRESS and SJS patients had a definite (>5) and very probable (>6) connection.

3.3. Frequency of HLA-B Alleles in PHT-Cases and Tolerant Controls

HLA-B genotyping data from PHT-CADRs cases showed higher frequencies (>5%) of HLA B*40:01 (40%), HLA B*55:01 (20%), HLA B*51:01 (18%), and HLA B*07:02 (10%) alleles and lower frequencies (<5) of HLA B*57:01 (4%), HLA B*52:01(2%), HLA B*15:01 (2%), HLA B*07:01, and HLA B*35:01(2%).In tolerant-controls, the following alleles were observed more frequently (>5%): HLA B*40:01 (28.33%), HLA B*55:01 (11.66%), HLA B*51:01 (11.66%), and HLA B*07:02 (6.66%), HLA B*52:01(6.66%), HLA B*15:01 (11.66%), and HLA B*35:01 (13.33%). On the other hand, HLA B*07:01 and HLA B*54:01 were reported at lower frequencies (Figure 2 and Supplementary Table S1).

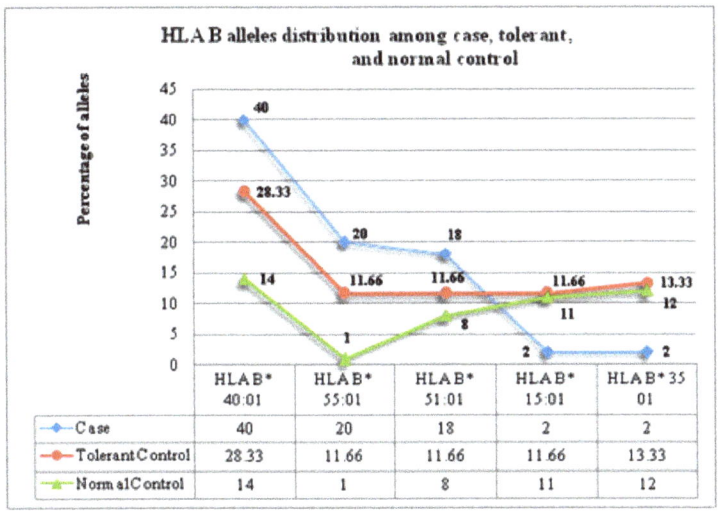

Figure 2. Frequently observed HLA B alleles among PHT-CADRs and PHT-tolerant controls.

3.4. Bivariate Analysis of HLA B Alleles and PHT-CADRs
3.4.1. SCARs

All six SCARs patients carried HLA B*51:01 allele against 7 out of 30 PHT-tolerant controls. In sub-group analysis, the association between PHT-DRESS was well demonstrated with both tolerant (OR = 21.93, 95% CI 1.013–474.9, p = 0.022) and normal controls (OR = 42.54, 95% CI 2.114–855.8, 0.003). The association between PHT-SJS and HLA B*51:01 was marginal with the PHT-tolerant control group (p = 0.072) and stronger with normal control group (p = 0.021), respectively. HLA B*40:01 was reported in all DRESS (3) and ED (1) cases against 14 out of 30 tolerant patients (28.33%), three of which were found to be homozygous. The association between PHT/DRESS and HLA B*40:01 was insignificant as the comparison made with PHT-tolerant group (p = 0.227) but found to be significant as the cases compared with normal control group ($p = 0.0001$). In this study, no other HLA B alleles were identified to be related to PHT-SCARs. The *HLA B*51:01* genetic marker to PHT-SCAR has a significant positive/negative predictive value (46/100).

3.4.2. Mild-Moderate Reactions

The *HLA B*40:01* allele was detected in 14 patients (73.68%) in the mild-moderate reaction group, and two PHT-MPE patients were homozygous for it. When compared to normal control, the association between *HLA B*40:01*/PHT-mild-moderate reactions, particularly MPE (OR = 10.45, 95% CI 3.299–29.34, $p = 0.0001$) and AFDE (OR = 25.65, 95% CI 1.172–552.8, $p = 0.028$), was found to be significant. The *HLA B*55:01* allele was the second most common among the mild-moderate reaction group. Only PHT-MPE patients had a greater frequency of this allele (33.33%), and homozygosity was found in one patient. The association between *HLA B*55:01* and PHT/MPE was stronger in both PHT-tolerant (OR = 4.929, 95% CI 1.322–17.33, $p = 0.022*$) and normal control group (OR = 204.0, 95% CI 27.72–2229, $p < 0.0001*$) with high positive/negative predictive value (56/79).

3.4.3. Overall PHT-Induced CADRs

*HLA B*51:01, HLA B*40:01,* and *HLA B*55:01* alleles were shown to have a significant association with overall PHT-CADRs when compared to normal controls, (*HLA B*51:01*; OR = 3.43, 95% CI 1.422–8.652, $p = 0.017$; *HLA B*40:01*, OR = 13.44, 95% CI 4.849–33.14, $p = <0.0001$; *HLA B*55:01*;OR = 76.50, 95% CI 10.40–841.9, $p < 0.0001$), but none of them were found to have a significant association with PHT-overall CADRs when compared to PHT-tolerant controls. The PHT-tolerant group showed higher frequencies of *HLA B*15:01* and *HLA B*35:01* than the case and normal control groups. For these alleles, the negative association with PHT-CADRs was found to be significant. (*HLA B*15:01*; OR = 0.1369, 95% CI of 0.0117–0.9204, $p = 0.0593$ and *HLA B*35:01*; OR = 0.1146, 95% CI 0.0099–0.7273, $p = 0.0307$) (Table 2).

3.4.4. CYP2C9*3

In the current study, the *CYP2C9*3* (AC) genotype was found in 12 out of 25 PHT-CADRs cases, but only two patients in the PHT-tolerant group had this allele, and the homozygous (CC) genotype was not found in either case or the tolerant control group (Table 3). The association testing was performed between case vs. PHT-tolerant and cases vs normal-control [23]. In both comparisons, the analysis revealed a stronger association between *CYP2C9*3* and overall PHT-CADRs (case vs. PHT-tolerant; OR = 12.92: 95% CI 2.777–61.46, $p = 0.0006$, case vs. normal control; OR = 5.385, 95% CI 1.917–13.67 $p = 0.0017$). SCARs (OR = 26.00, 95% CI2.855–1720, $p = 0.0043$) and mild-moderate reactions (OR = 9.455; 95% CI1.628–47.25, $p = 0.0086$) both showed a positive susceptibility association with *CYP2C9*3* in sub-group analysis. All three DRESS patients had this mutant allele in SCARs, and the relationship was found to be significant (OR = 74.20, 95% CI 2.922–1884, $p = 0.002$). This allele was observed in 5 MPE, 1 AFDE, 1 LDE, and 1 FDE patients with mild-moderate reactions. The MPE was found to have a substantial association with*CYP2C9*3* (OR = 6.500, 95% CI 1.008–35.01, $p = 0.039$) (Table 2).

Table 2. Bivariate analyses of association between HLA B alleles and CYP2C9*3 with PHT-CADRs.

HLA B Alleles	Phenotype (no of Cases)	Number of Cases			Case vs. Tolerant		Case vs. Healthy Population			
		Case n = 25 N (%)	Tolerant n = 30[HLA B]/28[CYP2C9*3] N (%)	General Population [R1 & R2] n = 463/82 N (%)	OR (95% CI)	p Value [a]	OR (95% CI)	p Value [a]	PPV/NPV	Sensitivity/ Specificity
				PHT-SCARs						
B*51/51: 01	SJS (2)	2 (100)		19 (13.86)	15.67 (0.6743–64.0)	0.07	30.38 (1.405–657.1)	0.02	22/100	100/76
	DRESS (3)	3 (100)	7 (23.33)		21.93 (1.013–474.9)	0.02	42.54 (2.114–855.8)	0.003	30/100	100/76
	ED (1)	1 (100)			9.40 (0.3452–56.0)	0.25	18.23 (0.716–463.8)	0.14	12.5/100	100/76
B*40/40:01	DRESS (3)	3 (100)	14 (46.66)	22 (16.05)	7.96 (0.3787–67.5)	0.22	35.93 (1.794–719.9)	0.005	17/100	100/53
	ED (1)	1 (100)			3.41 (0.1288–0.49)	0.48	15.40 (0.607–390.2)	0.16	6.6/100	100/53
B* 5101	SCARs (6)	6 (100)	7 (23.33)	19 (13.86)	40.73 (2.045–811.3)	0.0009	296.3 (16.11–5450)	<0.001	46/100	100/76
B* 4001	SCARs (6)	4 (66.66)	14 (46.66)	22 (16.05)	6.571 (1.157–37.69)	0.057	40.09 (8.70–213.6)	0.0001	36/92	66/76
				PHT-Mild-Moderate						
B* 40/40:01	MPE 15	10 (40)		22 (16.05)	2.286 (0.6742–7.887)	0.342	10.45 (3.299–29.34)	<0.001	41/76	66/53
	AFDE (2)	2 (50)	14 (28.33)		5.690 (0.2519–128.5)	0.483	25.65 (1.172–552.8)	0.02	12.5/100	100/53
	LDE (1)	1 (50)			3.414 (0.1288–90.49)	0.483	15.40 (0.607–390.2)	0.16	6.6/100	100/53
	FDE (1)	1 (50)			3.414 (0.1288–90.49)	0.483	15.40 (0.607–390.2)	0.16	6.6/100	100/53
B* 55/55:01	MPE (15)	9 (33.3)	07 (11.66)	1 (0.729)	4.929 (1.322–17.33)	0.022	204.0 (27.72–2229)	<0.001	56/79	60/76
B* 40/40:01	Mild-Mode CADRs19	14 (73.68)	14 (46.66)	22 (4.75)	3.200 (0. 885–10.34)	0.080	56.13 (18.42–147.5)	<0.001	50/70	73/53
B* 55/55:01	Mild-Mode CADRs19	9 (47.3)	07 (23.33)	1 (0.21)	2.957 (0.922–10.83)	0.119	415.8 (51.92–454)	<0.001	56/69	47/76
				PHT-Over all CADR						
B*51/51:01	CADRs	9 (36)	7 (23.33)	19 (13.8)	1.848 (0.5871–5.905)	0.377	3.493 (1.422–8.652)	0.01	56/58	36/76
B*40/40:01	CADRs	18 (72)	14 (46.66)	22 (16.05)	2.939 (0.9870–8.842)	0.098	13.44 (4.849–33.14)	<0.001	56/69	72/53
B*55/55:01	CADRs	10 (40)	07 (23.33)	1 (0.72)	1.848 (0.5871–5.905)	0.377	76.50 (10.40–841.9)	<0.001	58/60	40/76
B*57/57:01	CADRs	02 (8)	04 (13.33)	6 (4.37)	0.5652 (0.1013–2.643)	0.677	1.899 (0.369–8.216)	0.35	33/53	8/86

Table 2. Cont.

HLA B Alleles	Phenotype (no of Cases)	Number of Cases			Case vs. Tolerant		Case vs. Healthy Population			
		Case n = 25 N (%)	Tolerant n = 30^(HLA B)/28^(CYP2C9*3) N (%)	General Population^(R1 & R2) n = 463/82 N (%)	OR (95% CI)	p Value [a]	OR (95% CI)	p Value [a]	PPV/NPV	Sensitivity/Specificity
B*52/52:01	CADRs	02 (8)	04 (13.33)	11 (8.02)	0.5652 (0.1013–2.643)	0.677	0.996 (0.209–3.973)	>0.99	33/53	8/86
B*07/07:02	CADRs	05 (20)	04 (13.33)	26 (18.9)	1.625 (0.3967–5.800)	0.716	1.067 (0.4067–909)	>0.99	55/56	20/86
B*15/15:01	CADRs	01 (4)	07 (23.33)	11 (8.02)	0.1369 (0.0117–0.9204)	0.059	0.477 (0.042–3.005)	0.69	12.5/48	4/76
B*35/35.01	CADRs	01 (4)	08 (26.66)	22 (16.05)	0.1146 (0.009–0.7273)	0.030	0.2178 (0.020–.370)	0.20	11/47	4/73
				CYP2C9*3 carriers						
CYP2C9*3	Severe CADRs (6)	4 (66.6)	2 (7.14)	12 (14.63)	26.00 (2.855–1726)	0.0006	11.69 (2.386–63.63)	0.009	66/92	66/92
CYP2C9*3	DRESS(3)	3 (100)	2 (7.14)	12 (14.63)	74.20 (2.922–1884)	0.002	39.48 (1.920–811.9)	0.004	60/100	100/92
CYP2C9*3	M-Moder. (19)	8 (42.2)	2 (7.14)	12 (14.63)	9.455 (1.628–47.25)	0.008	2.917 (0.9178–0.969)	0.02	80/70	42/92
CYP2C9*3	MPE(15)	5 (33.33)	2 (7.14)	12 (14.63)	6.500 (1.008–35.01)	0.039	5.385 (1.917–13.67)	0.13	71/72	33/92
CYP2C9*3	Overall (25)	12 (48)	2 (7.14)	12 (14.63)	12.92 (2.777–61.46)	0.004	4.242 (1.378–12.89)	0.001	85/66	48/92

SJS, Steven Johnson syndrome; DRESS, drug reactions eosinophilia systemic syndrome; ED, exfoliative dermatitis; MPE, maculo-papular eruption; FDE, fixed drug eruption; LDE, lichenoid drug eruption; AFD, acneiform drug eruption; [a] Fisher's exact test was used for p calculation, R1 & R2 Percentages of HLA B alleles in Tamil population was taken from Leenam Dedhia et al. 2015 [22], and CYP2C9*3 distribution data was taken from Nahar R et al. 2013 [23] After Bonferroni correction, p-value 0.008 (<0.05/6—two tailed) were considered significant.

Table 3. Pooled data analysis for *HLA B*51:01* and PHT-CADRs.

Alleles	Phenotype	Present Study		Literatures		Total after Pooling		Before Pooling		After Pooling		PPV/NPV
		Case	Control	Case	Control	Case	Control	OR (95%CI)	p Value	OR (95%CI)	p Value	
HLA B*51:01 [R1]	SCARs	6/6	7/30	4/15	8/100	11/21	15/130	40.73 (2.045–811.3)	0.0009	6.273 (2.24–16.69)	0.0008	46/100 [a] 47/88 [b]
	MM	3/19	7/30	9/35	8/100	12/54	15/130	0.6161 (0.1563–2.603)	0.71	2.190 (0.939–4.97)	0.07	30/58 [a] 44/73 [b]
	Overall CADRs	9/25	7/30	13/50	8/100	22/75	15/130	0.848 (0.5871–0.377)	0.37	2.323 (1.122–5.899)	0.03	36/76 [a] 59/68 [b]

[R1] Percentage of *HLA B*51:01* in PHT-CADRs and tolerant control data was taken from Ihtisham et al. (2019). [a] Positive and negative predictive value before pooling. [b] Positive and negative predictive value after pooling. SCARs, severe cutaneous adverse drug reactions; OR, odds ratio; CI, confidence interval; MM reac, mild-moderate reactions that includes: MPE, maculo-papular Exanthema; FDE, fixed drug eruption; LDE, lichenoid drug eruption; AFDE, acneiform drug eruption.

3.5. Pooled Data Analysis

Prior to pooling, the association between *HLA B*51:01* and PHT-SCARs was shown to be stronger with broad CI (OR = 40.73, 95% CI 2.045–811.3, $p = 0.0009$) but not with overall PHT-CADRs (OR = 0.848, 95% CI 0.5871–0.377, $p = 0.377$). The number of CADRs increased to 75 after pooling, with 21 patients carrying *HLA B*51:01*, while the number of tolerant controls climbed to 130, with 15 *HLA B*51:01* carriers. *HLA B*51:01* and PHT-overall CADRs were found to have a significant relationship (OR = 2.323, 95% CI1.122–5.899, $p = 0.037$). Even after pooling the data, the connection between *HLA B* 51:01* and mild-moderate reactions is weaker ($p = 0.07$) (Table 3).

3.6. Multivariate Binary Logistic Regression Analysis

The multivariate binary logistic regression analysis showed a stronger association between *CYP2C9*3* and PHT-induced all kinds of CADRs, and it was the only predictor that was related to both severe and mild-moderate reactions (OR = 4.041, 95% CI 1.125–15.6, $p = 0.035$). In subgroup analysis, PHT-MPE was shown to be highly associated with *HLA B*55:01* (OR = 12.00, 95%CI 2.759–84.82, $p = 0.003$), and *CYP2C9*3* was the sole predictor variable with a significant association with PHT-SCARs (OR = 12.00, 95%CI 2.759–84.82, $p = 0.003$) (Table 4).

Table 4. Multivariate binary logistic regression analysis of PHT-CADRs and tolerant-control.

Predictor Variables	β	SE	OR	95% CI	p Value
PHT- All types of CADRs/tolerant Control					
CYP2C9*3	2.48	0.83	12	2.759–84.87	0.003
HLA B*51:01	0.48	0.67	1.61	0.429–6.104	0.47
PHT-SCARs/tolerant Control					
CYP2C9*3	2.52	1.22	12.4	1.138–136.2	0.003
HLA B*51:01	2.04	1.45	7.70	0.447–133.0	0.16
HLA B*40:01	−0.33	1.34	0.71	0.52–9.895	0.80
MPE/tolerant Control					
HLA B*55:01	1.39	0.66	4.04	1.125–15.67	0.03
HLAB*40:01	0.39	0.78	1.47	0.318–6.873	0.61
CYP2C9*3	1.57	1.05	4.89	0.617–37.79	0.13

β regression coefficient, SE, standard error; OR, odds ratio; CI, confidence interval; MPE, maculo-papularexanthema.

4. Discussion

In Asian populations, *HLA B*51:01* has been related to PHT-induced CADRs, particularly with PHT-SCARs [40,41]. A recent multicenter East Asian study that investigated the genetic predictors of PHT-hypersensitivity reported that concurrent testing of *HLA B* 13:01/HLA B* 15:02/HLA B*51:01* and *CYP2C9*3* would help in identifying individuals at risk of developing PHT-CADRs [42]. In India, one of the North Indian studies reported *HLA B*57:01* (OR = 11.00, 95% CI: 1.41–85.81, $p = 0.05$) and *HLA B*51:01* (OR = 6.90, 95% CI: 1.38–34.29, $p = 0.007$) as risk factors for CBZ-SJS and PHT-DRESS, respectively [20]. In the current study, the *HLA B*51:01* allele was found to be strongly associated with PHT-SCARs, especially DRESS, and the pooled data analysis corroborated this relationship with both SCARs and overall CADRs. However, this allele was presented in all of our SCAR patients (6/6), whereas only 4 of 15 patients in pooled data had this allele, which could be attributable to distribution variations. In Mumbai (central India), for example, it is more frequent among Patels (19.60%) and Iyers (17.60%), whereas it is less common among Marathas (4.84%) [43] and North Indian Hindus (3.5%) (Lucknow) [44]. Its distribution among South Indians, particularly Tamils, ranges between 8–12.5%.

A study from South India reported that *HLA B*07* was the most common allele (6–13%) in the HLA-B gene, and its association with cervical cancer along with *HLA DQ8* was found to be significant. The next common alleles reported in South Indians were the split antigens of the HLA B5 serotype, *HLA B* 51* (8–12.5%) and *HLA B* 52* (5–10%). Their association with different vasculitides was reported (HLA B*51 and Behchet'sdiseases, HLA B* 52, and Takayasu's arteritis) [45].

In this study, the association between *HLA B*40:01* and PHT-mild moderate reactions in particular, MPE, was found to be stronger when compared to normal healthy controls, confirming previous findings (Sukesm et al., 2020) [46], which confirmed *HLA B*40:01* as a risk factor for PHT-induced MPE (OR 3.647; 95% CI, 1.193–11.147; p = 0.023).This allele could be a drug-specific HLA genetic marker for PHT-MPE. However, a study with a larger cohort is needed to confirm this finding.

HLA B*55:01 was not shown to be susceptible to PHT-induced CADRs in any previous association studies that looked into the relationship between HLA and AEDs. The current study is the first to confirm this association in the South Indian-Tamil population. However, a Han-Chinese study also showed a correlation between *HLA B*55:01* and LTG-induced MPE (OR = 24.78, 95% CI 1.50–408.76, p = 0.08) [47]. This genotype has been linked to penicillin hypersensitivity and nevirapine-induced SCARs in addition to AEDs [48,49]. In this study, *HLA B*15:01* and *HLA B*35:01* were found in a higher percentage of PHT-tolerant people than in cases and normal controls. This finding is consistent with other Indian studies that indicated a higher prevalence of the *HLA B*15:01* allele in the control group than in the case group [23,24], whereas *HLA B*35:01* was associated with LTG-induced MPE [50]. In the Tamil population, *HLA B*15:01* and *HLA B*35:01* may be protective alleles for PHT-CADRs.

The mutant allele (AC) was present in 48 and 7.14 percent of cases and tolerant-control groups, respectively, with no homozygosity (CC), which is similar to a study that found no frequency of CC genotype in the South Indian Dravidian community [19]. The current investigation found a substantial link between the *CYP2C9*3* heterozygous condition and PHT-induced CADRs. In this investigation, patients with *CYP2C9*3* alleles were almost 13 times more vulnerable to PHT-CADRs than the tolerant group. This finding is comparable to that of a Thai study, which found that patients with *CYP2C9*3* have a 14.5 times higher incidence of PHT-SCARs. A subgroup analysis of this study within the SCARs group reveals a higher correlation between *CYP2C9*3* and PHT-induced DRESS, which was also corroborated in another Thai investigation [46,51,52].

There may be some limitations to this research. We did not rule out patients who were using CYP2C9 inhibitors, which could have contributed to the rise in PHT levels. Despite this, only three patients were prescribed VPA (CYP2C9 inhibitor), and no other known CYP2C9 inhibitors were prescribed in this group. Although a few studies have found a relationship between *CYP2C9*2* and PHT-CADRs, we did not investigate this allele in this study because it is extremely rare (1–2%) in the South Indian population. Another limitation of our research is the small sample size. The rare outcome of interest is the reason for it. In addition to genetic defects, clinical and non-clinical factors may play a role in the initiation of PHT-CADRs, and these should be examined alongside genetic variants.

5. Conclusions

CYP2C9*3 and *HLA B*51:01* were found to be associated with PHT-SCARs and PHT-DRESS. On the other hand, PHT-mild/moderate cutaneous reactions are linked with *HLA B*55:01* and *HLA B*40:01* in this study. This is the first study in South India, specifically among Tamils, to show a correlation between *HLA B*51:01*, *HLA B*55:01*, and *CYP2C9*3* alleles and PHT-CADRs. These alleles can be employed as genetic markers to identify individuals who are susceptible to PHT-CADRs and to ensure that PHT is as safe as possible for Tamil epileptic patients. Furthermore, our findings highlight the necessity of including the *HLA B*5101* and *CYP2C9*3* alleles into a pre-emptive genetic testing panel for Asians with PHT-CADRs.

Supplementary Materials: The following are available online at https://www.mdpi.com/article/10.3390/jpm11080737/s1, Figure S1: Frequently observed HLA B alleles among PHT-CADRs and PHT Tolerant; Table S1 Clinical characteristics and HLA-B and CYP2C9*3 genotyping of the patients with PHT-CADRs.

Author Contributions: S.J. was responsible for concept, study design, data collection, statistical analysis, and drafting and revising the manuscript. S.P. was responsible for concept and study design, supervised the study, revised the manuscript content, and approved the final manuscript. K.B. contributed to phenotype data of the study participants, laboratory consultation, and critically revised the manuscript content. C.S. contributed to study design, and supervised the study. T.C.V.A. contributed samples and case diagnosis. B.C. contributed to study design and revised the manuscript. All authors have read and agreed to the published version of the manuscript.

Funding: This work was done as part of a PhD study that was funded by the Graduate School, Prince of Songkla University, Hat Yai, Thailand-90110.

Institutional Review Board Statement: The study was conducted according to the guidelines of the Declaration of Helsinki, and approved by the Institutional Review Board (or Ethics Committee) of MEENAKSHI MISSION HOSPITAL AND RESEARCH CENTER (MMHRC/IEC/07/2018).

Informed Consent Statement: Informed consent was obtained from all subjects.

Acknowledgments: We would like to thank the staff members of the Neurology Department, Madurai Meenakshi Mission Hospital and Research Center, and staff members of the Department of Immunology, School of Biological Sciences, Madurai Kamaraj University Madurai, TN, India, for their assistance in conducting the study.

Conflicts of Interest: All authors declare no conflicts of interest.

Ethics Approval: The study protocol was approved by the Institutional Ethical Committee of the Meenakshi Mission Hospital and Research Center. (MMHRC/IEC/07/2018).

Abbreviations

ALDEN	Algorithm of drug causality for epidermal necrolysis
AEDs	Anti-epileptic drugs
CBZ	Carbamazepine
PHT	Phenytoin
DRESS	Drug reaction with eosinophilia and systemic symptoms
HLA	Human leukocyte antigen
MPE	Maculopapular exanthema
NPV	Negative predictive values
SCARs	Severe cutaneous adverse drug reactions
ED	Exfoliative dermatitis
AFDE	Acneiform drug eruption
FDE	Fixed drug eruption
LDE	Lichenoid drug eruption
CADRs	Cutaneous adverse drug reactions
VPA	Valproic acid
TEN	Toxic epidermal necrolysis

References

1. Twardowschy, C.A.; Germiniani, F.; Werneck, L.C.; Silvado, C.; De Paola, L. Pearls & Oysters: Soft-tissue necrosis as a result of intravenous leakage of phenytoin. *Neurology* **2009**, *73*, e94–e95. [PubMed]
2. Glick, T.H.; Workman, T.P.; Gaufberg, S.V. Preventing phenytoin intoxication: Safer use of a familiar anticonvulsant. *J. Fam. Pr.* **2004**, *53*, 197–202.
3. Błaszczyk, B.; Szpringer, M.; Czuczwar, S.J.; Lasoń, W. Single centre 20 years survey of antiepileptic drug-induced hypersensitivity reactions. *Pharmacol. Rep.* **2013**, *65*, 399–409. [CrossRef]
4. Chatterjee, S.; Ghosh, A.; Barbhuiya, J.; Dey, S. Adverse cutaneous drug reactions: A one year survey at a dermatology outpatient clinic of a tertiary care hospital. *Indian J. Pharmacol.* **2006**, *38*, 429–431. [CrossRef]

5. Patel, T.; Barvaliya, M.; Sharma, D.; Tripathi, C. A systematic review of the drug-induced Stevens-Johnson syndrome and toxic epidermal necrolysis in Indian population. *Indian J. Dermatol. Venereol. Leprol.* **2013**, *79*, 389–398. [CrossRef]
6. Chung, W.H.; Hung, S.I.; Hong, H.S. Medical genetics: A marker for Stevens-Johnson syndrome. *Nature* **2004**, *428*, 486. [CrossRef] [PubMed]
7. Karnes, J.H.; Rettie, A.E.; Somogyi, A.A.; Huddart, R.; Fohner, A.E.; Formea, C.M.; Lee, M.T.M.; Llerena, A.; Whirl-Carrillo, M.; Klein, T.E.; et al. Clinical Pharmacogenetics Implementation Consortium (CPIC) guideline for CYP2C9 and HLA-B genotypes and phenytoin dosing: 2020 Update. *Clin. Pharmacol. Ther.* **2020**, *109*, 302–309. [CrossRef]
8. Sukasem, C.; Sririttha, S.; Chaichan, C.; Nakkrut, T.; Satapornpong, P.; Jaruthamsophon, K.; Jantararoungtong, T.; Koomdee, N.; Medhasi, S.; Oo-Puthinan, S.; et al. Spectrum of cutaneous adverse reactions to aromatic antiepileptic drugs and human leukocyte antigen genotypes in Thai patients and meta-analysis. *Pharm. J.* **2021**, 1–9. [CrossRef]
9. Locharernkul, C.; Loplumlert, J.; Limotai, C.; Korkij, W.; Desudchit, T.; Tongkobpetch, S.; Kangwanshiratada, O.; Hirankarn, N.; Suphapeetiporn, K.; Shotelersuk, V. Carbamazepine and phenytoin induced Stevens-Johnson syndrome is associated with HLA-B*1502 allele in Thai population. *Epilepsia* **2008**, *49*, 2087–2091. [CrossRef]
10. Chang, C.-C.; Ng, C.-C.; Too, C.-L.; Choon, S.-E.; Lee, C.-K.; Chung, W.-H.; Hussein, S.H.; Lim, K.-S.; Murad, S. Association of HLA-B*15:13 and HLA-B*15:02 with phenytoin-induced severe cutaneous adverse reactions in a Malay population. *Pharm. J.* **2016**, *17*, 170–173. [CrossRef]
11. Thorn, C.F.; Whirl-Carrillo, M.; Leeder, J.S.; Klein, T.E.; Altman, R.B. PharmGKB summary: Phenytoin pathway. *Pharm. Genom.* **2012**, *22*, 466–470. [CrossRef] [PubMed]
12. Chung, W.-H.; Chang, W.-C.; Lee, Y.-S.; Wu, Y.-Y.; Yang, C.-H.; Ho, H.-C.; Chen, M.-J.; Lin, J.-Y.; Hui, R.C.-Y.; Ho, J.-C.; et al. Genetic variants associated with phenytoin-related severe cutaneous adverse reactions. *J. Am. Med. Assoc.* **2014**, *312*, 525–534. [CrossRef] [PubMed]
13. Rosemary, J.; Surendiran, A.; Rajan, S.; Shashindran, C.H.; Adithan, C. Influence of the CYP2C9 AND CYP2C19 polymorphisms on phenytoin hydroxylation in healthy individuals from south India. *Indian J. Med. Res.* **2006**, *123*, 665–670.
14. Agrawal, S.; Srivastava, S.K.; Borkar, M.; Chaudhuri, T.K. Genetic affinities of north and northeastern populations of India: Inference from HLA-based study. *Tissue Antigens* **2008**, *72*, 120–130. [CrossRef]
15. Joshi, C.G.; Patel, J.S.; Patel, M.M.; Koringa, P.G.; Shah, T.M.; Patel, A.K.; Tripathi, A.K.; Mathew, A.; Rajapurkar, M.M. Human leukocyte antigen alleles, genotypes and haplotypes frequencies in renal transplant donors and recipients from West Central India. *Indian J. Hum. Genet.* **2013**, *19*, 219–232. [CrossRef]
16. Coon, C.S. *Human Populations. The New Encyclopedia Britannica*, 15th ed.; Encyclopaedia Britannica: Chicago, IL, USA, 1983; Volume 14, pp. 839–848.
17. Mittal, K.K.; Naik, S.; Sansonetti, N.; Cowherd, R.; Kumar, R.; Wong, D.M. The HLA antigens in Indian Hindus. *Tissue Antigens* **1982**, *20*, 223–226. [CrossRef] [PubMed]
18. Shankarkumar, U.; Hla, A.B.C. Allele frequencies in a Parsi population from Western India. *Hum. Immunol.* **2004**, *65*, 992–993. [CrossRef]
19. Shankarkumar, U.; Hla, A.B.C. Allele frequencies in a Pawra population from Khandesh, India. *Hum. Immunol.* **2004**, *65*, 958. [CrossRef]
20. Nizamuddin, S.; Dubey, S.; Singh, S.; Sharma, S.; Mishra, A.; Harish, K.; Joshi, J.; Thangaraj, K. Genetic polymorphism of Cytochrome-P450-2C9 (CYP2C9) in Indian populations. *bioRxiv* **2017**. [CrossRef]
21. Ihtisham, K.; Ramanujam, B.; Srivastava, S.; Mehra, N.K.; Kaur, G.; Khanna, N.; Jain, S.; Kumar, S.; Kaul, B.; Samudrala, R.; et al. Association of cutaneous adverse drug reactions due to antiepileptic drugs with HLA alleles in a North Indian population. *Seizure* **2019**, *66*, 99–103. [CrossRef]
22. Devi, K. The association of HLA B*15:02 allele and Stevens-Johnson syndrome/toxic epidermal necrolysis induced by aromatic anticonvulsant drugs in a South Indian population. *Int. J. Dermatol.* **2017**, *57*, 70–73. [CrossRef]
23. Ramanujam, B.; Ihtisham, K.; Kaur, G.; Srivastava, S.; Mehra, N.K.; Khanna, N.; Singh, M.; Tripathi, M. Spectrum of cutaneous adverse reactions to Levetiracetam and human Leukocyte antigen typing in North-Indian patients. *J. Epilepsy Res.* **2016**, *6*, 87–92. [CrossRef] [PubMed]
24. Aggarwal, R.; Sharma, M.; Modi, M.; Garg, V.K.; Salaria, M. HLA-B*15 02 is associated with carbamazepine induced Stevens-Johnson syndrome in North Indian population. *Hum. Immunol.* **2014**, *75*, 1120–1122. [CrossRef]
25. Patel, T.K.; Thakkar, S.H.; Sharma, D.C. Cutaneous adverse drug reactions in Indian population: A systematic review. *Indian Dermatol. Online J.* **2014**, *5*, S76–S86. [CrossRef] [PubMed]
26. Shi, Y.W.; Min, F.L.; Zhou, D.; Qin, B.; Wang, J.; Hu, F.Y.; Cheung, Y.K.; Zhou, J.H.; Hu, X.S.; Zhou, J.Q.; et al. HLA-A*24:02 as a common risk factor for antiepileptic drug-induced cutaneous adverse reactions. *Neurology* **2017**, *88*, 2183–2191. [CrossRef] [PubMed]
27. Du-Thanh, A.; Kluger, N.; Bensalleh, H.; Guillot, B. Drug-induced acneiform eruption. *Am. J. Clin. Dermatology* **2011**, *12*, 233. [CrossRef]
28. Rita, V.; Nilofar, D.; Nidhi, J.; Rochit, S. A study of adverse cutaneous drug reactions (ACDR) owing to antiepileptics at a rural-based tertiary-care center, Gujarat. *Natl. J. Physiol. Pharm.Pharmacol.* **2016**, *6*, 140.
29. Roji, M.; Sebastian, M.; Lucca, J.M.; Pss, R Phenytoin induced oral Lichenoid eruption and melasma: A case report. *Indian J. Phurm. Pr.* **2018**, *11*, 55–57. [CrossRef]

30. Roujeau, J.C. The spectrum of Stevens-Johnson syndrome and toxic epidermal necrolysis: A clinical classification. *J.Invest. Dermatol.* **1994**, *102*, 28S–30S. [CrossRef]
31. Voora, L.; Shastry, C.; Bhandari, R.; Sukeerthi, D.; Rawal, K.B.; Chand, S. Phenytoin-induced Erythroderma. *J. Young Pharm.* **2019**, *11*, 320–321. [CrossRef]
32. Dedhia, L.; Gadekar, S.; Mehta, P.; Parekh, S. HLA haplotype diversity in the South Indian population and its relevance. *Indian J. Transplant.* **2015**, *9*, 138–143. [CrossRef]
33. Nahar, R.; Deb, R.; Saxena, R.; Puri, R.D.; Verma, I.C. Variability in CYP2C9 allele frequency: A pilot study of its predicted impact on warfarin response among healthy South and North Indians. *Pharmacol. Rep.* **2013**, *65*, 187–194. [CrossRef]
34. Naranjo, C.; Busto, U.; Sellers, E.; Sandor, P.; Ruiz, I.; Roberts, E.; Janecek, E.; Domecq, C.; Greenblatt, D.J. A method for estimating the probability of adverse drug reactions. *Clin. Pharmacol. Ther.* **1981**, *30*, 239–245. [CrossRef] [PubMed]
35. Kardaun, S.H.; Sidoroff, A.; Valeyrie-Allanore, L.; Halevy, S.; Davidovici, B.B.; Mockenhaupt, M.; Roujeau, J.C. Variability in the clinical pattern of cutaneous side-effects of drugs with systemic symptoms: Does a DRESS syndrome really exist? *Br.J. Dermatol.* **2007**, *156*, 609–611. [CrossRef] [PubMed]
36. Sassolas, B.; Haddad, C.; Mockenhaupt, M.; Dunant, A.; Liss, Y.; Bork, K.; Haustein, U.F.; Vieluf, D.; Roujeau, J.C.; Le Louet, H. ALDEN, an algorithm for assessment of drug causality in Stevens—Johnson syndrome and toxic epidermal necrolysis: Comparison with case-control analysis. *Clin. Pharmacol. Ther.* **2010**, *88*, 60–68. [CrossRef]
37. Welsh, K.; Bunce, M. Molecular typing for the MHC with PCR-SSP. *Rev. Immunogenet.* **1999**, *1*, 157–176.
38. Bunce, M.; O'neill, C.M.; Barnardo, M.C.N.M.; Krausa, P.; Browning, M.J.; Morris, P.J.; Welsh, K.I. Phototyping: Comprehensive DNA Typing for HLA A, B, C, DRB1, DRB3, DRB4, and DRB5 & DQB1 by PCR with 144 primers mixes utilizing sequence specific primers (PCR-SSP). *Tissue Antigens* **1995**, *46*, 355–367.
39. Tonks, S.; Marsh, S.G.E.; Bunce, M.; Bodmer, J.G. Molecular typing for HLA class I using ARMS-PCR: Further developments following the 12th international histocompatibility workshop. *Tissue Antigens* **1999**, *53*, 175–183. [CrossRef]
40. Kaniwa, N.; Sugiyama, E.; Saito, Y.; Kurose, K.; Maekawa, K.; Hasegawa, R.; Furuya, H.; Ikeda, H.; Takahashi, Y.; Muramatsu, M.; et al. Specific HLA types are associated with antiepileptic drug-induced Stevens-Johnson syndrome and toxic epidermal necrolysis in Japanese subjects. *Pharmacogenomics* **2013**, *14*, 1821–1831. [CrossRef]
41. Manuyakorn, W.; Likkasittipan, P.; Wattanapokayakit, S.; Suvichapanich, S.; Inunchot, W.; Wichukchinda, N.; Khongkhatithuml, C.; Thampratankul, L.; Kamchaisatian, W.; Benjaponpitak, S.; et al. Association of HLA genotypes with phenytoin induced severe cutaneous adverse drug reactions in Thai children. *Epilepsy Res.* **2020**, *162*, 106321. [CrossRef]
42. Su, S.-C.; Chen, C.-B.; Chang, W.-C.; Wang, C.-W.; Fan, W.-L.; Lu, L.-Y.; Nakamura, R.; Saito, Y.; Ueta, M.; Kinoshita, S.; et al. HLA alleles and CYP2C9*3 as predictors of Phenytoin hypersensitivity in East Asians. *Clin. Pharmacol. Ther.* **2018**, *105*, 476–485. [CrossRef]
43. Shankarkumar, U.; Ghosh, K.; Colah, R.B.; Gorakshakar, A.C.; Gupte, S.C.; Mohanty, D. HLA antigen distribution in selected caste groups from Mumbai, Maharastra, India. *J. Hum. Ecol.* **2002**, *13*, 209–215. [CrossRef]
44. Subramanian, V.S.; Selvaraj, P.; Narayanan, P.R.; Prabhakar, R.; Damodaran, C. Distribution of HLA (class I and class II) antigens in the native Dravidian Hindus of Tamil Nadu, south India. *Gene Geogr. Comput. Bull. Hum. Gene Freq.* **1995**, *9*, 15–24.
45. Narayan, S.; Maiers, M.; Halagan, M.; Sathishkannan, A.; Naganathan, C.; Madbouly, A.; Periathiruvadi, S. Human leukocyte antigen (HLA)-A, -B, -C, -DRB1 and -DQB1 haplotype frequencies from 2491 cord blood units from Tamil speaking population from Tamil Nadu, India. *Mol. Biol. Rep.* **2018**, *45*, 2821–2829. [CrossRef] [PubMed]
46. Sukasem, C.; Sririttha, S.; Tempark, T.; Klaewsongkram, J.; Rerkpattanapipat, T.; Puangpetch, A.; Boongird, A.; Chulavatnatol, S. Genetic and clinical risk factors associated with phenytoin-induced cutaneous adverse drug reactions in Thai population. *Pharmacoepidemiol. Drug Saf.* **2020**, *29*, 565–574. [CrossRef]
47. Shi, Y.-W.; Min, F.-L.; Liu, X.-R.; Zan, L.-X.; Gao, M.-M.; Yu, M.-J.; Liao, W.-P. Hla-B alleles and lamotrigine-induced cutaneous adverse drug reactions in the Han Chinese population. *Basic Clin. Pharmacol. Toxicol.* **2011**, *109*, 42–46. [CrossRef] [PubMed]
48. Krebs, K.; Bovijn, J.; Lepamets, M.; Censin, J.C.; Jürgenson, T.; Särg, D.; Abner, E.; Laisk, T.; Luo, L.; Skotee, L.; et al. Genome-wide study identifies association between HLA-B*55:01 and penicillin allergy. *Am. J. Hum. Genet.* **2020**, *107*, 612. [CrossRef] [PubMed]
49. Pavlos, R.; McKinnon, E.J.; Ostrov, D.A.; Peters, B.; Buus, S.; Koelle, D.; Chopra, A.; Schutte, R.; Rive, C.; Redwood, A.; et al. Shared peptide binding of HLA Class I and II alleles associate with cutaneous nevirapine hypersensitivity and identify novel risk alleles. *Sci. Rep.* **2017**, *7*, 8653. [CrossRef]
50. Peña-Balderas, A.M.; López-Revilla, R. Pharmacogenetics of adverse cutaneous reactions to lamotrigine. *Rev. Mex. Neuroci.* **2019**, *20*, 200–206. [CrossRef]
51. Tassaneeyakul, W.; Prabmeechai, N.; Sukasem, C.; Kongpan, T.; Konyoung, P.; Chumworathayi, P.; Tiamkao, S.; Khunarkornsiri, U.; Kulkantrakorn, K.; Saksit, N.; et al. Associations between HLA class I and cytochrome P450 2C9 genetic polymorphisms and phenytoin-related severe cutaneous adverse reactions in a Thai population. *Pharmacogenet. Genomics.* **2016**, *26*, 225–234. [CrossRef]
52. Yampayon, K.; Sukasem, C.; Limwongse, C.; Chinvarun, Y.; Tempark, T.; Rerkpattanapipat, T.; Kijsanayotin, P. Influence of genetic and non-genetic factors on phenytoin-induced severe cutaneous adverse drug reactions. *Eur. J. Clin. Pharmacol.* **2017**, *73*, 855–865. [CrossRef] [PubMed]

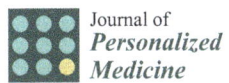

Article

Application of a Pharmacogenetics-Based Precision Medicine Model (5SPM) to Psychotic Patients That Presented Poor Response to Neuroleptic Therapy

Lorena Carrascal-Laso [1], Manuel Ángel Franco-Martín [1,*], María Belén García-Berrocal [2], Elena Marcos-Vadillo [2], Santiago Sánchez-Iglesias [3], Carolina Lorenzo [3], Almudena Sánchez-Martín [4], Ignacio Ramos-Gallego [5], M Jesús García-Salgado [2] and María Isidoro-García [2,6]

1. Servicio de Psiquiatría, Hospital Provincial de Zamora, IBSAL, 49071 Zamora, Spain; lorenacarraslaso@gmail.com
2. Farmacogenética y Medicina de Precisión, Servicio de Bioquímica, Hospital Universitario de Salamanca, IBSAL, 37007 Salamanca, Spain; mbgarcia@saludcastillayleon.es (M.B.G.-B.); elemarcos@hotmail.com (E.M.-V.); mjgarciasal@saludcastillayleon.es (M.J.G.-S.); misidoro@saludcastillayleon.es (M.I.-G.)
3. Servicio de Psiquiatría, Hospital Universitario de Salamanca, IBSAL, 37007 Salamanca, Spain; sisanchez@saludcastillayleon.es (S.S.-I.); carolinalorenzo@usal.es (C.L.)
4. Pharmacogenetics Unit, Pharmacy Department, University Hospital Virgen de las Nieves, UGC Provincial de Farmacia de Granada, Avda. Fuerzas Armadas, 18014 Granada, Spain; almuweb06@gmail.com
5. Departamento de Fisiología y Farmacología, Universidad de Salamanca, 37007 Salamanca, Spain; ignramos@usal.es
6. Departamento de Medicina, Universidad de Salamanca, 37007 Salamanca, Spain
* Correspondence: mfrancom@saludcastillayleon.es

Received: 4 November 2020; Accepted: 15 December 2020; Published: 18 December 2020

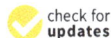

Abstract: Antipsychotics are the keystone of the treatment of severe and prolonged mental disorders. However, there are many risks associated with these drugs and not all patients undergo full therapeutic profit from them. The application of the 5 Step Precision Medicine model(5SPM), based on the analysis of the pharmacogenetic profile of each patient, could be a helpful tool to solve many of the problematics traditionally associated with the neuroleptic treatment. In order to solve this question, a cohort of psychotic patients that showed poor clinical evolution was analyzed. After evaluating the relationship between the prescribed treatment and pharmacogenetic profile of each patient, a great number of pharmacological interactions and pharmacogenetical conflicts were found. After reconsidering the treatment of the conflictive cases, patients showed a substantial reduction on mean daily doses and polytherapy cases, which may cause less risk of adverse effects, greater adherence, and a reduction on economic costs.

Keywords: antipsychotic agents; pharmacogenetics; cytochrome P-450 enzyme system; psychotic disorders; precision medicine

1. Introduction

The pharmacological tools of the severe mental disorders have been historically scarce until the appearance of the first antipsychotic, which had been used in surgical practice as a sedative agent categorized as an antihistaminic (chlorpromazine) [1]. Its application in psychotic patients was considered a resounding success because of its efficacy on positive symptoms, which led to a drastic reduction in admissions to mental institutions and in the use of more aggressive therapies such as lobotomy or electro convulsive therapy (ECT). These substances were initially defined as "chemical lobotomies" and had a wide repertoire of extrapyramidal effects, among others [2].

Second-generation anti-psychotics, entail a lower incidence of extrapyramidal side effects [3,4]. Same way as typical antipsychotics, second-generation antipsychotics bind the dopamine type 2 (D2) receptors, but the latter act selectively on the mesolimbic pathway due to its lower D2 receptor affinity, avoiding extrapyramidal effects when administered in low doses, and have antagonistic effects on the 5-hydroxytryptamine (5-HT) receptors in the cerebral area, which could explain the improvement in negative symptomatology and reduced drug-induced extrapyramidal symptoms [5].

However, empiricism continued to be frequent in clinical practice, with therapeutic decisions based primarily on strategies of trial and error, which prolong the time during which the patient would not receive effective therapy. This practice tends to result in polytherapy, in an effort to cover the entire spectrum of receptors when the search for an efficient monotherapy seems to be unsuccessful [6]. Antipsychotic polytherapy, is not supported by scientific evidence and involves a greater risk of side effects and therapeutic failure [7–10]. Adverse effects of a specific therapy may cause a special impact on the adherence to the treatment and the therapeutic success [9,10].

Precision Medicine derives from the creation of a diagnostic/prognostic approach, based on genetic, clinical, and environmental information relative to the patient, that makes possible to forecast the response to treatment and opt for the optimal therapeutic option [11,12]. The application of such strategies to routine psychiatric clinical practice may allow solving the problems related to adverse effects that condition the clinical evolution [13,14]. One of the more widespread hypotheses to explain this interindividual variable response to treatment directs the question to a pharmacokinetic cause. Therefore, it is proposed that the metabolism of the neuroleptics administered to the patient could explain these differences [15–17].

In our environment, the most commonly used atypical antipsychotics are metabolized mainly through the cytochrome P 450 (CYP450) system [18]. The superfamily CYP450 is a set of highly polymorphic genes, which suggests a possible strong genetic variability among individuals and, consequently, a potential strong phenotypic variability, which translates into different enzymatic activity on the drugs administered to the individual [15,19–22]. In addition, the therapeutic target of these drugs is found in the central nervous system, meaning they must pass through the blood-brain barrier [23], therefore, the genes involved in the absorption and transport process should be considered [24]. On the other hand, some major side effects related to antipsychotic administration could possibly be related to polymorphism of genes associated with neurotransmitters signaling or catabolic pathways, such as the cathechol-O-methyltransferase (COMT), and the dopamine receptor (DRD) family [25,26].

Application of precision medicine can help to decrease adverse events; however, so far it is mostly driven to specific drugs and oriented to genotype of the patient without considering drug-phenoconversion. This is a phenomenon that could cause genotypic extensive metabolizers to behave as phenotypic poor metabolizers [27]. In this sense, we have developed the 5SPM (5 step precision medicine) model [28] that simultaneously evaluates the effects of the pharmacological drug–drug and gene–drug interaction in the complete polypharmacy context of the prescription of each patient. The hypothesis of this study is that the application of 5SPM will lead to a reduction in the dosage of the drug used and in the number of polytherapy cases avoiding adverse effects and therapeutic failure.

2. Materials and Methods

2.1. Study Sample

A cohort of 188 patients from the psychiatry units of the Complejo Asistencial de Zamora (Zamora, Spain), Hospital Universitario Rio Hortega (Valladolid, Spain) and Hospital Universitario de Salamanca (Salamanca, Spain), was used for this study, and was analyzed in the Unidad de Medicina de Precisión of the latter. Patients gave informed consent for pharmacogenetic analysis according to the ethics committee of the Hospital Universitario de Salamanca (CEIC ref.: 107/12/2016). Criteria of inclusion were listed as: suffering from a prolonged serious mental illness, poor response to conventional treatment, which eventually results in polypharmacy, with its consequent adverse effects and little support by clinical guides in the matter. Patients who did not receive antipsychotic therapy and were under 16 years of age were excluded. Information was collected on the patient's diagnosis, current psychopharmacotherapy, and the dose/day used. Likewise, the age, gender, pharmacological history, and significant adverse effects related to antipsychotic therapy or its interactions with concomitant therapy that had been recorded in the patient's medical history were collected. Clinical and pharmacological data was recorded between 2013 and 2019.

Step Precision Medicine

The 5SPM method consisting of a five-step precision medicine protocol was applied, including: (1) obtaining of clinical, epidemiological, and therapeutical data, including current prescriptions, diagnosis and therapeutic response; (2) analysis of pharmacological interactions based on the drug-specific pharmacokinetic pathways of drugs included in the study by processing databases such as Pharmacogenomic Knowledgebase (PharmGKB) [29], PubMed-NCBI [30], Charite's SuperCYP-Transformer [31], and the Pharmacogene Variation (PharmVar) Consortium [32]. The potential drug—drug and gene drug interaction were analyzed from the previous databases to evaluate the probability of drug-phenoconversion (3) pharmacogenetic analysis of the genes chosen in the study. The genetic markers were selected considering the genes that code enzymes involved in their metabolism (4) correction of pharmacotherapy applied to the patient based on the data obtained by the previous three steps, resolving those cases in which: one or more prescribed drugs were metabolized by an enzyme that had an inefficient phenotype, a pharmacological interaction with influence on the plasma levels of one of the drugs involved was found, or when there was a potential phenoconversion effect due to one or more of the prescribed drugs, fixing those cases in which, there was a detriment to the patient; and (5) the study of results and a reassessment of the model by verifying the evolution of the patients involved (Figure 1, Figure S1). Pharmacogenetic testing (PGx) was performed using the AmpliChip CYP450 Test (Roche Molecular Diagnostics, Pleasanton, CA, USA) [33], the Autogenomics platform, MassARRAY 4.2 (Agena, India), and probe-based assays using the LightCycler platform (Roche Diagnostics, Basel, Switzerland) testing was performed following the directives of the European Molecular Genetics Management Network for DNA handling, with the requisite controls. The application of quality norms followed the UNE-EN-ISO 15189:2007 Normative in the Accredited Section of Molecular Genetics and Pharmacogenetics of the Clinical Biochemistry Service of the University Hospital in Salamanca. The normative included training and qualification of personal, preanalytical, analytical and postanalytical control, blinding, repeating measurements, and internal and external validity.

The genes studied were the ones encoding enzymes 1A2, 2B6, 2C9, 2C19, 2D6, 3A4, 3A5 of the CYP450 cytochrome family. The CYP450 superfamily is composed of highly polymorphic genes (see PharmVar.org). The usual approach to the relationship between genotypic variability and the metabolism of CYP450 substrates is based on the definition of metabolic phenotypes with their characteristic pharmacokinetic implications based on different genetic mechanisms. Poor metabolizers (PM) were associated with two inactive alleles. The combination of two reduced-activity alleles or a reduced-activity with an inactive allele or an inactive allele with an active allele results in an intermediate metabolizer (IM). An individual with two wt-like alleles was labelled as an extensive metabolizer (EM). The presence of a duplication in the absence of inactive or reduced activity alleles results in an ultrarapid metabolizer (UM) [34,35].

Antipsychotic dose comparison was made using chlorpromazine as a reference [36]; chlorpromazine equivalents were calculated by using dose converters to establish a unique chlorpromazine dose value (mg/day) for each patient, before and after the clinical intervention, even if the patient was prescribed with antipsychotic polytherapy.

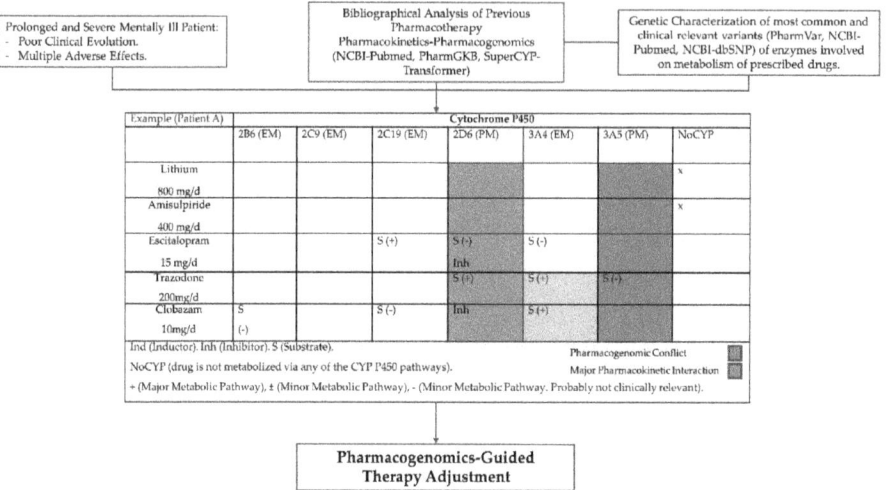

Figure 1. Practical application of the precision medicine model.

2.2. Statistics

Descriptive statistics were used to determine the central tendency and dispersion. Normality of the distribution was assessed using Kolmogorov–Smirnov test. Statistical power was calculated for sample size using Interactive Statistical Calculation Pages. Wilcoxon Paired Signed Test was used as a paired difference test to determine the difference in distribution of numerical non-gaussian variables before and after the application of PGx testing (i.e., chlorpromazine dose), Mcnemar Test was used to determine the paired homogeneity on nominal data. Statistical power calculation to test the primary hypothesis (reduction of clorpromazine-corrected antipsychotic dose via reduction of each patient's daily dose and the number of antipsychotic prescribed) was done assuming a mean initial chlorpromazine dose of 600 mg/d with an standard deviation of 1050 mg/d and a minimum clinically important difference of 200 mg/d, obtaining a value greater than 0.80 for an α value of 0.05.

3. Results

3.1. Demographics

The results are presented for a total of 188 patients, whose clinical data were collected between 2013 and 2019. The average age of the total study participants was 47.21 (±12.93) years (24–84), with 59.57% of the patients being female ($n = 112$). The distribution in diagnostics is presented in Table 1; the most common diagnosis was paranoid schizophrenia (Diagnostic and Statistical Manual of Mental Disorders, Fifth Edition, DSM-V, F20), which occurred in 67.02% of the cases ($n = 126$). Tobacco smoking was present in 51.38% of the patients ($n = 93$).

Table 1. Demographic data.

Variable	Value
PATIENTS	
Total number of patients included:	188
- Average age	47 (±13)
- Male: Female (%)	59.58:37.77

Table 1. Cont.

Variable	Value
DIAGNOSTIC	
DSM-V *	n (%)
DSM-V *	n (%)
F03—Dementia	1 (0.53)
F19—Substance-Related Disorder	12 (6.38)
F20—Schizophrenia	126 (67.02)
F22—Persistent Delusional Disorder	2 (1.06)
F23—Brief and Acute Psychotic Disorder	1 (0.53)
F25—Schizoaffective Disorder	13 (6.92)
F31—Bipolar Disorder	25 (13.30)
F33—Major Depressive Disorder	1 (0.53)
F60—Specific Personality Disorders	2 (1.06)
F61—Mixed Personality Disorder	1 (0.53)
F79—Intellectual Disability	2 (1.06)

* All the pathologies are referred to the official standard nomenclature of the Diagnostic and Statistical Manual of Mental Disorders 5th-edition (DSM-V).

3.2. Pharmacological Interactions

Data on drug prescribing prior to and after pharmacogenetic analysis are presented in Table 2. A total 343 antipsychotics (Table 2) were prescribed, for an average of 1.82 antipsychotics (range: 1 to 4) per patient, which in the course of this study and after the pharmacogenetic analysis, were reduced to 239, averaging to 1.27 antipsychotics per patient (range 1 to 3), meaning a 30.32% ($p < 0.05$) reduction. 20.75% of patients had more than five drugs prescribed, situation that was reduced to 10.64% ($p < 0.05$) and 71.28% of patients more than one neuroleptic, which goes down to 26.60% ($p < 0.05$) after the 5SPM application. On average, each patient has 14.55 less drugs prescribed and 23.63 less antipsychotics prescribed after the PGx-guided pharmacotherapy adjustment (Table 3) ($p < 0.05$).

Table 2. Antipsychotics prescriptions before/after PGx testing.

Antipsychotic	Presentation	
	Oral (n Before/After PGx)	IM (n Before/After PGx)
Amisulpride	14/7	
Aripiprazole	38/21	13/26
Asenapine	20/16	
Olanzapine	56/40	
Paliperidone	18/12	23 */66 *
Quetiapine	71/20	
Risperidone	44/2	5/0

PGx: Pharmacogenetic Analysis. * 5 (Before PGx) and 10 (After PGx) patients were prescribed coadjutant oral Paliperidone.

Two or more drugs mainly metabolized by the same enzyme prescribed to the patients were considered as an interaction regardless of the number of drugs involved and was counted independently for each CYP450 member. A total of 173 pharmacological interactions were discovered in the pharmacotherapy of the sample, including neuroleptics and concomitant therapy, both psychiatric and non-psychiatric. The cytochrome through which more conflicts occur was CYP3A4 ($n = 67$), followed by 3A5 ($n = 27$) and 1A2 ($n = 27$). Taking only neuroleptic therapy into account, 78 interactions were tested, most of which occur through cytochromes CYP3A4 ($n = 27$), CYP3A5 ($n = 27$), and CYP1A2 ($n = 17$). Following the modification of pharmacotherapy motivated by the pharmacogenetic study, these interactions were reduced to 135 (CYP3A4, 57; CYP2D6, 22; CYP2C9, 19) and 25 (CYP3A4, 10; CYP3A5, 10; CYP1A2, 5), achieving a reduction in pharmacological interactions of 26.10% ($p < 0.05$) and. 67.95% ($p < 0.05$), respectively (Figure 2).

Table 3. Drug prescriptions.

Variable	Value
DRUG PRESCRIPTIONS (Pre-PGx Testing/Post-PGx Testing)	
Total Number of drugs (n):	635/478
- Average drugs	3.67/3.11
- Average Antipsychotics	1.82/1.27
- More than 5 drugs prescribed (% of total)	20.75/10.64
- More than 1 antipsychotic prescribed (% of total)	71.28/26.60
- Average Within-Patient Drug Variation (%)	−14.55
- Average Within-Patient Antipsychotic Variation (%)	−23.63
Medication classes (% of total)	
A. Digestive system and metabolic	7.24/8.55
B. Blood and hematopoietic organs	0.32/0.00
C. Cardiovascular system	0.95/2.14
D. Dermatologic medications	0.00/0.00
E. Genitourinary apparatus and sex hormones	0.63/0.43
H. Systemic hormone preparations excluded hormones	2.68/4.06
J. Anti-infectious in general for systemic use	0.00/0.00
L. Antineoplastic and immunomodulatory agents	0.16/0.21
M. Skeletal muscle	0.00/0.00
N. Nervous system (Total)	87.72/86.74
N1. Antipsychotics	54.02/51.06
P. antiparasitic products, insecticides, and repellents	0.00/0.00
R. respiratory system	0.00/0.00
S. organs of the senses	0.00/0.00
V. various	0.32/0.00

PGx: Pharmacogenetic Analysis.

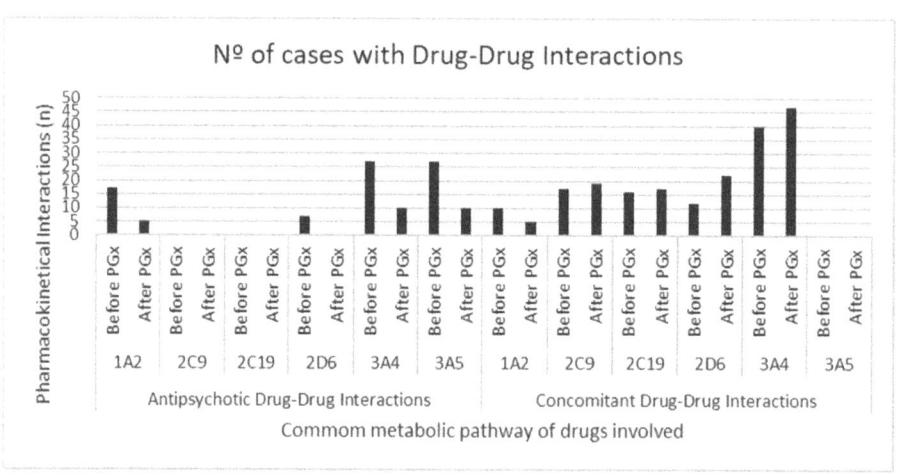

Figure 2. Number of conflicts found associated with each one of the Cytochrome P 450 (CYP450) members studied, before and after pharmacogenetic testing, including neuroleptic and concomitant therapy. PGx: Pharmacogenetic Analysis.

For approximately one quarter of the patients receiving polytherapy treatment, it involves the coadministration of olanzapine in infratherapeutic doses for hypnotic purposes, or coadministration of quetiapine for the same purpose. Therefore, there was a small percentage (less than 10%) who truly receives neuroleptic polytherapy as such (Table 4).

Table 4. Infratherapeutic dosage percentage.

	Pre-PGx (%)	Post-PGx (%)
Amisulpride (<400 mg)	14	86
Aripiprazole (<10 mg)	16	4
Asenapine (<5 mg)	0	0
Olanzapine (<10 mg)	11	45
Paliperidone (<6 mg)	46	72
Quetiapine (<400 mg)	66	95
Risperidone (<2 mg)	6	0

The criteria to decide what was considered to be the "minimum therapeutic dose" was based on their respective datasheets and the Sthal's Prescriber Guide. PGx: Pharmacogenetic Analysis.

3.3. Drug-Gene Conflicts

The presence of the alleles listed in Table 5 of the CYP1A2, CYP2B6, CYP2C9, CYP2C19, CYP2D6, CYP3A4, and CYP3A5 genes was analyzed in the Pharmacogenetics and Precision Medicine Unit of the University Hospital of Salamanca. Table 6 shows the frequency of occurrence of the estimated phenotypes from the detection of the different alleles in the sample. Notice that as a Precision Medicine-approach the model is adapted to the specific situation of the patient. Each patient was genotyped, selecting in each case the SNPs that could predict the metabolization of the prescribed therapy. Since each prescription can be different, SNPs can be different between patients.

Table 5. Pharmacogenetic testing. Genes and alleles included in the study.

Gene	Alleles
1A2	*1F
2B6	*6
2C9	*1 (WT), *2, *3
2C19	*1 (WT), *2, *4, *17
2D6	*1 (WT), *2, *3, *4, *5, *6, *7, *8, *9, *10, *12, *14, *17, *29, *41, *46
3A4	*1B
3A5	*3C

Alleles listed using the PharmVar Haplotype nomenclature. *: Allele. WT: Wild Type.

Table 6. Phenotype profile.

	n	PM	IM	EM	UM	HI
CYP1A2	179	-	-	13.97% (n = 25)		86.03% (n = 154)
CYP2B6	166	9.04% (n = 15)	40.96% (n = 68)	50% (n = 83)	-	
CYP2C9	183	7.10% (n = 13)	35.52% (n = 65)	57.38% (n = 105)	-	
CYP2C19	186	3.23% (n = 6)	20.43% (n = 38)	47.85% (n = 89)	27.96% (n = 52)	
CYP2D6	183	3.78% (n = 7)	5.95% (n = 11)	85.95% (n = 159)	3.24% (n = 6)	
CYP3A4	188	1.06% (n = 2)	7.45% (n = 14)	91.49% (n = 172)	-	
CYP3A5	187	87.85% (n = 159)	13.81% (n = 25)	1.66% (n = 3)	-	

Allele Frequencies of the sample were similar to the NCBI dbSNP ALFA Project Frequencies [37]. PM: Poor Metabolizer. IM: Intermediate Metabolizer. EM: Extensive Metabolizer. UM: Ultrarapid Metabolizer. HI: Higher Inducibility.

The CYP1A2 gene was studied in 179 patients, with the most prevalent phenotype being HI (Higher Inducibility) (86.03%, $n = 154$). Among the 166 patients who were tested for the CYP2B6 gene, the most common phenotype was EM (Extensive Metabolizer) (50.00%, n. 83). In reference to the CYP2C9 and CYP2C19 genes ($n = 183$, $n = 186$), the majority phenotype was EM (57.38%, $n = 105$; 47.85%, $n = 89$). Most patients had an EM phenotype (85.95%, $n = 159$; 91.49%, $n = 172$) with respect to CYP2D6 cytochromes ($n = 183$) and CYP3A4 ($n = 188$), and PM (Poor Metabolizer) phenotype (87.85%, $n = 159$) was the most frequent with respect to CYP3A5 cytochrome ($n = 187$).

In total, taking into account the liver metabolism, mediated through the previously mentioned CYP450 system members, from both antipsychotic therapy (Table 7) [18,31,38] and concomitant therapy, 458 conflicts were discovered between the patient's prescription and genotype, with most conflicts associated with concomitant therapy occurring through cytochrome CYP3A5 ($n = 57$), and those primarily related to the metabolism of neuroleptics occurring through CYP1A2 ($n = 80$); taking into account the minor metabolizers of the studied antipsychotics, the cytochrome with the highest number of incidences found was CYP3A5 ($n = 93$) (Figure 3). The number of prescriptions of antipsychotics to patients with non-efficient metabolic phenotypes is summarized in Table 8. Following the conduct of the pharmacogenetic study, the total drug-gene conflicts were reduced by 11.02% ($p < 0.05$), based on a reduction in conflicts between neuroleptic therapy and the patient genotype of 19.80% ($p < 0.05$) considering all possible interactions, and 39.02% ($p < 0.05$) considering those that had a noticeable potential impact on the plasma levels of the drug involved. Moreover, with drug-drug interactions, there were more gene-drug interactions associated with non-psychiatric concomitant therapy.

Table 7. Antipsychotic therapy CYP450-mediated metabolism.

	Major Metabolizer	Minor Metabolizer	Product
Olanzapine ^	CYP1A2	CYP2D6 *,#	Inactive
Aripiprazole	CYP2D6 #,‡, CYP3A4	CYP3A5 *	Active
Risperidone	CYP2D6 #	CYP3A4 #	Active (Paliperidone)
Amisulpride		NO CYP	
Clozapine	CYP1A2 #, CYP3A4 #,‡	CYP2C19 *,#, CYP2C9 *,#, CYP2D6 #, CYP3A5 *,#	Reduced Activity, Inactive (CYP1A2/CYP3A4)
Paliperidone		NO CYP	
Quetiapine	CYP3A4	CYP3A5 *, CYP2D6 *,#	Inactive
Asenapine	CYP1A2	CYP2D6 †	Inactive
Levomepromazine	CYP3A4 #	CYP1A2	Inactive

* Almost null influence on plasma levels, # substrate inhibition, † suicide inhibition, ‡ inductor, ^ inhibits CYP3A4.

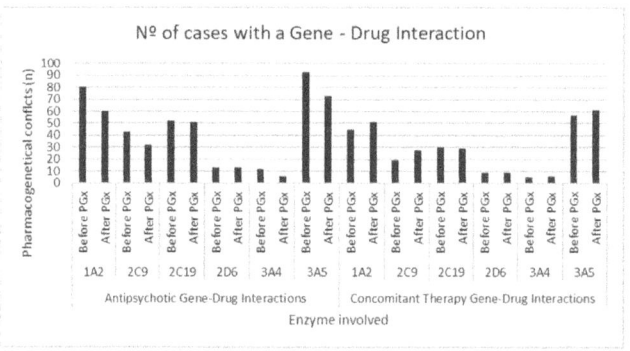

Figure 3. Number of conflicts between the patients' genotype and the prescribed pharmacotherapy associated with each member of the CYP450 system studied. PGx: Pharmacogenetic Analysis.

Table 8. Number of cases (and percentage of the total of individuals presenting each specific phenotype) prescribed with and antipsychotic metabolized by an altered pathway.

n before PGx/ n after PGx (%)	1A2 HI	2D6 PM	2D6 IM	2D6 UM	3A4 PM	3A4 IM	3A5 PM	3A5 IM
Aripiprazole	-	1 (14.3)/ 1 (14.3)	1 (9.1)/ 2 (18.2)	1 (16.7)/ 0 (0)	1 (50)/0 (0)	7 (50)/ 3 (21.4)	42 (26.4)/ 42 (26.4)	8 (32)/ 5 (20)
Asenapine	11 (7.1)/ 11 (7.1)	1 (14.3)/ 1 (14.3)	2 (18.2)/ 2 (18.2)	0 (0)/0 (0)	-	-	-	-
Clozapine	34 (22.1)/ 21 (13.6)	1 (14.3)/ 2 (28.6)	1 (9.1)/ 1 (9.1)	2 (33.3)/ 1 (16.7)	0 (0)/ 1 (50)	4 (28.6)/ 2 (14.3)	31 (19.5)/ 21 (13.2)	7 (28)/ 4 (16)
Olanzapine	51 (33.1)/ 31 (20.1)	3 (42.9)/ 3 (42.9)	4 (36.4)/ 4 (36.4)	1 (16.7)/ 1 (16.7)	-	-	-	-
Quetiapine	-	2 (28.6)/ 0 (0)	2 (18.2)/ 1 (9.1)	3 (50)/ 1 (16.7)	1 (50)/ 0 (0)	5 (35.7)/ 1 (7.1)	59 (37.1)/ 16 (10.1)	11 (44)/ 4 (16)
Risperidone	-	2 (28.6)/ 0 (0)	2 (18.2)/ 0 (0)	3 (50)/ 0 (0)	0 (0)/ 0 (0)	0 (0)/0 (0)	-	-

HI: Higher Inducibility. PM: Poor Metabolizer. IM: Intermediate Metabolizer. UM: Ultrarapid Metabolizer.

3.4. Clinical Impact

The number of prescriptions for the most widely used atypical neuroleptic drugs, together with the prescribed minimum, maximum, and mean dose (mg/day), prior to and after intervention using method 5SPM, are listed in Tables 9 and 10. It is frequent to see doses beyond the recommended upper limit registered in the pharmacological data sheet of each drug, as frequently prescribe doses were increased by 20–30% before making the decision of considering the pharmacotherapy as a failure and choosing other neuroleptic [39]. As can be seen, the prescription of oral drugs whose metabolism is related to enzymes frequently altered in the study population, is reduced by between 20 and 100%, in favor of intramuscular prescriptions that either do not have liver metabolism, such as Paliperidone, which increases by 186.95%, or whose main route of metabolism is associated with an enzyme that usually has no alterations, such as Aripiprazole, whose prescriptions increase by 100%, predominantly metabolized by CYP3A4.

Table 9. Mean, Min, and Max Daily Dose prescribed to the study population.

	Pre-PGx			Post-PGx			Variation		
	Mean Dose (mg/d)	Min Dose (mg/d)	Max Dose (mg/d)	Mean Dose (mg/d)	Min Dose (mg/d)	Max Dose (mg/d)	Mean Dose (mg/d)	Min Dose (mg/d)	Max Dose (mg/d)
Olanzapine	16.38	2.5	45	10.5	2.5	40	−0.36	0	−0.11
Aripiprazole	14.79	3	30	14.06	3	30	−0.05	0	0
Risperidone	5.39	1	28.33	5.5	5	6	0.02	4	−0.79
Amisulpride	514.29	100	1000	224.57	100	400	−0.56	0	−0.6
Clozapine	325	100	700	253.85	100	400	−0.22	0	−0.43
Paliperidone	7.08	3	14	5.89	3	9	−0.17	0	−0.36
Quetiapine	304.01	10	1200	199.5	40	600	−0.34	3	−0.5
Asenapine	11.75	5	20	10	5	20	−0.15	0	0

Stahl Prescriber Guide dose ranges (mg/d): amisulpride (400–800), aripiprazole (15–20), asenapine (10–20), clozapine (300–450), olanzapine (10–20), quetiapine (400–800), risperidone (2–8). PGx: Pharmacogenetic Analysis.

To establish comparisons at the prescribed mean dose of antipsychotic drugs, chlorpromazine was established as a reference drug. The average dose of the different antipsychotics used in the sample per patient, and the average dose of chlorpromazine associated with them, is shown in Figure 4. The reduction by 50.88% ($p < 0.05$) of the mean dose of chlorpromazine per patient in mg/d following the application of the pharmacogenetic study is noteworthy, as an average each patient was prescribed 36.40 less chlorpromazine-corrected antipsychotic dose (384.94 mg/d) (Table 11) ($p < 0.05$). Likewise, the proportion of patients above 800 mg/d was reduced from 34.95% to 1.61% ($p < 0.05$), and the proportion of patients below 300 mg/d increases from 15.05% to 33.87% ($p < 0.05$). A reduction of more than 20% in the dose of chlorpromazine was observed in 78.19% of the sample, achieving a reduction of more than 60% in 23.40% of the sample ($p < 0.05$).

Table 10. % of prescriptions of the different antipsychotics and presentations.

% Prescriptions	PrePGx	PostPGx	Variation
Olanzapine	29.8	21.3	−28.6
Aripiprazole (Oral)	20.2	11.2	−44.7
Aripiprazole (IM)	6.9	13.8	+100.0
Risperidone	23.4	1.1	−95.5
Risperidone (IM)	2.7	0	−100.0
Clozapine	20.2	13.8	−31.6
Quetiapine	37.8	10.6	−71.8
Asenapine	10.6	8.5	−20.0
Amisulpride	7.4	3.7	−50.0
Paliperidone (Oral)	9.6	6.4	−33.3
Paliperidone (IM)	12.2	35.1	+186.9

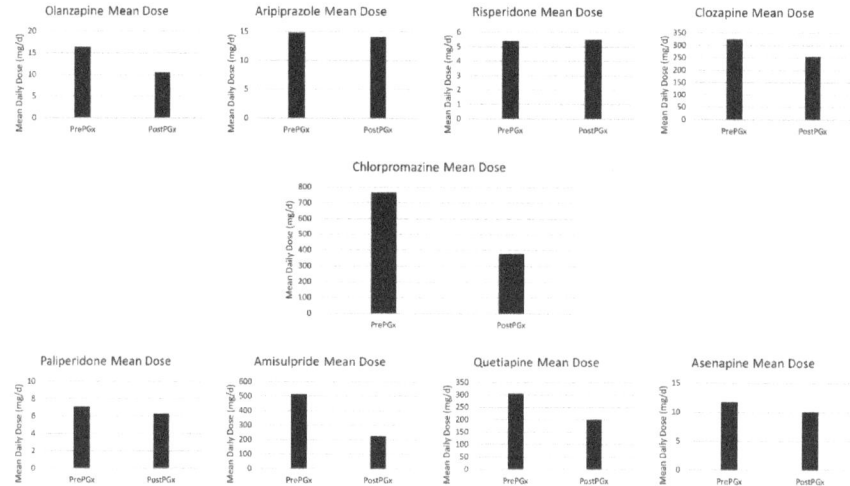

Figure 4. Antipsychotics mean dose and chlorpromazine conversion.

Table 11. Within-patient variation on antipsychotic daily dose.

	Excluding Therapy Switches		Including Therapy Switches	
Antipsychotic	Mean Variation (%) (CI 95%)	Standard Deviation	Mean Variation (%) (CI 95%)	Standard Deviation
Olanzapine	−30.69 (−35.34, −26.04)	32.54	−30.75 (−42.43, −19.07)	81.71
Aripiprazole	6.37 (−0.24, 12.98)	46.22	−3.22 (−15.19, 8.75)	83.76
Risperidone	0	0	−94 (−98.44, −89.56)	31.05
Amisulpride	−25 (−28.57, −21.43)	25	−39.48 (−51.88, −27.08)	86.73
Clozapine	−23.6 (−27.51, −19.69)	27.33	−27.54 (−39.87, −15.21)	86.24

Table 11. Cont.

Antipsychotic	Excluding Therapy Switches		Including Therapy Switches	
	Mean Variation (%) (CI 95%)	Standard Deviation	Mean Variation (%) (CI 95%)	Standard Deviation
Paliperidone	−3.7 (−8.32, 0.92)	32.3	40.33 (29.86, 50.79)	73.21
Quetiapine	−24.38 (−30.38, −18.38)	41.95	−73.2 (−81.04, −65.36)	54.87
Asenapine	−13.89 (−16.78, −10.99)	20.23	−16.12 (−28.79, −3.44)	88.67
	Mean Variation (%) (CI 95%)	Standard Deviation		
Chlorpromazine Conversion	−36.4 (−42.12, −30.68)	40.02		

Mean relative within-patient difference in daily dose comparing itself before and after the application of the *5-step Precision Medicine* (5SPM) model. CI: Confidence Interval

4. Discussion

A patient with prolonged severe mental illness usually has a heterogeneous and highly variable symptomatology, including positive, negative, affective, and cognitive symptomatology, which usually induces the prescriber to opt for the use of the combination of several drugs. However, polypharmacy is not a practice supported by scientific evidence and often carries an increased risk of adverse effects [8], which may imply less adherence to treatment and consequent therapeutic failure, with a higher number of hospital admissions and emergency care, and subsequently increased economic and personal expenditure [19].

It is necessary to know the adverse effects profile of neuroleptic treatment in order to perform a risk-benefit balance and thereby facilitate the individualization of the therapy. Polytherapy treatment is considered "justifiable" by some authors given the presence of a profile of adverse effects that hinders adherence to treatment by the patient, or that is detrimental to an underlying pathology of the individual, or when the therapeutic response has not been effective with the antipsychotics available for the specific case of the subject [40]. Consequently, knowledge of the pharmacogenetic profile of the patients becomes more relevant, so that monotherapy adapted to their metabolism can predominantly be applied, suitable for the treatment of symptomatic exacerbations and maintenance, reducing the presence of adverse effects [15].

This study is a retrospective descriptive analysis of 188 patients suffering from a prolonged serious mental illness, poor response to conventional treatment, which eventually results in polypharmacy, to whom the 5SPM model was applied. A PGx analysis was carried out aiming to study the main cytochromes involved in both the metabolism of the most commonly used atypical antipsychotics in their clinical centers, as well as in the metabolism of concomitant. It is important to clarify that, even being the application of the 5SPM Model intended as a multidisciplinary effort, the adjustment made on these patients' pharmacotherapy was mediated by the Psychiatry Department, therefore we discovered more interactions in the sample regarding non-psychiatric concomitanttherapy.

After making corrections on patient pharmacotherapy as part of the 5SPM model, our study revealed a significant reduction in the mean dose of antipsychotic (approximately 50%), which is justified both by the reduction in doses of neuroleptic administered, and by the reduction in approximately 60% of patients receiving two or more antipsychotics.

The pharmacogenetic profile of the population (CYP1A2 HI: 0.86; CYP2D6 EM: 0.85; CYP3A4 EM: 0.91) could explain the need to apply a higher dose with its consequent adverse effects in patients treated with olanzapine [41], clozapine [42], or asenapine [43], all related to CYP1A2, while favoring the use of aripiprazole or risperidone in those who have a wt-like haplotype in CYP2D6 [44–49] and CYP3A4 [44,50] cytochromes, a situation frequently found in our population.

The significant decrease in the mean dose of neuroleptic per patient should be discussed, together with the fact of the increase in the prescription of paliperidone and aripiprazole IM (DEPOT), the use of which doubles and almost triples from the beginning of the study. Aripiprazole is a neuroleptic whose metabolism develops predominantly in the liver, through the CYP450 system, specifically by CYP2D6 and CYP3A4 cytochromes which, in the vast majority of our patients (more than 80%), presented an EM phenotype, favoring its use. Paliperidone is an active metabolite of risperidone that has no liver metabolism. This, together with the fact that they are injectable presentations, favors the prevention of side effects and adherence to treatment, with its consequent positive effect when assessing therapeutic success. As mentioned above, there is a decrease in the use of olanzapine (Oral), aripiprazole (Oral), risperidone (Oral and IM), clozapine (Oral), quetiapine (Oral), asenapine (Oral), and paliperidone (Oral) in favor of these long-lasting injectable presentations, presenting better compliance, a potential decrease in hospital admissions, and a reduction in adverse effects. The preference in the use of these antipsychotics is largely determined by the profile of adverse effects associated with them, influenced by the rational approach that this study proposes. In our sample, DEPOT antipsychotics are prescribed frequently as monotherapy and the patients are administered a standardized dose by sanitary personnel, ensuring treatment compliance. Furthermore, gastrointestinal absorption variables, not always totally controlled in this type of patients (such as alcohol consumption), are nullified. One of the main problems of polytherapy is the potential presence of pharmacological interactions, which may lead to an alteration of the biological availability of one of the drugs involved, with the consequent alteration of the therapeutic effect on its target and the presence of possible adverse effects. Drug-induced phenoconversion during routine clinical practice remains a major public health issue (27). This phenomenon needs to be well addressed by precision medicine approaches focused in the drugs in the context of the patient prescription and oriented not only to genotype but considering drug–drug and gene–drug interactions. In fact phenoconversion has been previously called the Achilles' heel of personalized medicine reporting three principal concerns; drugs susceptible to phenoconversion, co-medications that can cause phenoconversion, and dosage amendments that need to be applied during and following phenoconversion (27).

The application of 5SPM has helped us to significantly reduce interaction in our patients, either by an increase in the use of drugs not metabolized by the CYP450 system, the decrease in polytherapy previously exposed, or the possible didactic role on medical personnel that the implementation of pharmacogenetic analysis may have provided, regarding the role of the CYP450 system in antipsychotic metabolism. This methodology has led to the discovery of a large number of cases in which there was a problem in the pharmacotherapy due to the metabolism mainly mediated by CYP1A2. In the vast majority of cases, the dose administered per patient has been reduced, as well as cases of polytherapy. It should be noted that the use of DEPOT presentations of drugs such as paliperidone (not metabolized by the CYP450 system) or aripiprazole (whose predominant pathway within the CYP450 system is CYP3A4, which presents a wt-like genotype in the vast majority of the study population) has been the solution for the majority of problematic cases, because of the pharmacogenetic profile of the sample, even considering that each patient was studied individually attending its personal genetic implications. In conclusion, the success achieved in reducing the average dose of antipsychotic administered per patient, which has in turn facilitated the avoidance of a large number of adverse effects and potentially reduced the cost per patient, may be due to the combination of applying a methodology such as 5SPM, focused on the genetic and environmental circumstances of the patient alongside the rise of DEPOT prescriptions, which facilitate adherence to treatment and the use of standardized doses.

Supplementary Materials: The following are available online at http://www.mdpi.com/2075-4426/10/4/289/s1. Figure S1: 5 Step precision medicine model.

Author Contributions: Conceptualization, M.J.G.-S., M.Á.F.-M., and M.I.-G.; methodology, L.C.-L., I.R.-G., M.I.-G.; software, L.C.-L., I.R.-G.; validation, M.I.-G., M.B.G.-B., E.M.-V.; formal analysis, L.C.-L., I.R.-G.; investigation, L.C.-L., I.R.-G.; resources, S.S.-I., C.L., M.Á.F.-M.; data curation, L.C.-L.; writing—original draft preparation, L.C.-L., I.R.-G.; writing—review and editing, M.I.-G., A.S.-M.; visualization, L.C.-L., I.R.-G., M.I.-G.; supervision,

M.I.-G.; project administration, M.Á.F.-M., M.J.G.-S., and M.I.-G.; funding acquisition, M.Á.F.-M. and M.I.-G. All authors have read and agreed to the published version of the manuscript.

Funding: This research received no external funding.

Conflicts of Interest: The authors declare no conflict of interest. The funders had no role in the design of the study; in the collection, analyses, or interpretation of data; in the writing of the manuscript, or in the decision to publish the results.

References

1. Turner, T. Chlorpromazine: Unlocking psychosis. *BMJ* **2007**, *334* (Suppl. 1), s7. Available online: https://www.bmj.com/content/334/suppl_1/s7 (accessed on 4 November 2020). [CrossRef] [PubMed]
2. Pieters, T.; Majerus, B. The introduction of chlorpromazine in Belgium and the Netherlands (1951–1968); tango between old and new treatment features. *Stud. Hist. Philos. Sci. Part C Stud. Hist. Philos. Biol. Biomed. Sci.* **2011**, *42*, 443–452. [CrossRef] [PubMed]
3. Naber, D.; Haasen, C.; Perro, C. Clozapine: The first atypical antipsychotic. In *Atypical Antipsychotics*; Springer Science and Business Media LLC: Berlin/Heidelberg, Germany, 2000; pp. 145–162. Available online: https://link.springer.com/chapter/10.1007/978-3-0348-8448-8_8 (accessed on 4 November 2020).
4. Lally, J.; MacCabe, J.H. Antipsychotic medication in schizophrenia: A review. *Br. Med. Bull.* **2015**, *114*, 169–179. Available online: https://pubmed.ncbi.nlm.nih.gov/25957394/ (accessed on 4 November 2020). [CrossRef] [PubMed]
5. Heuvel, L.L.V.D. Stahl's essential psychopharmacology: Neuroscientific basis and practical applications (4th edition). *J. Child Adolesc. Ment. Health* **2014**, *26*, 157–158. Available online: https://www.tandfonline.com/doi/abs/10.2989/17280583.2014.914944 (accessed on 4 November 2020). [CrossRef]
6. Shenoy, S.; Amrtavarshini, R.; Bhandary, R.P.; Praharaj, S.K. Frequency, reasons, and factors associated with antipsychotic polypharmacy in Schizophrenia: A retrospective chart review in a tertiary hospital in India. *Asian J. Psychiatry* **2020**, *51*, 102022. Available online: https://linkinghub.elsevier.com/retrieve/pii/S1876201820301337 (accessed on 4 November 2020). [CrossRef]
7. Lin, S.K. Antipsychotic Polypharmacy: A Dirty Little Secret or a Fashion? *Int. J. Neuropsychopharmacol.* **2020**, *23*, 125–131. Available online: https://academic.oup.com/ijnp/article/23/2/125/5684986 (accessed on 4 November 2020). [CrossRef]
8. Yamanouchi, Y.; Sukegawa, T.; Inagaki, A.; Inada, T.; Yoshio, T.; Yoshimura, R.; Iwata, N. Evaluation of the individual safe correction of antipsychotic agent polypharmacy in Japanese patients with chronic schizophrenia: Validation of safe corrections for antipsychotic polypharmacy and the high-dose method. *Int. J. Neuropsychopharmacol.* **2014**, *18*. Available online: https://pubmed.ncbi.nlm.nih.gov/25522380/ (accessed on 4 November 2020). [CrossRef]
9. Kamei, H.; Yamada, H.; Hatano, M.; Hanya, M.; Yamada, S.; Iwata, N. Effectiveness in Switching from Antipsychotic Polypharmacy to Monotherapy in Patients with Schizophrenia: A Case Series. *Clin. Psychopharmacol. Neurosci.* **2020**, *18*, 159–163. [CrossRef]
10. Kasteridis, P.; Ride, J.; Gutacker, N.; Aylott, L.; Dare, C.; Doran, T.; Gilbody, S.; Goddard, M.; Gravelle, H.; Kendrick, T.; et al. Association Between Antipsychotic Polypharmacy and Outcomes for People With Serious Mental Illness in England. *Psychiatr. Serv.* **2019**, *70*, 650–656. Available online: https://pubmed.ncbi.nlm.nih.gov/31109263/ (accessed on 4 November 2020). [CrossRef]
11. König, I.R.; Fuchs, O.; Hansen, G.; Von Mutius, E.; Kopp, M.V. What is precision medicine? *Eur. Respir. J.* **2017**, *50*, 1700391. [CrossRef]
12. Carrasco-Ramiro, F.; Peiró-Pastor, R.; Aguado, B. Human genomics projects and precision medicine. *Gene Ther.* **2017**, *24*, 551–561. [CrossRef] [PubMed]
13. Beckmann, J.S.; Lew, D. Reconciling evidence-based medicine and precision medicine in the era of big data: Challenges and opportunities. *Genome Med.* **2016**, *8*, 1–11. Available online: https://pubmed.ncbi.nlm.nih.gov/27993174/ (accessed on 4 November 2020). [CrossRef] [PubMed]
14. Liperoti, R.; Bernabei, R.; Onder, G. Managing Antipsychotic Medications in Schizophrenia: Comprehensive Assessment and Personalized Care to Improve Clinical Outcomes and Reduce Costs. *J. Clin. Psychiatry* **2015**, *76*, e1159–e1160. Available online: http://www.psychiatrist.com/jcp/article/pages/2015/v76n09/v76n0922.aspx (accessed on 4 November 2020). [CrossRef] [PubMed]

15. Osmanova, D.Z.; Freidin, M.B.; Fedorenko, O.Y.; Pozhidaev, I.V.; Boiko, A.S.; Vyalova, N.M.; Tiguntsev, V.V.; ooa, .; Loonen, A.J.M.; Semke, A.V.; et al. A pharmacogenetic study of patients with schizophrenia from West Siberia gets insight into dopaminergic mechanisms of antipsychotic-induced hyperprolactinemia. *BMC Med. Genet.* **2019**, *20*, 35–44. Available online: https://pubmed.ncbi.nlm.nih.gov/30967134/ (accessed on 4 November 2020). [CrossRef]
16. Lee, B.S.; McIntyre, R.S.; Gentle, J.E.; Park, N.S.; Chiriboga, D.A.; Lee, Y.; Singh, S.; McPherson, M.A. A computational algorithm for personalized medicine in schizophrenia. *Schizophr. Res.* **2018**, *192*, 131–136. Available online: https://pubmed.ncbi.nlm.nih.gov/28495491/ (accessed on 4 November 2020). [CrossRef]
17. Li, N.; Cao, T.; Wu, X.; Tang, M.; Xiang, D.; Cai, H. Progress in genetic polymorphisms related to lipid disturbances induced by atypical antipsychotic drugs. *Front. Pharmacol. Front. Media* **2020**, *10*. Available online: /pmc/articles/PMC7011106/?report=abstract (accessed on 4 November 2020). [CrossRef]
18. Urichuk, L.; Prior, T.I.; Dursun, S.; Baker, G. Metabolism of Atypical Antipsychotics: Involvement of Cytochrome P450 Enzymes and Relevance for Drug-Drug Interactions. *Curr. Drug Metab.* **2008**, *9*, 410–418. Available online: http://www.eurekaselect.com/openurl/content.php?genre=article&issn=1389-2002&volume=9&issue=5&spage=410 (accessed on 4 November 2020). [CrossRef]
19. Herbild, L.; Andersen, S.E.; Rasmussen, H.B.; Jürgens, G.; Werge, T. Does Pharmacogenetic Testing for CYP450 2D6 and 2C19 Among Patients with Diagnoses within the Schizophrenic Spectrum Reduce Treatment Costs? *Basic Clin. Pharmacol. Toxicol.* **2013**, *113*, 266–272. [CrossRef]
20. Lu, Y.F.; Goldstein, D.B.; Angrist, M.; Cavalleri, G. Personalized medicine and human genetic diversity. *Cold Spring Harb. Perspect Med.* **2014**, *4*. Available online: https://pubmed.ncbi.nlm.nih.gov/25059740/ (accessed on 4 November 2020). [CrossRef]
21. Pina-Camacho, L.; Díaz-Caneja, C.M.; Saiz, P.A.; Bobes, J.; Corripio, I.; Grasa, E. Estudio farmacogenético del tratamiento a largo plazo con antipsicóticos de segunda generación y sus efectos adversos metabólicos (Estudio SLiM): Justificación, objetivos, diseño y descripción de la muestra. *Rev. Psiquiatr. Salud. Ment.* **2014**, *7*, 166–178. Available online: https://pubmed.ncbi.nlm.nih.gov/25440735/ (accessed on 4 November 2020). [CrossRef]
22. Ravyn, D.; Ravyn, V.; Lowney, R.; Nasrallah, H.A. CYP450 Pharmacogenetic treatment strategies for antipsychotics: A review of the evidence. *Schizophr. Res.* **2013**, *149*, 1–14. [CrossRef] [PubMed]
23. Javaid, J.I. Clinical pharmacokinetics of antipsychotics. *J. Clin. Pharmacol.* **1994**, *34*, 286–295. Available online: https://pubmed.ncbi.nlm.nih.gov/7911807/ (accessed on 4 November 2020). [CrossRef] [PubMed]
24. Moons, T.; De Roo, M.; Claes, S.; Dom, G. Relationship between P-glycoprotein and second-generation antipsychotics. *Pharmacogenomics* **2011**, *12*, 1193–1211. Available online: https://pubmed.ncbi.nlm.nih.gov/21843066/ (accessed on 4 November 2020). [CrossRef] [PubMed]
25. Zivković, M.; Mihaljević-Peles, A.; Bozina, N.; Sagud, M.; Nikolac-Perkovic, M.; Vuksan-Cusa, B.; Muck-Seler, D. The Association Study of Polymorphisms in DAT, DRD2, and COMT Genes and Acute Extrapyramidal Adverse Effects in Male Schizophrenic Patients Treated With Haloperidol. *J. Clin. Psychopharmacol.* **2013**, *33*, 593–599. [CrossRef]
26. Gassó, P.; Mas, S.; Bernardo, M.; Alvarez, S.; Parellada, E.; Lafuente, A. A common variant in DRD3 gene is associated with risperidone-induced extrapyramidal symptoms. *Pharm. J.* **2009**, *9*, 404–410. Available online: https://pubmed.ncbi.nlm.nih.gov/19506579 (accessed on 4 November 2020). [CrossRef]
27. Shah, R.R.; Smith, R.L. Addressing phenoconversion: The Achilles' heel of personalized medicine. *Br. J. Clin. Pharmacol.* **2015**, *79*, 222–240. [CrossRef]
28. Isidoro-García, M.; Sanchez-Martin, A.; Garcia-Berrocal, B. Impact of New Technologies on Pharmacogenomics. *Curr. Pharm. Pers. Med.* **2017**, *14*, 74–85. [CrossRef]
29. PharmGKB. Available online: https://www.pharmgkb.org/ (accessed on 4 November 2020).
30. Available online: https://pubmed.ncbi.nlm.nih.gov/ (accessed on 4 November 2020).
31. Hoffmann, M.F.; Preissner, S.C.; Nickel, J.; Dunkel, M.; Preissner, R.; Preissner, S. The Transformer database: Biotransformation of xenobiotics. *Nucleic Acids Res.* **2014**, *42*, D1113–D1117. Available online: https://pubmed.ncbi.nlm.nih.gov/24334957/ (accessed on 4 November 2020). [CrossRef]
32. Gaedigk, A.; Ingelman-Sundberg, M.; Miller, N.A.; Leeder, J.S.; Whirl-Carrillo, M.; Klein, T.E.; the PharmVar Steering Committee. The Pharmacogene Variation (PharmVar) Consortium: Incorporation of the Human Cytochrome P450 (CYP) Allele Nomenclature Database. *Clin. Pharmacol. Ther.* **2018**, *103*, 399–401. Available online: http://www.ncbi.nlm.nih.gov/pubmed/29134625 (accessed on 4 November 2020). [CrossRef]

33. De Leon, J.; Susce, M.T.; Murray-Carmichael, E. The AmpliChipTM CYP450 Genotyping Test. *Mol. Diagn Ther.* **2012**, *10*, 135–151. [CrossRef]
34. Waring, R.H. Cytochrome P450: Genotype to phenotype. *Xenobiotica* **2020**, *50*, 9–18. Available online: https://pubmed.ncbi.nlm.nih.gov/31411087/ (accessed on 4 November 2020). [CrossRef] [PubMed]
35. Samer, C.; Lorenzini, K.I.; Rollason, V.; Daali, Y.; Desmeules, J.A. Applications of CYP450 Testing in the Clinical Setting. *Mol. Diagn. Ther.* **2013**, *17*, 165–184. Available online: http://link.springer.com/10.1007/s40291-013-0028-5 (accessed on 4 November 2020). [CrossRef]
36. Venkatasubramanian, G.; Danivas, V. Current perspectives on chlorpromazine equivalents: Comparing apples and oranges! *Indian J. Psychiatry* **2013**, *55*, 207–208. Available online: https://www.ncbi.nlm.nih.gov/pmc/articles/PMC3696254/ (accessed on 12 October 2020). [CrossRef] [PubMed]
37. Phan, Y.L.; Jin, H.; Zhang, W.; Qiang, E.; Shekhtman, D.; Shao, D.; Revoe, R.; Villamarin, E.; Ivanchenko, M.; Kimura, Z.Y.; et al. *ALFA: Allele Frequency Aggregator*; National Center for Biotechnology Information, U.S. National Library of Medicine, U.S.: Rockville Pike, Bethesda, MD, USA, 2020. Available online: www.ncbi.nlm.nih.gov/snp/docs/gsr/alfa/ (accessed on 4 November 2020).
38. Sheehan, J.J.; Sliwa, J.; Amatniek, J.; Grinspan, A.; Canuso, C. Atypical Antipsychotic Metabolism and Excretion. *Curr. Drug Metab.* **2010**, *11*, 516–525. Available online: https://pubmed.ncbi.nlm.nih.gov/20540690/ (accessed on 4 November 2020). [CrossRef] [PubMed]
39. Samara, M.T.; Klupp, E.; Helfer, B.; Rothe, P.H.; Schneider-Thoma, J.; Leucht, S. Increasing antipsychotic dose for non response in schizophrenia. *Cochrane Database Syst. Rev.* **2018**, *5*, CD011883. [CrossRef] [PubMed]
40. Huffman, J.C.; Chang, T.E.; Durham, L.E.; Weiss, A.P. Antipsychotic polytherapy on an inpatient psychiatric unit: How does clinical practice coincide with Joint Commission guidelines? *Gen. Hosp. Psychiatry* **2011**, *33*, 501–508. [CrossRef] [PubMed]
41. Söderberg, M.M.; Haslemo, T.; Molden, E.; Dahl, M.-L. Influence of CYP1A1/CYP1A2 and AHR polymorphisms on systemic olanzapine exposure. *Pharmacogenet. Genom.* **2013**, *23*, 279–285. Available online: http://www.ncbi.nlm.nih.gov/pubmed/23492908 (accessed on 4 November 2020). [CrossRef]
42. Kohlrausch, F.B.; Gama, C.S.; Lobato, M.I.; Belmontedeabreu, P.S.; Gesteira, A.; Barros-Angueira, F.; Carracedo, Á.; Hutz, M.H. Molecular diversity at theCYP2D6locus in healthy and schizophrenic southern Brazilians. *Pharmacogenomics* **2009**, *10*, 1457–1466. Available online: http://www.ncbi.nlm.nih.gov/pubmed/19761369 (accessed on 4 November 2020). [CrossRef]
43. Correll, C.U.; Citrome, L.; Haddad, P.M.; Lauriello, J.; Olfson, M.; Calloway, S.M. The use of long-acting injectable antipsychotics in Schizophrenia: Evaluating the evidence. *J. Clin. Psychiatry Physicians* **2020**, *77*, 3–24. Available online: https://pubmed.ncbi.nlm.nih.gov/27732772/ (accessed on 4 November 2020). [CrossRef]
44. Belmonte, C.; Ochoa, D.; Román, M.; Saiz-Rodríguez, M.; Wojnicz, A.; Gómez-Sánchez, C.I.; Martin-Vilchez, S.; Abad-Santos, F. Influence of CYP2D6, CYP3A4, CYP3A5 and ABCB1 Polymorphisms on Pharmacokinetics and Safety of Aripiprazole in Healthy Volunteers. *Basic Clin. Pharmacol. Toxicol.* **2018**, *122*, 596–605. Available online: https://pubmed.ncbi.nlm.nih.gov/29325225/ (accessed on 4 November 2020). [CrossRef]
45. Novalbos, J.; López-Rodríguez, R.; Roman, M.; Gallego-Sandín, S.; Ochoa, D.; Abad-Santos, F. Effects of CYP2D6 Genotype on the Pharmacokinetics, Pharmacodynamics, and Safety of Risperidone in Healthy Volunteers. *J. Clin. Psychopharmacol.* **2010**, *30*, 504–511. [CrossRef] [PubMed]
46. Nagai, G.; Mihara, K.; Nakamura, A.; Suzuki, T.; Nemoto, K.; Kagawa, S. Prolactin concentrations during aripiprazole treatment in relation to sex, plasma drugs concentrations and genetic polymorphisms of dopamine D2 receptor and cytochrome P450 2D6 in Japanese patients with schizophrenia. *Psychiatry Clin. Neurosci.* **2012**, *66*, 518–524. [CrossRef] [PubMed]
47. Patteet, L.; Vincent, H.; Kristof, M.; Bernard, S.; Manuel, M.; Hugo, N. Genotype and co-medication dependent CYP2D6 metabolic activity: Effects on serum concentrations of aripiprazole, haloperidol, risperidone, paliperidone and zuclopenthixol. *Eur. J. Clin. Pharmacol.* **2015**, *72*, 175–184. [CrossRef] [PubMed]
48. Jukic, M.M.; Smith, R.L.; Haslemo, T.; Molden, E.; Ingelman-Sundberg, M. Effect of CYP2D6 genotype on exposure and efficacy of risperidone and aripiprazole: A retrospective, cohort study. *Lancet Psychiatry* **2019**, *6*, 418–426. Available online: http://www.ncbi.nlm.nih.gov/pubmed/31000417 (accessed on 4 November 2020). [CrossRef]

49. Nemoto, K.; Mihara, K.; Nakamura, A.; Nagai, G.; Kagawa, S.; Suzuki, T.; Kondo, T. Effects of escitalopram on plasma concentrations of aripiprazole and its active metabolite, dehydroaripiprazole, in Japanese patients. *Pharmacopsychiatry* **2014**, *47*, 101–104. Available online: http://onlinelibrary.wiley.com/o/cochrane/clcentral/articles/321/CN-01051321/frame.html (accessed on 4 November 2020). [CrossRef]
50. Van der Weide, K.; van der Weide, J. The Influence of the CYP3A4*22 Polymorphism on Serum Concentration of Quetiapine in Psychiatric Patients. *J. Clin. Psychopharmacol.* **2014**, *34*, 256–260. Available online: http://www.ncbi.nlm.nih.gov/pubmed/24525658 (accessed on 4 November 2020). [CrossRef]

Publisher's Note: MDPI stays neutral with regard to jurisdictional claims in published maps and institutional affiliations.

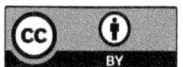

© 2020 by the authors. Licensee MDPI, Basel, Switzerland. This article is an open access article distributed under the terms and conditions of the Creative Commons Attribution (CC BY) license (http://creativecommons.org/licenses/by/4.0/).

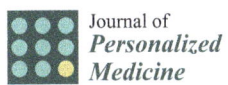

Article

Impact of Drug-Gene-Interaction, Drug-Drug-Interaction, and Drug-Drug-Gene-Interaction on (es)Citalopram Therapy: The PharmLines Initiative

Muh. Akbar Bahar [1,2,*], Pauline Lanting [3], Jens H. J. Bos [1], Rolf H. Sijmons [3], Eelko Hak [1] and Bob Wilffert [1,4]

1. Department of PharmacoTherapy, -Epidemiology & -Economics, University of Groningen, 9713 AV Groningen, The Netherlands; h.j.bos@rug.nl (J.H.J.B.); e.hak@rug.nl (E.H.); b.wilffert@rug.nl (B.W.)
2. Faculty of Pharmacy, Universitas Hasanuddin, Makassar 90245, Indonesia
3. Department of Genetics, Groningen, University Medical Center Groningen, University of Groningen, 9713 AV Groningen, The Netherlands; p.lanting@umcg.nl (P.L.); r.h.sijmons@umcg.nl (R.H.S.)
4. Department of Clinical Pharmacy and Pharmacology, University Medical Center Groningen, University of Groningen, 9713 AV Groningen, The Netherlands
* Correspondence: akbarbahar@unhas.ac.id; Tel.: +31-50-3632954

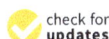

Received: 9 October 2020; Accepted: 14 November 2020; Published: 28 November 2020

Abstract: We explored the association between CYP2C19/3A4 mediated drug-gene-interaction (DGI), drug-drug-interaction (DDI) and drug-drug-gene-interaction (DDGI) and (es)citalopram dispensing course. A cohort study was conducted among adult Caucasians from the Lifelines cohort (167,729 participants) and linked dispensing data from the IADB.nl database as part of the PharmLines Initiative. Exposure groups were categorized into (es)citalopram starters with DGI, DDI and DDGI. The primary outcome was drug switching and/or dose adjustment, and the secondary was early discontinuation after the start of (es)citalopram. Logistic regression modeling was applied to estimate adjusted odd ratios with their confidence interval. We identified 316 (es)citalopram starters with complete CYP2C19/3A4 genetic information. The CYP2C19 IM/PM and CYP3A4 NM combination increased risks of switching and/or dose reduction (OR: 2.75, 95% CI: 1.03–7.29). The higher effect size was achieved by the CYP2C19 IM/PM and CYP3A4 IM combination (OR: 4.38, 95% CI: 1.22–15.69). CYP2C19/3A4 mediated DDIs and DDGIs showed trends towards increased risks of switching and/or dose reduction. In conclusion, a DGI involving predicted decreased CYP2C19 function increases the need for (es)citalopram switching and/or dose reduction which might be enhanced by co-presence of predicted decreased CYP3A4 function. For DDI and DDGI, no conclusions can be drawn from the results.

Keywords: (es)citalopram; drug-gene-interaction; drug-drug-interaction; drug-drug-gene-interaction; the PharmLines initiative

1. Introduction

Selective serotonin re-uptake inhibitors (SSRIs) such as citalopram and escitalopram ((es)citalopram) are among the first-line pharmacological options for depression in Europe and the US, and the use of SSRIs has increased considerably over the years [1,2]. However, reports showed that less than 50% of (es)citalopram users achieved disease symptom remission during their first treatment episode, and prognosis appeared unpredictable [3,4]. Such variable effectiveness may be explained by a large inter-individual pharmacokinetic variability among patients treated with (es)citalopram [5,6]. This variability is known to be caused partly by differences in metabolic activity of drug metabolizing Cytochrome P450 (CYP) enzymes [7].

(Es)citalopram is primarily metabolized by the combination of CYP2C19 and CYP3A4 enzymes, and to a lesser extent by CYP2D6 enzyme [8,9]. Genetic polymorphisms are known to affect the catalytic activity of these enzymes. Some studies have investigated the role of *CYP2C19* and *CYP2D6* polymorphisms on the exposure as well as the clinical impact of (es)citalopram [7,10]. Such interaction between the drug treatment and genetic variation is referred to as drug-gene interaction (DGI) [11]. To the best of our knowledge, no previous studies have explored the impact of the DGI related to CYP3A4 polymorphisms, or its combination with *CYP2C19* polymorphisms, in (es)citalopram treatment. In addition, the concomitant administration of CYP2C19, CYP3A4, and/or CYP2D6 (CYP2C19/3A4/2D6) modulator drugs (inhibitor/inducer) produces a drug-drug-interaction (DDI) with (es)citalopram by affecting blood concentrations and hence modifying its effectiveness [12].

To make it even more complicated for treating physicians, (es)citalopram treatment may be affected by both genetics and drugs that modulate the activity of the metabolic pathways at the same time which potentially affect blood concentration even more unpredictably than DGI and DDI alone [13]. In other words, a drug-drug-gene-interaction (DDGI) is encountered when a DGI coincides with a DDI [14,15]. Generally, DDGIs show more pharmacokinetic diversity than DDIs and DGIs alone, since DDGIs concern several modes of interactions [15,16]. For example, a DDGI may involve the co-existence of a genetic polymorphism and a CYP-inhibitor for one CYP-enzyme or the co-presence of a genetic polymorphism in one or two metabolic pathways and a CYP modulator in another pathway [14,15].

Due to restricted study populations in trials and scarcity of health care databases with a possibility to link genetic and drug dispensing data, large-scale real-world pharmacogenetic studies are lacking on the impact of pharmacogenetic and drug interactions in general. Consequently, recent guidelines have only provided specific recommendations on the management of (es)citalopram-related DGIs and DDIs separately, but a knowledge gap remains regarding the pharmacotherapeutic management of DDGIs [17,18]. The PharmLines Initiative enables the unique linkage of genetic and drug data to perform an inception cohort study in a large population cohort which we used to explore the impact of DDIs, DGIs (specifically *CYP2C19/3A4* polymorphisms), and DDGIs on short-term first-time (es)citalopram therapy [19]. To mirror treatment success, proxy outcomes such as drug switching, dose adjustment, and an early discontinuation after the first prescription of (es)citalopram are used [20,21].

2. Methods

2.1. Study Design, Setting and Data Sources

This retrospective cohort study was performed using data from the PharmLines Initiative which links the Lifelines cohort and the University of Groningen prescription IADB.nl database, two large databases in the Northern part of the Netherlands [19].

The Lifelines cohort is a three-generation prospective cohort covering 167,729 Dutch participants from the Northern provinces of the Netherlands [22,23]. It was established with the aim to study 'complex interactions between environmental, phenotypic and genomic factors in the development of chronic diseases and healthy ageing' [22,23]. The participants from the Lifelines cohort generally represent the characteristics of the adult population of the Northern part of the Netherlands [24]. More comprehensive information about the Lifelines cohort can be found in the publications of Stolk et al. and Scholtens et al. [22,23].

The University of Groningen prescription database IADB.nl collected over 1.2 million prescriptions from 72 pharmacies. The information about gender, date of birth and four-digit postal codes (optional) from 730,000 recorded anonymous patients are available [25]. The prescription information of each participant is recorded such as dispensing date, Anatomical Therapeutic Chemical code (ATC code), quantity, duration, and DDD (defined daily dose) [25]. The participants recorded in the IADB.nl are found to be representative of the general population in the Netherlands as whole [25]. The IADB.nl is a reliable database and has been used in many pharmacoepidemiological studies [26–28]

The linking process of these two databases was facilitated by a trusted third party, the Statistic Netherlands. The linkage was performed at the individual level and relied on combined information of postal code, date of birth, and gender. Once the selection process was completed, identifiers from each database were cleared and then, a new unique identifier (pseudoID) was assigned. Using the pseudoID, genetic and prescription information of the participants from the Lifelines cohort and the IADB.nl, respectively, could be combined. Details on the linking process has been published elsewhere [19].

2.2. Study Population

Adult Lifelines participants (Caucasian, 18 years and older) with available genetic information (CYP2C19 and CYP3A4 genes) and who had their first citalopram (N06AB04) or escitalopram (N06AB10) prescription recorded in the PharmLines Iniative were eligible. Those who were not prescribed any (es)citalopram for at least 180 days before starting their drug dispensing were included. If there were several periods of (es)citalopram dispensing, only the first dispensing period was included in the analysis. Date of the first (es)citalopram prescription was regarded as an index date which indicates the start of follow-up.

2.3. Genotyping

Genotyping for single-nucleotide polymorphism (SNP) of CYP2C19 and CYP3A4 genes in the Lifelines cohort was performed using the Illumina CytoSNP-12v2 array [22]. The genotype data was imputed by using the Genome of the Netherlands reference panel [22]. The quality of genotyping data was checked using the following requirements i.e., (i) the p-value of Hardy-Weinberg equilibrium distribution was $> 1 \times 10^{-4}$, (ii) call rate of 95%, and (iii) minor allele frequency (MAF) was > 0.001 [22]. Additionally, principal component analysis was used to detect statistical outliers [22]. More detailed information on the genotyping process can be found in the publication of Scholtens et al. (2014) [22].

CYP2C19 and CYP3A4 genotypes were translated to haplotypes, which were used to predict corresponding phenotypes (Tables 1–4). Relevant haplotypes were selected and genotypes were translated to predicted phenotypes based on available information from the Dutch Pharmacogenetics Working Group (DPWG). Corresponding predicted phenotypes include poor metabolizer (PM), intermediate metabolizer (IM), and normal metabolizer (NM) for CYP2C19 and CYP3A4, and ultra-rapid metabolizer (UM) for CYP2C19.

Table 1. Pipeline translation table for CYP2C19 with haplotypes and their Single Nucleotide Polymorphisms (SNPs) information.

Haplotype Name	Gene	rsID	Reference Sequence	Variant. Start	Variant. Stop	Reference. Allele	Variant. Allele	Type
CYP2C19*1	CYP2C19	rs3758581	10	96602622	96602622	G	-	single
CYP2C19*1	CYP2C19	rs12769205	10	96535123	96535123	A	-	single
CYP2C19*1	CYP2C19	rs28399504	10	96522462	96522462	A	-	single
CYP2C19*1	CYP2C19	rs41291556	10	96535172	96535172	T	-	single
CYP2C19*1	CYP2C19	rs11188072	10	96519060	96519060	C	-	single
CYP2C19*2	CYP2C19	rs12769205	10	96535123	96535123	A	G	single
CYP2C19*4	CYP2C19	rs28399504	10	96522462	96522462	A	G	single
CYP2C19*5/7	CYP2C19	rs3758581	10	96602622	96602622	G	A	single
CYP2C19*8	CYP2C19	rs41291556	10	96535172	96535172	T	C	single
CYP2C19*17	CYP2C19	rs11188072	10	96519060	96519060	C	T	single

Table 2. Pipeline translation table for CYP3A4 with haplotypes and their SNP information.

Haplotype. Name	Gene	rsID	Reference Sequence	Variant. Start	Variant. Stop	Reference. Allele	Variant. Allele	Type
CYP3A4*1A	CYP3A4	rs2740574	7	99382095	99382095	T	-	single
CYP3A4*1A	CYP3A4	rs2242480	7	99361465	99361465	C	-	single
CYP3A4*1A	CYP3A4	rs35599367	7	99366315	99366315	G	-	single
CYP3A4*1B	CYP3A4	rs2740574	7	99382095	99382095	T	C	single
CYP3A4*1G	CYP3A4	rs2242480	7	99361465	99361465	C	T	single
CYP3A4*22	CYP3A4	rs35599367	7	99366315	99366315	G	A	single

Table 3. The translation of CYP2C19 and CYP3A4 haplotypes to their predicted metabolic activity.

Gene	Haplotype	Metabolic Function	Reference
CYP2C19	CYP2C19*1	Normal	[29]
	CYP2C19*2	No	[29]
	CYP2C19*4	No	[29]
	CYP2C19*5/7	No	[29]
	CYP2C19*8	No	[29]
	CYP2C19*17	Increased	[29]
CYP3A4	CYP3A4*1A	Normal	[29]
	CYP3A4*1B	Normal	[30]
	CYP3A4*1G	Decreased	[31]
	CYP3A4*22	Decreased	[29]

Table 4. The translation of CYP2C19 and CYP3A4 haplotype combinations to their predicted phenotypes.

CYP2C19	No	Normal	Increased	CYP3A4	Decreased	Normal
No	PM	IM	IM	Decreased	PM	IM
Normal	IM	NM	NM	Normal	IM	NM
Increased	IM	NM	UM			

NM: Normal Metabolizer. IM: Intermediate Metabolizer. PM: Poor Metabolizer. UM: Ultrarapid Metabolizer.

2.4. Definition of Exposures

The exposure groups were defined as (es)citalopram users with a DGI, DDI, or DDGI. Participants who were predicted to be CYP2C19 UM, IM, or PM and/or CYP3A4 IM or PM and were prescribed (es)citalopram without co-prescription of CYP2C19/3A4/2D6 modulators (inhibitors/inducers) were classified as experiencing a DGI. For statistical power reasons, IM and PM groups were pooled into a combined IM/PM group, but we provided a sensitivity analysis for the separated IM and PM groups (Supplementary Materials S2).

Participants were classified to have a DDI when they were predicted as normal metabolizers (NM) of CYP2C19 and CYP3A4, and at the same time were co-prescribed a CYP2C19 and/or CYP3A4 and/or CYP2D6 modulator during the (es)citalopram treatment within a follow-up time frame of 90 days. A list of clinically relevant CYP2C19/3A4/2D6 modulators was based on *Commentaren Medicatiebewaking* (Health Base, NL) and the Flockhart table^{TM} (Supplementary S1) [32,33]. Only non-SSRI drugs were included as CYP2C19/3A4/2D6 modulators since our study population consists of first-time (es)citalopram users and it is uncommon to combine this with another SSRI drug in the early phase of drug treatments [34].

DDGI was defined as the occurrence of a DGI and DDI at the same time in which (es)citalopram patients with a CYP2C19/3A4 predicted deviating phenotype received a CYP2C19/3A4/2D6 modulator. The non-exposed reference group was defined as (es)citalopram users with a predicted normal

CYP2C19/3A4 and who were not prescribed any CYP2C19/3A4/2D6 modulator during first-time (es)citalopram treatment.

2.5. Study Outcomes

Study outcomes were drug switching, dose adjustment, and early discontinuation. The incidence of these outcomes within the time frame of a 90 day follow-up after the index date were identified. This time frame was used since the acute phase treatment of SSRIs is considered to be between 6 and 12 weeks after the start of drug treatment. A previous report indicated that about 70% of antidepressant users stopped their therapy within 90 days [35]. However, since interactions commonly have an immediate effect, the presence of the outcomes within the time frame of a 45 day follow-up after the index date were also explored (Supplementary S3) [21]. Drug switching was defined as patients having an early discontinuation of (es)citalopram as well as the prescription of another antidepressant, regardless of the class, within 120 days after the index date. The follow-up time frame was expanded for dispensing of other antidepressants from 90 to 120 days after the index date in order to accommodate the possible time gap between the dispensing of (es)citalopram and the new antidepressant [36,37]. Meanwhile, dose adjustment was defined as having a dose reduction or a dose elevation for at least 25% of the first dose within 90 days after the index date. Early discontinuation was defined as discontinuing the prescription of (es)citalopram within 90 days after the index date, having no further re-prescription of (es)citalopram for at least 180 days after the stop date as well as no switching as described previously. In the preliminary analysis the effects of exposure on drug switching and dose reduction were in the same direction, therefore the outcomes were combined. Analysis on the separated outcomes are provided in the Supplementary S2.

2.6. Co-Variates

The following co-variates were recorded to compare groups: age, gender, dose of (es)citalopram at the index date, number of co-prescriptions, and pre-defined drugs as a proxy for certain co-existing comorbidities (Supplementary S1). (Es)citalopram users had to have at least two prescriptions of these proxy medications within six months before or after the index date to be assumed as having a chronic condition of the potential comorbidities [38]. The presence of NSAIDs co-prescription during (es)citalopram prescription was checked within the time frame of 90 days since the combination of NSAIDs and SSRIs was reported to increase the risk of gastrointestinal bleeding [39]. The potential comorbidities were clustered into one group, namely 'potential comorbidities,' in order to increase the power of the calculation. The distribution for each potential comorbidity was compared separately between outcomes and none of them were statistically significant different ($p < 0.05$). Lastly, the distribution of the number of CYP2C19/3A4/2D6 modulator prescriptions during the use of (es)citalopram was compared, since a previous study indicated that the higher the number of CYP2C19/3A4/2D6 modulator prescriptions, the more alteration in the clearance of (es)citalopram [12].

2.7. Statistical Analysis

The Chi-square (or Fisher's exact test) and Mann-Whitney test were used to compare distribution of categorical and skewed distributed continuous variables between outcomes, respectively. Co-variates which differed significantly ($p < 0.05$) were entered into final multivariate logistic regression model to obtain adjusted odds ratio as measure of association (OR). We also provided adjusted p-values for false discovery rates due to multiple comparisons using the Benjamini-Hochberg method (q-values, with a $q < 0.05$ as the significance threshold). Since some participants did not have dosing information, a complete case analysis in cases of dosing comparison as well as dose adjustment analysis were performed. The baseline characteristics were compared between participants with complete information and participants without dosing information (Supplementary S2).

3. Results

Overall, 316 (es)citalopram users (median 45 years, 63% women) with *CYP2C19* and *CYP3A4* genetic information were available (Figure 1). Baseline characteristics of patients are displayed in Table 5. There were 32.6%, 7.3% and 4.4% of participants to have predicted CYP2C19 IM, PM, and UM, respectively, and there were 17.7% and 1.9% of our sample to have predicted CYP3A4 IM and PM, respectively. After combining both genetic information (regardless the presence of another exposure such as CYP modulators), we found that about 56% of the patients had at least one predicted deviating phenotype of CYP2C19 or CYP3A4. There were about 33%, 6%, 11%, and 4% of the participants having predicted CYP2C19 IM/PM + CYP3A4 NM, CYP2C19 IM/PM + CYP3A4 IM/PM, CYP2C19 NM + CYP3A4 IM/PM, and CYP2C19 UM + CYP3A4 NM/IM, respectively.

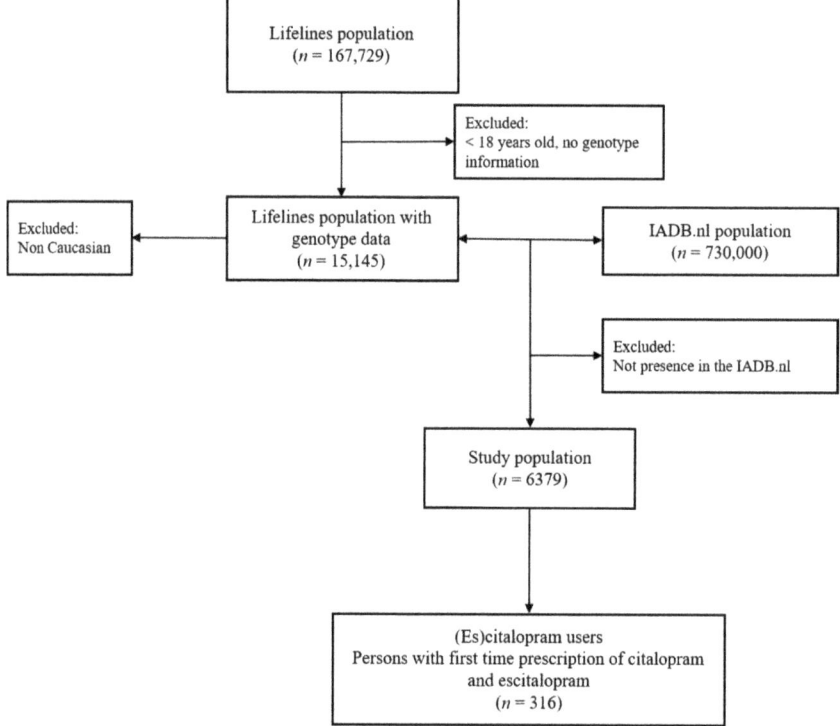

Figure 1. Selection of (es)citalopram first time users.

Table 5. Characteristics of patients starting (es)citalopram ($n = 316$).

Variabels	N	%
Gender (*n* women, %)	200	63.3
Age in years, median (IQR)	45	14
CYP2C19 Phenotypes		
CYP2C19 NM (*n*, %)	176	55.7
CYP2C19 IM (*n*, %)	103	32.6
CYP2C19 PM (*n*, %)	23	7.3
CYP2C19 UM (*n*, %)	14	4.4

Table 5. Cont.

Variabels	N	%
CYP3A4 Phenotypes		
CYP3A4 NM (n, %)	254	80.4
CYP3A4 IM (n, %)	56	17.7
CYP3A4 PM (n, %)	6	1.9
Combination of CYP2C19 & CYP3A4 Phenotypes		
CYP2C19 NM + CYP3A4 NM (n, %)	140	44.3
CYP2C19 IM/PM + CYP3A4 NM (n, %)	104	32.9
CYP2C19 IM/PM + CYP3A4 IM/PM (n, %)	20	6.3
CYP2C19 NM + CYP3A4 IM/PM (n, %)	36	11.4
CYP2C19 UM + CYP3A4 NM/IM (n, %)	14	4.4
Type of CYP modulator combination		
No inhibitor or inducer of CYP2C19/3A4/2D6	260	82.3
CYP2C19 inhibitor alone (n, %)	44	13.9
CYP3A4 inhibitor alone (n, %)	4	1.3
CYP2D6 inhibitor alone (n, %)	6	1.9
CYP2C19 inhibitor + CYP2D6 inhibitor (n, %) *	1	0.3
CYP2C19 inhibitor + CYP3A4 inducer (n, %) *	1	0.3
DDD at start of citalopram and escitalopram		
DDD < 1 (n, %)	25	7.9
DDD >= 1 (n, %)	197	62.3
No dose information (n, %)	94	29.7
Potential comorbidities		
No comorbidity (n, %)	65	20.6
1–2 potential comorbidities (n, %)	216	68.3
≥3 potential comorbidities (n, %)	35	11.1
Number of co-prescriptions during (es)citalopram		
1–3 type of drugs (n, %)	247	78.2
>3 type of drugs (n, %)	69	21.8
Number of CYP modulator during (es)citalopram		
No CYP modulator (n, %)	260	82.3
1 CYP modulator (n, %)	27	8.5
≥2 CYP modulator (n, %)	29	9.2
Combined exposures		
No exposures		
CYP2C19 NM + CYP3A4 NM + No CYP Modulator (n, %)	111	35.1
DDI		
CYP2C19 NM + CYP3A4 NM + Yes CYP Modulator (n, %)	29	9.2
DGI		
CYP2C19 IM/PM + CYP3A4 NM + No CYP Modulator (n, %)	89	28.2
CYP2C19 IM/PM + CYP3A4 IM/PM + No CYP Modulator (n, %)	20	6.3
CYP2C19 NM + CYP3A4 IM/PM + No CYP Modulator (n, %)	29	9.2
CYP2C19 UM + CYP3A4 NM/IM + No CYP Modulator (n, %)	11	3.5
DDGI (n, %)	27	8.5

* Excluded. NM: Normal Metabolizer. IM: Intermediate Metabolizer. PM: Poor Metabolizer. UM: Ultrarapid Metabolizer. DDD: Defined Daily Dose. CYP: Cytochrome P450.

Regardless of the number of prescribed CYP modulators, about 18% of the participants were exposed to CYP-modulators during (es)citalopram prescription and most of them were CYP2C19 inhibitors (13.9%). No combination of (es)citalopram with CYP2C19/3A4 inducer alone was identified. Two patients exposed to a combination of CYP modulators (one patient with a CYP2C19 and a CYP2D6 inhibitor, and one patient with a CYP2C19 inhibitor and a CYP3A4 inducer) were excluded since the number was too small to analyze. More than 60% of the participants had at least 20 mg citalopram or 10 mg escitalopram daily ($\geq$ 1 Defined Daily Dose/DDD) at the start of their prescriptions. About 68% of the population had 1 to 2 potential comorbidities and about 78% of them used one to three different type of drugs during (es)citalopram prescription.

The more concomitant the CYP modulator used during (es)citalopram prescription, the more alteration in the (es)citalopram produced [12]. In our sample, we only found less than 10% of them using at least two concomitant CYP modulator at the same pathway. After looking on the combination of exposures (*CYP2C19/3A4* genotypes and CYP modulators) among our study population, we found that 9%, 47%, and 8.5% of participants were exposed to DDIs, DGIs, and DDGIs, respectively. Frequency of each type of DDGIs is presented in Table 6.

Table 6. Frequency of DDGI (overlapping condition of DDI and DGI).

CYP2C19 Phenotype	CYP3A4 Phenotype	CYP2C19 Inhibitor	CYP3A4 Inhibitor	CYP2D6 Inhibitor	CYP2C19 Inducer	CYP3A4 Inducer	N	%
One pathway								
UM/IM/PM	NM	Y	N	N	N	N	14	51.8
Two pathways								
IM	IM	Y	N	N	N	N	2	7.4
IM	NM	N	Y	N	N	N	2	7.4
IM	NM	N	N	Y	N	N	2	7.4
NM	IM/PM	Y	N	N	N	N	6	22.2
NM	IM	N	N	Y	N	N	1	3.7
SUM							27	

NM: Normal Metabolizer. IM: Intermediate Metabolizer. PM: Poor Metabolizer. UM: Ultrarapid Metabolizer. Y: Yes. N: No.

There were 25 (7.9%), 7 (2.2%), 80 (25%), and 47 (15%) of (es)citalopram users experiencing drug switching, dose reduction, dose elevation, and early discontinuation, respectively. Number of co-prescriptions seemed to influence the rate of switching ($p = 0.02$). Female gender and a higher dose at the index date are less prevalent in the subgroup that experienced dose elevation of (es)citalopram ($p = 0.003$ and 0.002, respectively) (Table 7).

In our dataset, participants with a predicted CYP2C19 IM phenotype had an increased risk of drug switching and/or dose reduction (aOR: 3.16, 95% CI: 1.41–7.09) but CYP2C19 PM did not show a comparable result (aOR: 0.54, 95% CI: 0.07–4.52) (Table 8). Meanwhile, both CYP2C19 IM and PM had a comparable trend on the risk of early discontinuation (aOR: 0.35, 95% CI: 0.15–0.79 and aOR: 0.41, 95% CI: 0.09–1.89, respectively) (Table 9).

Furthermore, there was an indication showing that co-presence of CYP3A4 IM/PM in individuals with CYP2C19 IM/PM increased the risk of switching and/or dose reduction of (es)citalopram to a larger extent than the combination of CYP2C19 IM/PM and CYP3A4 NM (aOR: 4.38, 95% CI: 1.22–15.69 and aOR: 2.75, 95% CI: 1.03–7.29, respectively). This effect might be facilitated by the combination of CYP2C19 IM and CYP3A4 IM since there was only one participant with CYP2C19 PM and no participants with CYP3A4 PM experiencing switching or dose reduction (Table 8). Meanwhile, CYP3A4 IM/PM in the co-presence of CYP2C19 NM did not seem to influence the risk of switching and/or dose reduction (aOR: 1.02, 95% CI: 0.19–5.24). No participants with the CYP2C19 UM and CYP3A4 NM/IM combination experienced drug switching and/or dose reduction and no significant association with early discontinuation as well as with dose elevation was observed (Tables 8–10).

DDIs seemed to increase the risk of drug switching and/or dose reduction (aOR: 2.82, 95% CI: 0.49–15.97), which was mainly facilitated by the co-presence of CYP2C19 inhibitors, but seemingly not to increase the risk of dose elevation and early discontinuation (Tables 8–10).

DDGIs also seemed to increase the risk of drug switching and/or dose reduction (aOR: 2.33, 95% CI: 0.42–12.78). However, there were only two participants with DDGIs experiencing drug switching or dose reduction, consisting of one participant with a DDGI affecting one pathway and the other one with a DDGI affecting two pathways (Supplementary S2). Consequently, a separated analysis of DDGIs based on the number of pathways affected produced comparable effect sizes (DDGI affecting one pathway: aOR: 2.52, 95% CI: 0.26–24.61; DDGI affecting two pathways: aOR: 2.17, 95% CI: 0.23–20.67).

Overall, there were no associations between the exposures and any outcomes tested reaching the statistical significance threshold of a false discovery rate-adjusted p-value ($q > 0.05$).

Analysis using a time frame of 45 days after the index date produced comparable results. CYP2C19 IM increased the risk of switching and the effect size was also larger in combination with CYP3A4 IM/PM (aOR: 6.41, 95% CI: 1.19–34.40) than with CYP3A4 NM (aOR: 2.66, 95% CI: 0.65–10.96). CYP2C19 IM seemingly increased the risk of dose reduction (aOR: 2.69, 95% CI: 0.43–16.96). Lastly, DDIs and DDGIs have a tendency to increase the risk of dose reduction and switching, respectively. Detailed data can be found in Supplementary S3.

Table 7. Baseline comparisons.

Variables	Switching *			Decreased Dose #			Increased Dose #			Discontinuation *		
	Yes (n = 25)	No (n = 279)	p-Value	Yes (n = 7)	No (n = 213)	p-Value	Yes (n = 80)	No (n = 140)	p-Value	Yes (n = 47)	No (n = 257)	p-Value
Gender (n Women)	15	177	0.73	5	133	1.00	40	98	0.003	29	163	0.82
Age in years (median, IQR)	41	45	0.68	39	42	0.38	43.5	41	0.92	48	44	0.03
DDD at start (n DDD ≥1)	18	177	1.00	7	188	1.00	64	131	0.002	31	164	0.57
Potential comorbidities (n Yes)												
No comorbidity (n)	3	60	0.18	3	36	0.22	16	23	0.79	9	54	0.71
1–2 potential comorbidities (n)	21	185		4	152		55	101		34	172	
≥3 potential comorbidities (n)	1	34		0	25		9	16		4	31	
N of co-prescriptions												
1–3 (n)	24	213	0.02	7	166	0.35	63	110	0.97	38	199	0.60
>3 (n)	1	66		0	47		17	30		9	58	
N of CYP modulator prescriptions												
No (n)	22	229	0.92	6	177	0.73	69	114	0.62	41	210	0.64
1 (n)	2	25		1	18		5	14		4	23	
≥2 (n)	1	25		0	18		6	12		2	24	

* No start/stop date = 10: # no dose information = 94. NM: Normal Metabolizer. IM: Intermediate Metabolizer. PM: Poor Metabolizer. UM: Ultrarapid Metabolizer. DDD: Defined Daily Dose. CYP: Cytochrome P450. N: Number. IQR: Interquartile Range.

Table 8. Association between DDI, DGI, and DDGI with drug switching and/or dose reduction.

Variables	Switching and/or Dose Reduction		Univariate Analysis			Multivariate Analysis		
	Yes (n = 31, %)	No (n = 273, %)	OR (95%CI)	p-Value	q-Value	aOR (95%CI)	p-Value	q-Value
CYP2C19 & CYP3A4 predicted phenotypes								
CYP2C19 predicted phenotypes *								
CYP2C19 NM	12 (38.7)	157 (57.5)	Ref.			Ref.		
CYP2C19 IM	18 (58.1)	82 (30)	2.87 (1.32–6.25)	0.01	0.08	3.16 (1.41–7.09)	0.005	0.06
CYP2C19 PM	1 (3.2)	20 (7.3)	0.65 (0.08–5.30)	0.69	0.90	0.54 (0.07–4.52)	0.57	0.68
CYP2C19 UM	0 (0)	14 (5.1)	NA			NA		

Table 8. Cont.

Variables	Switching and/or Dose Reduction			Univariate Analysis			Multivariate Analysis		
	Yes (n = 31, %)	No (n = 273, %)		OR (95%CI)	p-Value	q-Value	aOR (95%CI)	p-Value	q-Value
CYP3A4 predicted phenotypes **									
CYP3A4 NM	23 (74.2)	220 (80.6)		Ref.			Ref.		
CYP3A4 IM	8 (25.8)	47 (17.2)		1.63 (0.69–3.86)	0.27	0.54	1.37 (0.55–3.39)	0.50	0.67
CYP3A4 PM	0 (0)	6 (2.2)		NA			NA		
Combination of predicted phenotypes ***									
CYP2C19 NM + CYP3A4 NM	9 (29)	125 (45.8)		Ref.			Ref.		
CYP2C19 IM/PM + CYP3A4 NM	14 (45.2)	85 (31.1)		2.29 (0.95–5.52)	0.07	0.17	2.35 (0.96–5.76)	0.06	0.14
CYP2C19 IM/PM + CYP3A4 IM/PM	5 (16.1)	17 (6.2)		4.08 (1.22–13.63)	0.02	0.08	3.46 (1.02–11.75)	0.05	0.14
CYP2C19 NM + CYP3A4 IM/PM	3 (9.7)	32 (11.7)		1.30 (0.33–5.09)	0.70	0.90	1.11 (0.28–4.43)	0.88	0.96
CYP2C19 UM + CYP3A4 NM/IM	0 (0)	14 (5.1)		NA			NA		
CYP modulator #									
No inhibitor/inducer of CYP2C19/3A4/2D6	27 (87.1)	224 (82.1)		Ref.			Ref.		
CYP2C19 inhibitor	4 (12.9)	40 (14.7)		0.83 (0.27–2.49)	0.74	0.90	2.36 (0.67–8.32)	0.18	0.36
CYP3A4 inhibitor	0 (0)	4 (1.5)		NA			NA		
CYP2D6 inhibitor	0 (0)	5 (1.8)		NA			NA		
Combined exposures ^									
No exposures									
CYP2C19 NM + CYP3A4 NM + No CYP Modulator	7 (22.6)	101 (37)		Ref.			Ref.		
DDI									
CYP2C19 NM + CYP3A4 NM + Yes CYP Modulator	2 (6.5)	24 (8.8)		1.20 (0.24–6.16)	0.83	0.90	2.82 (0.49–15.97)	0.24	0.41
DGI									
CYP2C19 IM/PM + CYP3A4 NM + No CYP Modulator	13 (41.9)	71 (26)		2.64 (1.00–6.95)	0.05	0.15	2.75 (1.03–7.29)	0.04	0.14
CYP2C19 IM/PM + CYP3A4 IM/PM + No CYP Modulator	5 (16.1)	15 (5.5)		4.81 (1.35–17.12)	0.02	0.08	4.38 (1.22–15.69)	0.02	0.12
CYP2C19 NM + CYP3A4 IM/PM + No CYP Modulator	2 (6.5)	26 (9.5)		1.11 (0.22–5.66)	0.90	0.90	1.02 (0.19–5.24)	0.98	0.98
CYP2C19 UM + CYP3A4 NM/IM + No CYP Modulator	0 (0)	11 (4)		NA			NA		
DDGI									
DDGI	2 (6.5)	25 (9.2)		1.15 (0.23–5.89)	0.86	0.90	2.33 (0.42–12.78)	0.33	0.49

Adjusted for: * CYP3A4 phenotypes, CYP modulator & N of co-prescriptions; ** CYP2C19 phenotypes, CYP modulator & N of co-prescriptions; *** CYP2C19 & CYP3A4 phenotypes & N of co-prescriptions; ^ N of co-prescriptions. NM: Normal Metabolizer. IM: Intermediate Metabolizer. PM: Poor Metabolizer. UM: Ultrarapid Metabolizer. DDI: Drug-Drug Interaction. DGI: Drug-Gene Interaction. DDGI: Drug-Drug-Gene Interaction (overlapping condition of DDI and DGI, please see Table 6: Frequency of DDGI). CYP: Cytochrome P450. NA: Not Available. OR: Odds Ratio. aOR: Adjusted Odds ratio. CI: Confidence Interval. Ref.: Reference.

Table 9. Association between DDI, DGI, and DDGI with early discontinuation.

Variables	Early Discontinuation Yes (n = 47, %)	No (n = 257, %)	Univariate Analysis OR (95%CI)	p-Value	q-Value	Multivariate Analysis aOR (95%CI)	p-Value	q-Value
CYP2C19 & CYP3A4 predicted phenotypes								
CYP2C19 phenotypes *								
CYP2C19 NM	33 (70.2)	136 (52.9)	Ref.			Ref.		
CYP2C19 IM	9 (19.1)	91 (35.4)	0.41 (0.19–0.89)	0.03	0.45	0.35 (0.15–0.79)	0.01	0.15
CYP2C19 PM	2 (4.3)	19 (7.4)	0.43 (0.09–1.96)	0.28	0.50	0.41 (0.09–1.89)	0.25	0.54
CYP2C19 UM	3 (6.4)	11 (4.3)	1.12 (0.29–4.26)	0.86	0.86	1.24 (0.32–4.88)	0.75	0.75
CYP3A4 phenotypes **								
CYP3A4 NM	36 (76.6)	207 (80.5)	Ref.			Ref.		
CYP3A4 IM	11 (23.4)	44 (17.1)	1.44 (0.68–3.04)	0.34	0.51	1.29 (0.59–2.84)	0.51	0.59
CYP3A4 PM	0 (0)	6 (2.3)	NA			NA		
Combination of predicted phenotypes ***								
CYP2C19 NM + CYP3A4 NM	24 (51.1)	110 (42.8)	Ref.			Ref.		
CYP2C19 IM/PM + CYP3A4 NM	10 (21.3)	89 (34.6)	0.52 (0.23–1.13)	0.09	0.45	0.45 (0.20–1.02)	0.06	0.35
CYP2C19 IM/PM + CYP3A4 IM/PM	1 (2.1)	21 (8.2)	0.22 (0.03–1.70)	0.15	0.45	0.17 (0.02–1.39)	0.10	0.36
CYP2C19 NM + CYP3A4 IM/PM	9 (19.1)	26 (10.1)	1.59 (0.66–3.81)	0.30	0.50	1.43 (0.58–3.53)	0.44	0.59
CYP2C19 UM + CYP3A4 NM/IM	3 (6.4)	11 (4.3)	1.25 (0.32–4.83)	0.75	0.80	1.43 (0.36–5.69)	0.61	0.65
CYP modulator #								
No inhibitor/inducer of CYP2C19/3A4/2D6	41 (87.2)	210 (81.7)	Ref.			Ref.		
CYP2C19 inhibitor alone	6 (12.8)	38 (14.8)	0.81 (0.32–2.04)	0.65	0.80	0.68 (0.26–1.75)	0.42	0.59
CYP3A4 inhibitor alone	0 (0)	4 (1.6)	NA			NA		
CYP2D6 inhibitor alone	0 (0)	5 (1.9)	NA			NA		
Combined exposures ^								
No exposures								
CYP2C19 NM + CYP3A4 NM + No CYP Modulator	20 (42.6)	88 (34.2)	Ref.			Ref.		

Table 9. *Cont.*

Variables	Early Discontinuation		Univariate Analysis			Multivariate Analysis		
	Yes (n = 47, %)	No (n = 257, %)	OR (95%CI)	p-Value	q-Value	aOR (95%CI)	p-Value	q-Value
DDI								
CYP2C19 NM + CYP3A4 NM + Yes CYP Modulator	4 (8.5)	22 (8.6)	0.80 (0.25–2.58)	0.71	0.80	0.67 (0.20–2.21)	0.51	0.59
DGI								
CYP2C19 IM/PM + CYP3A4 NM + No CYP Modulator	9 (19.1)	75 (29.2)	0.53 (0.23–1.23)	0.14	0.45	0.44 (0.19–1.06)	0.07	0.35
CYP2C19 IM/PM + CYP3A4 IM/PM + No CYP Modulator	1 (2.1)	19 (7.4)	0.23 (0.03–1.83)	0.17	0.45	0.19 (0.02–1.53)	0.12	0.36
CYP2C19 NM + CYP3A4 IM/PM + No CYP Modulator	8 (17)	20 (7.8)	1.76 (0.68–4.56)	0.25	0.50	1.52 (0.57–4.04)	0.41	0.59
CYP2C19 UM + CYP3A4 NM/IM + No CYP Modulator	3 (6.4)	8 (3.1)	1.65 (0.40–6.78)	0.49	0.67	1.89 (0.45–8.07)	0.39	0.59
DDGI	2 (4.3)	25 (9.7)	0.35 (0.08–1.61)	0.18	0.45	0.38 (0.08–1.75)	0.21	0.53

Adjusted for: * CYP3A4 phenotypes, CYP modulator & age; ** CYP2C19 phenotypes, CYP modulator & age; *** CYP2C19 & CYP3A4 phenotypes & age; ^ age. NM: Normal Metabolizer. IM: Intermediate Metabolizer. PM: Poor Metabolizer. UM: Ultrarapid Metabolizer. DDI: Drug-Drug interaction. DGI: Drug-Gene Interaction. DDGI: Drug-Drug-Gene Interaction (overlapping condition of DDI and DGI, please see Table 6: Frequency of DDGI). CYP: Cytochrome P450. NA: Not Available. OR: Odds Ratio. aOR: Adjusted Odds ratio. CI: Confidence Interval. Ref.: Reference.

Table 10. Association between DDI, DGI, and DDGI with dose elevation.

Variables	Dose Elevation		Univariate Analysis			Multivariate Analysis		
	Yes (n = 80, %)	No (n = 140, %)	OR (95%CI)	p-Value	q-Value	aOR (95%CI)	p-Value	q-Value
CYP2C19 & CYP3A4 predicted phenotypes								
CYP2C19 predicted phenotypes *								
CYP2C19 NM	51 (63.7)	67 (47.9)	Ref.			Ref.		
CYP2C19 IM	23 (28.7)	56 (40)	0.54 (0.29–0.99)	0.05	0.45	0.59 (0.31–1.12)	0.11	0.54
CYP2C19 PM	4 (5)	10 (7.1)	0.53 (0.16–1.77)	0.29	0.61	0.56 (0.16–2.02)	0.38	0.54
CYP2C19 UM	2 (2.5)	7 (5)	0.37 (0.07–1.88)	0.23	0.61	0.35 (0.07–1.85)	0.22	0.54
CYP3A4 predicted phenotypes **								
CYP3A4 NM	61 (76.3)	114 (81.4)	Ref.			Ref.		
CYP3A4 IM	17 (21.3)	24 (17.1)	1.32 (0.66–2.65)	0.43	0.61	1.48 (0.70–3.12)	0.30	0.54
CYP3A4 PM	2 (2.5)	2 (1.4)	1.87 (0.26–13.59)	0.54	0.66	1.27 (0.15–10.64)	0.82	0.87

Table 10. Cont.

Variables	Dose Elevation Yes (n = 80, %)	Dose Elevation No (n = 140, %)	Univariate Analysis OR (95%CI)	p-Value	q-Value	Multivariate Analysis aOR (95%CI)	p-Value	q-Value
Combination of predicted phenotypes ***								
CYP2C19 NM + CYP3A4 NM	40 (50)	56 (40)	Ref.			Ref.		
CYP2C19 IM/PM + CYP3A4 NM	21 (26.3)	52 (37.1)	0.56 (0.29–1.08)	0.08	0.45	0.69 (0.35–1.36)	0.28	0.54
CYP2C19 IM/PM + CYP3A4 IM/PM	6 (7.5)	14 (10)	0.60 (0.21–1.69)	0.34	0.61	0.57 (0.19–1.68)	0.31	0.54
CYP2C19 NM + CYP3A4 IM/PM	11 (13.8)	11 (7.9)	1.40 (0.55–3.54)	0.48	0.63	1.66 (0.62–4.49)	0.31	0.54
CYP2C19 UM + CYP3A4 NM/IM	2 (2.5)	7 (5)	0.40 (0.08–2.03)	0.27	0.61	0.41 (0.08–2.18)	0.29	0.54
CYP modulator #								
No inhibitor/inducer of CYP2C19/3A4/2D6	69 (86.3)	114 (81.4)	Ref.			Ref.		
CYP2C19 inhibitor alone	9 (11.3)	21 (15)	0.71 (0.31–1.63)	0.42	0.61	0.80 (0.33–1.95)	0.63	0.76
CYP3A4 inhibitor alone	2 (2.5)	2 (1.4)	1.65 (0.23–11.99)	0.62	0.70	2.75 (0.37–20.74)	0.33	0.54
CYP2D6 inhibitor alone	0 (0)	3 (2.1)	NA			NA		
Combined exposures ^								
No exposures								
CYP2C19 NM + CYP3A4 NM + No CYP Modulator	33 (41.3)	46 (32.9)	Ref.			Ref.		
DDI								
CYP2C19 NM + CYP3A4 NM + Yes CYP Modulator	7 (8.8)	10 (7.1)	0.98 (0.34–2.83)	0.96	0.96	1.03 (0.34–3.12)	0.96	0.96
DGI								
CYP2C19 IM/PM + CYP3A4 NM + No CYP Modulator	18 (22.5)	42 (30)	0.59 (0.29–1.22)	0.16	0.61	0.69 (0.33–1.45)	0.33	0.54
CYP2C19 IM/PM + CYP3A4 IM/PM + No CYP Modulator	6 (7.5)	13 (9.3)	0.64 (0.22–1.87)	0.42	0.61	0.64 (0.21–1.91)	0.42	0.55
CYP2C19 NM + CYP3A4 IM/PM + No CYP Modulator	10 (12.5)	9 (6.4)	1.55 (0.57–4.23)	0.39	0.61	1.60 (0.56–4.56)	0.37	0.54
CYP2C19 UM + CYP3A4 NM/IM + No CYP Modulator	2 (2.5)	4 (2.9)	0.69 (0.12–4.03)	0.69	0.73	0.72 (0.12–4.35)	0.72	0.82
DDGI	4 (5)	16 (11.4)	0.35 (0.11–1.14)	0.08	0.45	0.48 (0.14–1.61)	0.23	0.54

Adjusted for: * CYP3A4 phenotypes, CYP modulator, gender & dose at start; ** CYP2C19 phenotypes, CYP modulator, gender & dose at start; *** CYP modulator, gender & dose at start; # CYP2C19 & CYP3A4 phenotypes, gender & dose at start; ^ gender & dose at start. NM: Normal Metabolizer. IM: Intermediate Metabolizer. PM: Poor Metabolizer. UM: Ultrarapid Metabolizer. DDI: Drug–Drug interaction. DGI: Drug–Gene Interaction. DDGI: Drug–Drug–Gene Interaction (overlapping condition of DDI and DGI, please see Table 6: Frequency of DDGI) CYP: Cytochrome P450. NA: Not Available. OR: Odds Ratio. aOR: Adjusted Odds ratio. CI: Confidence Interval. Ref.: Reference.

4. Discussion

In this explorative inception cohort study, we presented for both CYP2C19 and CYP3A4 the associations of DGI, DDI, and DDGI and the risk of switching or dose adjustments and early discontinuation in the first treatment episode of (es)citalopram. In our relatively small samples, we found an indication that participants with DGI involving predicted CYP2C19 IM tended to experience switching and/or dose reduction, instead of early discontinuation, regardless of the CYP3A4 predicted phenotype. For participants with DGI involving predicted CYP3A4 IM/PM, no influence on switching and/or dose reduction was found. Yet, the effect of CYP2C19 IM might be enhanced by the presence of CYP3A4 IM. DDI and DDGI might be associated with an increased risk of switching or dose reduction, but the associations were not significant with wide confidence intervals.

We found that participants with CYP2C19 IM were more likely to experience switching than those with NM. This is consistent with the study reported by Mrazek et al. which showed that individuals with CYP2C19 reduced catalytic function were less tolerant to citalopram than those with increased catalytic function [40]. We also found that (es)citalopram users with CYP2C19 IM tended to experience dose reductions more than those with CYP2C19 NM. Decreasing the maximum daily dose of (es)citalopram in patients with CYP2C19 IM by 25% of the normal maximum dose is recommended by the DPWG [41]. As a note, we possibly managed to find some associations on CYP2C19 IM and the outcomes because we had a large enough number of (es)citalopram users with the genotype (about 33% of the cohort).

Unfortunately, we did not find any significant association between patients with CYP2C19 PM and UM to the outcomes which was probably due to a limited sample size. Some clinical studies reported that patients with CYP2C19 PM were exposed to (es)citalopram blood concentration to a greater extent than CYP2C19 IM and that patients with CYP2C19 UM had a lower exposure to (es)citalopram compared to CY2C19 NMs [7]. Jukic et al. using about 2000 genotyped persons from the Oslo population found that escitalopram users with CYP2C19 UM and PM (33% of the study population) had a three times higher odds of switching to another antidepressant than those with CYP2C19 NM [20].

To the best of our knowledge, this is the first study to examine the impact of CYP3A4 alone and in combination with CYP2C19 on (es)citalopram treatment. Decreased function of CYP3A4 in the CYP2C19 NM participants did not seem to influence the outcomes, but might have increased the effect of CYP2C19 IM. A comparable trend of effects has been reported for CYP2D6. The effect of the CYP2D6 variant in individuals with CYP2C19 NM on the AUC of citalopram was limited. However, when there was a co-presence of CYP2C19 *1/*2 (IM), the influence of CYP2D6 *1/*4 (IM) became stronger [10].

In our dataset, there were about nine percent of (es)citalopram users exposed to potential DDIs. This might be because about 79% of our study population had at least one comorbidity and therefore, they used other drug(s) which might potentially interact with (es)citalopram. In the Lifelines population, the most prevalent potential CYP2C19 mediated DDI was citalopram and omeprazole [42]. Omeprazole was reported to increase s-citalopram plasma concentration by about 50% to 120% [43,44]. Therefore, it has been recommended that patients with omeprazole or esomeprazole should have a dose adjustment of (es)citalopram [45].

Although we did not find any significant associations between DDGI and the outcomes, this study is the first to explore the impact of complex DDGI on the (es)citalopram treatment at the population level. Generally, DDGI may come in two main scenarios [14,15]. Firstly, it may only affect one metabolic pathway of a drug, for example overlapping conditions between a CYP2C19 UM/IM/PM and a CYP2C19 inhibitor in (es)citalopram users. In this scenario, we might expect that the level of blood concentration of (es)citalopram in an individual with a CYP2C19 UM and a CYP2C19 inhibitor might be different from an individual with a CYP2C19 IM and a CYP2C19 inhibitor [15]. This is because the more the number of active allelic variants in the CYP450, the more difficult for their phenotypes to be converted by the co-presence of inhibitors [46]. The second main scenario is the alteration of two or even three metabolic pathways of a drug. The alteration can be a result of the presence of deviating genotypes in one/two metabolic pathway(s) and the co-presence of CYP modulator in one/two other pathway(s). In this scenario, each possible combination of co-inhibition produced by genetic variation and CYP modulators might result in variation of (es)citalopram concentration in the blood [15]. Therefore, the effect of DDGI can vary depending on the scenario of interactions, the metabolic contribution of the inhibited pathway(s), and the potency of CYP modulators [15]. In this study, since we had only two patients with DDGI experiencing switching (Supplementary S2), we could not explore more about the impact of the different scenarios on the outcomes. It is plausible because the number of patients with DDI and DGI were limited, we could expect that the number of patients exposed to DDGI is even less. Hence, further study with a larger dataset is needed to provide solid evidence about the impact of DDGI in clinical practice which can be used to support the lack of pharmacotherapeutic management of DDGI in the current guidelines.

Since genotyping is still not a part of routine clinical testing, prescribers often have no indication about the genotype of the patients at the time of prescription. Consequently, the presence of DGI and DDGI related to (es)citalopram, exposing 56% of our study population, is potentially missed by health practitioners. Therefore, in order to avoid DGI and DDGI complex interaction, pre-emptive genotyping, inclusion of genetic information in electronic health records as well as a sophisticated computerized drug interaction surveillance system are needed in clinical practice.

Several potential limitations need to be discussed. First, we did not have data on the blood concentration of (es)citalopram as the best indicator to show the effect of interactions. Consequently, we could not ascertain the effect of DDI/DGI/DDGI on the citalopram metabolism and validate the associations between the exposures and the outcomes. In addition, we did not have information about the genotype status of *CYP2D6*. Therefore, we could not assess the combined effects of *CYP2C19/3A4/2D6* polymorphisms on (es)citalopram efficacy. *CYP2D6* is the most polymorphic CYP enzyme and the prevalence of people with CYP2D6 IM and PM genotypes in the Caucasian population is 40% and 10%, respectively [47]. Therefore, there might be some persons with *CYP2D6* polymorphisms among our participants. Despite its minor metabolic contribution on (es)citalopram disposition, *CYP2D6* polymorphism might corroborate the alteration of citalopram clearance in the presence of *CYP2C19* polymorphism [10]. It was reported in a small DGI study among healthy persons that one participant with CYP2C19 PM and CYP2D6 PM taking citalopram developed severe side effects and was withdrawn early before the study was completed [48]. Therefore, there was a possibility that the co-presence of combined *CYP2C19/3A4/2D6* polymorphisms might produce a substantial effect on citalopram disposition.

Furthermore, though, our study population from the PharmLines database is rather large (6379 participants), the statistical power of the study is relatively low to detect significant associations between multiple exposures as DGI, DDI, DDGI and outcomes. Therefore, the results of this study should be interpreted as hypothesis-generating rather than confirmative to explore potential effects of DGI, DDI, and DDGI on the prognosis of (es)citalopram treatment. Much larger studies are required to further confirm our findings. Lastly, about 30% of our dataset had no information about the dose of (es)citalopram. The missingness may probably not be related to other variables since it may be because pharmacists or pharmacy technicians forgot to include the dose information before sending the prescription data to the IADB.nl. In the baseline comparisons, we found that patients without dosing information were significantly older than those with complete information (Supplementary S2). Hence, we might underestimate the effect of age on the dose adjustments of (es)citalopram. Among those with complete information, age seemed not to influence the dose elevation or reduction of (es)citalopram (Table 7).

5. Conclusions

In conclusion, the predicted CYP2C19 IM phenotype increased the need of drug switching and/or dose reduction, and the co-presence of CYP3A4 IM enhanced these effects. Therefore, when patients receive (es)citalopram, it is important to not only consider the genetic information for CYP2C19 but also the genetic status of CYP3A4 as well.

Despite the fact that DDI and DDGI showed trends towards increased risks of switching and/or dose reduction, no conclusions can be drawn from the results because there were great uncertainties surrounding the estimates. Therefore, further real-world studies with larger samples are needed to confirm the results.

Supplementary Materials: The following are available online at http://www.mdpi.com/2075-4426/10/4/256/s1, Table S1: List of comorbidities; Table S2.1: Separated analysis of drug switching and dose reduction; Table S2.2: Differentiation of DDGI affecting one and two pathways; Table S2.3: Sensitivity Analysis for specific combination of CYP2C19 & CYP3A4 Phenotypes; Table S2.4: Demographics of participants, discriminated between complete and missing dose information; Table S3.1: Frequency of DDGI for time frame of 45 days; Table S3.2: Baseline comparisons for time frame of 45 days; Table S3.3: Association between exposures and outcomes for time frame of 45 days.

Author Contributions: Conceptualization: M.A.B., P.L., J.H.J.B., R.H.S., E.H. and B.W.; Data curation, M.A.B., P.L. and J.H.J.B.; Formal analysis, M.A.B.; Investigation, M.A.B., P.L. and J.H.J.B.; Methodology, M.A.B., E.H. and B.W.; Project administration, J.H.J.B.; Resources, P.L. and J.H.J.B.; Software, J.H.J.B.; Supervision, R.H.S., E.H. and B.W.; Writing—original draft, M.A.B. and B.W.; Writing—review & editing, P.L., J.H.J.B., R.H.S. and E.H. All authors have read and agreed to the published version of the manuscript.

Funding: The Lifelines Biobank initiative has been made possible by funds from FES (Fonds Economische Structuurversterking), SNN (Samenwerkingsverband Noord Nederland) and REP (Ruimtelijk Economisch Programma). The IADB.nl is funded by the University of Groningen. Muh. Akbar Bahar obtained a DIKTI scholarship from the Ministry of Research, Technology and Higher Education of Indonesia. The funding organizations had no role and influence in the study design and results.

Acknowledgments: The authors wish to acknowledge the services of the Lifelines Cohort Study, the contributing research centres delivering data to Lifelines, and all the study participants, and the participating IADB.nl pharmacies for kindly providing their data for research.

Conflicts of Interest: The authors declare no conflict of interest.

References

1. Abbing-Karahagopian, V.; Huerta, C.; Souverein, P.C.; De Abajo, F.; Leufkens, H.G.M.; Slattery, J.; Alvarez, Y.; Miret, M.; Gil, M.; Oliva, B.; et al. Antidepressant prescribing in five European countries: Application of common definitions to assess the prevalence, clinical observations, and methodological implications. *Eur. J. Clin. Pharmacol.* **2014**, *70*, 849–857. [CrossRef]
2. Kaplan, C.; Zhang, Y. Assessing the comparative-effectiveness of antidepressants commonly prescribed for depression in the US Medicare population. *J. Ment. Health Policy Econ.* **2012**, *15*, 171–178.
3. Li, G.; Shen, Y.; Luo, J.; Li, H. Efficacy of escitalopram monotherapy in the treatment of major depressive disorder: A pooled analysis of 4 Chinese clinical trials. *Medicine* **2017**, *96*, e8142. [CrossRef]
4. Trivedi, M.H.; Rush, A.J.; Wisniewski, S.R.; Nierenberg, A.A.; Warden, D.; Ritz, L.; Norquist, G.; Howland, R.H.; Lebowitz, B.; McGrath, P.J.; et al. Evaluation of outcomes with citalopram for depression using measurement-based care in STAR* D: Implications for clinical practice. *Am. J. Psychiatry* **2006**, *163*, 28–40. [CrossRef]
5. Fredricson Overo, K. Kinetics of citalopram in man; plasma levels in patients. *Prog. Neuropsychopharmacol. Biol. Psychiatry* **1982**, *6*, 311–318. [CrossRef]
6. Jin, Y.; Pollock, B.G.; Frank, E.; Cassano, G.B.; Rucci, P.; Müller, D.J.; Kennedy, J.L.; Forgione, R.N.; Kirshner, M.; Kepple, G.; et al. Effect of age, weight, and CYP2C19 genotype on escitalopram exposure. *J. Clin. Pharmacol.* **2010**, *50*, 62–72. [CrossRef]
7. Chang, M.; Tybring, G.; Dahl, M.L.; Lindh, J.D. Impact of cytochrome P450 2C19 polymorphisms on citalopram/escitalopram exposure: A systematic review and meta-analysis. *Clin. Pharmacokinet.* **2014**, *53*, 801–811. [CrossRef] [PubMed]
8. Rochat, B.; Amey, M.; Gillet, M.; Meyer, U.A.; Baumann, P. Identification of three cytochrome P450 isozymes involved in N-demethylation of citalopram enantiomers in human liver microsomes. *Pharmacogenetics* **1997**, *7*, 1–10. [CrossRef] [PubMed]

9. von Moltke, L.L.; Greenblatt, D.J.; Giancarlo, G.M.; Granda, B.W.; Harmatz, J.S.; Shader, R.I. Escitalopram (S-citalopram) and its metabolites in vitro: Cytochromes mediating biotransformation, inhibitory effects, and comparison to R-citalopram. *Drug Metab. Dispos.* **2001**, *29*, 1102–1109. [PubMed]
10. Fudio, S.; Borobia, A.M.; Piñana, E.; Ramírez, E.; Tabarés, B.; Guerra, P.; Carcas, A.; Frías, J. Evaluation of the influence of sex and CYP2C19 and CYP2D6 polymorphisms in the disposition of citalopram. *Eur. J. Pharmacol.* **2010**, *626*, 200–204. [CrossRef] [PubMed]
11. Westervelt, P.; Cho, K.; Bright, D.R.; Kisor, D.F. Drug-gene interactions: Inherent variability in drug maintenance dose requirements. *Pharm. Ther.* **2014**, *39*, 630–637.
12. Wenzel-Seifert, K.; Brandl, R.; Hiemke, C.; Haen, E. Influence of concomitant medications on the total clearance and the risk for supra-therapeutic plasma concentrations of Citalopram. A population-based cohort study. *Pharmacopsychiatry* **2014**, *47*, 239–244. [CrossRef] [PubMed]
13. Thirumaran, R.K.; Heck, J.W.; Hocum, B.T. CYP450 genotyping and cumulative drug–gene interactions: An update for precision medicine. *Future Med.* **2016**. [CrossRef] [PubMed]
14. Verbeurgt, P.; Mamiya, T.; Oesterheld, J. How common are drug and gene interactions? Prevalence in a sample of 1143 patients with CYP2C9, CYP2C19 and CYP2D6 genotyping. *Pharmacogenomics* **2014**, *15*, 655–665. [CrossRef] [PubMed]
15. Bahar, M.A.; Setiawan, D.; Hak, E.; Wilffert, B. Pharmacogenetics of drug–drug interaction and drug–drug–gene interaction: A systematic review on CYP2C9, CYP2C19 and CYP2D6. *Pharmacogenomics* **2017**, *18*, 701–739. [CrossRef] [PubMed]
16. Malki, M.A.; Pearson, E.R. Drug–drug–gene interactions and adverse drug reactions. *Pharm. J.* **2019**, *20*, 355–366. [CrossRef] [PubMed]
17. Hicks, J.K.; Bishop, J.R.; Sangkuhl, K.; Müller, D.J.; Ji, Y.; Leckband, S.G.; Leeder, J.S.; Graham, R.L.; Chiulli, D.L.; LLerena, A.; et al. Clinical Pharmacogenetics Implementation Consortium (CPIC) guideline for CYP2D6 and CYP2C19 genotypes and dosing of selective serotonin reuptake inhibitors. *Clin. Pharmacol. Ther.* **2015**, *98*, 127–134. [CrossRef]
18. Swen, J.J.; Nijenhuis, M.; de Boer, A.; Grandia, L.; Maitland-van der Zee, A.H.; Mulder, H.; Rongen, G.A.P.J.M.; Van Schaik, R.H.N.; Schalekamp, T.; Touw, D.J.; et al. Pharmacogenetics: From bench to byte—An update of guidelines. *Clin. Pharmacol. Ther.* **2011**, *89*, 662–673. [CrossRef]
19. Sediq, R.; van der Schans, J.; Dotinga, A.; Alingh, R.A.; Wilffert, B.; Bos, J.H.; Schuiling-Veninga, C.C.; Hak, E. Concordance assessment of self-reported medication use in the netherlands three-generation lifelines Cohort study with the pharmacy database iaDB. nl: The Pharmlines initiative. *Clin. Epidemiol.* **2018**, *10*, 981. [CrossRef]
20. Jukić, M.M.; Haslemo, T.; Molden, E.; Ingelman-Sundberg, M. Impact of CYP2C19 genotype on escitalopram exposure and therapeutic failure: A retrospective study based on 2087 patients. *Am. J. Psychiatry* **2018**, *175*, 463–470. [CrossRef]
21. Bijl, M.J.; Visser, L.E.; Hofman, A.; Vulto, A.G.; Van Gelder, T.; Stricker, B.H.C.; Van Schaik, R.H. Influence of the CYP2D6* 4 polymorphism on dose, switching and discontinuation of antidepressants. *Br. J. Clin. Pharmacol.* **2008**, *65*, 558–564. [CrossRef] [PubMed]
22. Scholtens, S.; Smidt, N.; Swertz, M.A.; Bakker, S.J.; Dotinga, A.; Vonk, J.M.; Van Dijk, F.; van Zon, S.K.; Wijmenga, C.; Wolffenbuttel, B.H.; et al. Cohort Profile: LifeLines, a three-generation cohort study and biobank. *Int. J. Epidemiol.* **2014**, *44*, 1172–1180. [CrossRef] [PubMed]
23. Stolk, R.P.; Rosmalen, J.G.; Postma, D.S.; de Boer, R.A.; Navis, G.; Slaets, J.P.; Ormel, J.; Wolffenbuttel, B.H. Universal risk factors for multifactorial diseases. *Eur. J. Epidemiol.* **2008**, *23*, 67–74. [CrossRef] [PubMed]
24. Klijs, B.; Scholtens, S.; Mandemakers, J.J.; Snieder, H.; Stolk, R.P.; Smidt, N. Representativeness of the LifeLines cohort study. *PLoS ONE* **2015**, *10*, e0137203. [CrossRef]
25. Visser, S.T.; Schuiling-Veninga, C.C.; Bos, J.H.; de Jong-van den Berg Lolkje, T.W.; Postma, M.J. The population-based prescription database IADB. nl: Its development, usefulness in outcomes research and challenges. *Expert Rev. Pharm. Outcomes Res.* **2013**, *13*, 285–292.
26. Bahar, M.; Hak, E.; Bos, J.H.; Borgsteede, S.D.; Wilffert, B. The burden and management of cytochrome P450 2D6 (CYP2D6)-mediated drug–drug interaction (DDI): Co-medication of metoprolol and paroxetine or fluoxetine in the elderly. *Pharmacoepidemiol. Drug Saf.* **2017**, *26*, 752–765. [CrossRef]